The 12-Lead ECG in Acute Myocardial Infarction

The 12-Lead ECG in Acute Myocardial Infarction

TIM PHALEN

with 181 *illustrations*

Line drawings (except 12-leads) by Kimberly Battista
Photographs by Vincent Knaus

Mosby Lifeline

St. Louis Baltimore Boston Carlsbad Chicago Naples New York Philadelphia Portland
London Madrid Mexico City Singapore Sydney Tokyo Toronto Wiesbaden

Mosby Lifeline
Dedicated to Publishing Excellence

A Times Mirror Company

Senior Vice President: David T. Culverwell
Publisher: David Dusthimer
Executive Editor: Claire Merrick
Editor: Julie Scardiglia
Assistant Editor: John Goucher
Production Manager: Chris Baumle
Production Editor: Susie Coladonato
Electronic Production Coordinator: Pamela Merritt
Manufacturing Manager: Bill Winneberger
Design Manager: Nancy McDonald
Design: Design Concept, Inc.

Printed in the United States of America

Printing/Binding by: Courier Companies, Inc.

Mosby-Year Book, Inc.
11830 Westline Industrial Drive
St. Louis, Missouri 63146

Library of Congress catalog card number: 95-81496

International Standard Book Number 0-8151-6752-0
97 98 99/9 8 7 6 5 4 3 2

Dedication

To my Dad
James T. Phalen

Foreword

The greatest health malady in developed countries remains coronary artery disease. It robs more adults of life and health than any other disorder. Treatment plans this past decade shifted from watchful waiting (with treating symptoms) to aggressive interventions. Clinical outcomes improved dramatically with the modern interventions. Early ECG information isn't just for someone with chest pain, it assists to diagnose and speed treatment for acute ischemic conditions, electrolyte imbalance, poisonings and a host of other medical problems. Physicians rely upon all health care team members to avoid delays obtaining appropriate patient data.

Here's a book shaped by what its audience needs to know about ECGs. Tim Phalen studied how people learn. He also noticed how they fail to learn. What started as a much Xeroxed classroom syllabus has emerged as a fresh learning approach. Current texts about ECGs either overwhelm you with excessive detail, or just offer an elementary introduction. When faced with a mammoth project, like comprehending ECGs, we tend to take on too much, too soon. These chapters build fundamental concepts into a systematic, powerful approach. As you progress through the book, electrical cardiac messages begin to form patterns and start making sense. Optimal electrocardiography acquisition is tricky. Plain language describes technical aspects required for getting clean signals thereby reducing misinterpretations. It's all here. This way works. Understanding electrocardiography becomes not just a needed expertise; it's an enjoyable pursuit!

You hold in your hand a key to unlock mysteries imparted through the 12-lead electrocardiogram. If you want to decode "voices" from a passionate organ, turn the page. It's irresistible.

Judith Reid Graves

Preface

The challenge in providing a simplified method of 12-lead ECG acquisition and infarct recognition lies in determining which information is absolutely necessary for effective recognition and treatment of AMI. If too much "nice to know" information is provided the reader is quickly overwhelmed. If a text supplies an inadequate amount of information, it is of little benefit to the reader's clinical practice. In writing this book I have attempted to walk that fine line and avoid both of these outcomes.

Each chapter contains information that emergency cardiac care providers need to know. The format is designed to present the information in an easy to understand, step-by-step method. Through the use of tables, illustrations, and a large number of practice 12-lead ECGs, the reader is exposed to new information, provided with examples, and then given the opportunity to apply this new knowledge. A summary is provided at the end of each chapter for quick review of important information. Once the main body of the text has been completed, the reader should be proficient in the fundamentals of infarct recognition and management.

The author recognizes that the transition from interpreting ECGs in a textbook to actually using 12-lead ECG interpretive skills in clinical practice is a big step. Therefore, the last three chapters are intended to assist the reader in that effort. Because the ability to recognize certain conditions that can mimic an infarct is an important clinical skill, Chapter 7 is devoted to some of the more common infarct impostors. A systematic approach to ECG interpretation is always necessary and Chapter 8 provides a five-step approach for the recognition of myocardial infarction on the ECG and offers the opportunity to apply this approach through the use of five case studies. To further develop these skills and to keep them current, Chapter 9 contains 50 full-size, practice 12-lead ECGs, with their interpretations on the flip side of the page.

All of the material in this text was classroom-tested and presented in various forms to thousands of paramedics and nurses. I know that every cardiac care provider can master all of the learning objectives required to integrate the 12-lead ECG into their clinical practice. I hope that this text provides you with a practical jumpstart towards infarct recognition and management, convinces you that 12-leads don't have to be intimidating, and encourages you to go on and learn even more advanced electrocardiography.

Tim Phalen

Acknowledgments

I wish to thank some of the people that have been so helpful to me in the completion of this project:

The reviewers, **Edgar Batsford, Marlene Beckman, Randall W. Benner, Gary Rushworth, James H. Sandlin,** and **Paul Werfel,** who spent many hours evaluating the manuscript, artwork, and tracings. Your thoughtfulness and comments have greatly improved this text. In particular, I wish to thank **Dr. Henry J.L. Marriott** for generously agreeing to review the text in its final version.

Gary Denton, early in my career your example showed me that there is no limit to what a paramedic can learn. As a friend you have always provided me with encouragement and direction.

Everyone that has provided me with ECG tracings. I especially wish to thank **Lani Clark** who provided the tracings which made the final chapter possible.

The thousands of emergency cardiac care providers that have attended one of my presentations. Through your feedback and comments, you told me exactly what you "needed to know" and what was "nice to know."

Kim Battista and **Vincent Knaus**, what a great job you did in translating my notes and feeble sketches into wonderful artwork and photographs.

Physio Control Corporation, for providing the equipment used in 12-lead acquisition photographs.

Claire Merrick of Mosby Lifeline, cutter of red tape. You made things happen for me when they needed to happen. Literally, this book would not be a reality without your help and support.

Julie Scardiglia and **John Goucher** of Mosby Lifeline, if it weren't for you two there is no doubt that I'd still be trying to make one last change to the book. You are both great to work with. Julie, I also want you to know how much I appreciate the special attention that you gave to this project. Thanks for your faith in me.

My wife **LeAnne**, you have been incredibly patient and understanding during the months that I kept vanishing into the back office to write this book. I love you, and I thank God that you are sharing your life with me.

Tim Phalen

Contents

Introduction: The Need for 12-Leads

A Change in Responsibilities

Until very recently, little could be done to treat myocardial infarction. Before the 1960s, treatment consisted primarily of bed rest. Then, in recognition of the fact that many infarct deaths are really dysrhythmia deaths, coronary care units were formed to continuously monitor patients in the hope that life-threatening dysrhythmias could be quickly identified and treated. This concept led to reduced mortality and was adopted by most hospitals.

Since a great many infarct deaths occurred outside of the hospital, the concept of the coronary care unit was extended to the prehospital setting. In the late 1960s and early 1970s, many communities began to equip their rescue squads with monitor/defibrillators, and train their staff to recognize and treat lethal dysrhythmias. While both the coronary care unit and prehospital defibrillation have proven to be effective strategies in reducing cardiac related deaths, neither actually treats the underlying cause, which is an occlusion of the coronary artery.

In the 1970s, percutaneous transluminal coronary angioplasty (PTCA) and emergency coronary artery by-pass graft (CABG) surgery offered the first available means by which the infarct process could be halted. While studies have demonstrated both methods to be effective in the treatment of AMI, in many hospitals neither option could be provided. Thus, although a direct "treatment" of myocardial infarction did exist, it was not always available. Accordingly, in many areas of the country, dysrhythmia suppression continued to be the primary thrust of infarct treatment.

In the 1980s, studies began to show that thrombolytic drugs could also be used to reduce the mortality seen with myocardial infarction. Several investigators, examining large patient populations, demonstrated reductions in mortality and morbidity when these agents were used in the early hours of infarction. These results were confirmed in subsequent studies and a clearer recognition of the time dependence of these benefits emerged. The advantage of thrombolytic agents over PTCA and CABG is basic: The availability and efficacy of thrombolytic drugs brings to every emergency department a treatment that has the potential to stop the process of infarction and restore coronary circulation.

It is precisely because a very effective treatment for myocardial infarction is available to physicians that the nonphysician, emergency cardiac care provider must learn to recognize infarction. Early identification of infarction is crucial because the benefits of thrombolytic therapy are time dependent. The adage "time is muscle" refers to the necessity of infarcting patients to be identified early so thrombolytic therapy can be initiated as soon as possible. To accomplish this task, emergency cardiac care providers must become skilled at recognizing the infarct patient.

Door-to-Drug Time

The label most commonly applied to the interval between a patient's arrival at the emergency department and the administration of thrombolytic therapy is the phrase "door-to-drug" time. This phrase encompasses all of the steps and processes that must be accomplished to identify AMI patients and begin thrombolytic treatment. Now that thrombolytic therapy is available, it is the responsibility of every emergency department to quickly identify the infarcting patient and provide treatment with the shortest possible door-to-drug time.

Why the rush? Studies investigating the efficacy of thrombolytic therapy have demonstrated that the extent of myocardial salvage is dependent upon the time interval between the onset of the infarction and the administration of thrombolytic agents. The investigations have also shown that not only is it a case of "the sooner the better" but that much more myocardial salvage (and decreased mortality) occur when thrombolytic agents are administered very early in the infarction. Therefore, every moment of the first 2 hours are precious and the savings of even a few minutes at each step can combine to make a significant change in patient outcome. One study documented a 99% survival rate when infarct patients received thrombolytic agents within 70 minutes of symptom onset. Contrast that figure with the 90 minutes required to administer thrombolytic agents noted in some studies. Clearly, if the maximal benefit of thrombolysis is to be achieved, emergency departments must be adept at screening chest pain patients and rapidly treating myocardial infarction.

One of the primary methods to speed the recognition of myocardial infarction rests in the ability of the nonphysicians to recognize myocardial infarction. Specifically, this means that nurses, paramedics, and other emergency cardiac care providers must be adept at recognizing myocardial infarction. To accomplish this goal, emergency cardiac care providers must rely on more than just the clinical presentation when attempting to identify infarct patients. They also must be able to recognize the pattern of infarction on the 12-lead ECG. Once infarction has been recognized, or at least strongly suspected, information can be quickly gathered and presented to the physician for immediate review. This new aspect of cardiac care is so significant that two large national organizations, the recently formed National Heart Attack Alert Program (NHAAP), and the American Heart Association (AHA) have specific recommendations about the 12-lead ECG.

The NHAAP recommends that a 12-lead ECG be available in the emergency department and that ". . . nurses should be provided with a standing order to obtain a 12-lead ECG on any patient suspected of having myocardial ischemia or AMI." In addition, nurses should be trained to acquire the 12-lead and to recognize the ECG changes indicative of acute myocardial infarction. In fact, NHAAP believes that "obtaining the 12-lead ECG on patients with suspected heart attack should be considered part of the patient's vital signs."

The Emergency Cardiac Care Committee of the AHA has also assessed the situation. Both organizations agree that eligible patients should receive thrombolytic therapy within a short time after arriving at the emergency department. The recommendation of the AHA is that patients be treated within 30–60 minutes of their arrival. The NHAAP recommends that emergency departments strive to treat all AMI patients within 30 minutes of arrival. The 12-lead ECG is a crucial component to the rapid recognition of AMI.

While the 12-lead ECG is a routine part of the evaluation of the chest pain patient in the emergency department, it is relatively new to the prehospital environment. Because "time is muscle," the concept of prehospital 12-leads initially received attention because it was thought that prehospital thrombolysis may save the most muscle. However, the studies that investigated prehospital administration of thrombolytic agents found little or no benefit in urban settings. One of the principal reasons that little benefit was noted in these studies was that the prehospital 12-lead ECG produced a substantial reduction in door-to-drug time within the emergency department. In fact, without one drop of thrombolytic agent administered outside the hospital, reductions in the range of 20, 40 and even 60 minutes have been reported. Therefore, the prehospital 12-lead ECG is a very effective method for reducing door-to-drug time within the emergency department.

Purpose

The future is clear: Emergency cardiac care providers must become familiar with 12-lead ECG acquisition techniques, and must learn to identify acute myocardial infarction on the ECG.

This text provides nurses, paramedics, and other emergency cardiac care providers with an opportunity to become proficient in recognizing myocardial infarction on the ECG and helps them confidently apply their knowledge to their clinical practice.

1

ECG Basics

CHAPTER

OBJECTIVES

- Understand that the cardiac monitor is a voltmeter.
- Identify the leads that constitute the standard 12-lead ECG.
- Express time in both seconds and milliseconds.
- Define the proper anatomic position for the placement of chest and limb leads.
- Determine which portion of the heart that each lead "sees."
- Recognize the various components of the QRS complex.
- Classify Q waves as either physiologic or pathologic.
- Identify the J point and ST segment deviations.
- Identify normal and abnormal values for the QRS duration.
- Distinguish patterns of normal and abnormal R wave progression.

The Cardiac Monitor is Just a Voltmeter

Every emergency care provider is familiar with the admonition, "Treat your patient, not the monitor." In keeping with the spirit of that advice, it is worthwhile to discuss early on in the text the limitations of the ECG. A useful way to appreciate the ECG's limitations is to think of the cardiac monitor as a simple voltmeter.

The voltmeter analogy demonstrates that the basic function of the ECG is to detect current flow as measured on the patient's skin. That's it. No matter how sophisticated the cardiac monitor, no matter how many additional features the monitor may include, the electrocardiogram is just a display of the electrical activity recorded on the body's surface. The ECG monitor is not a magic window that allows the clinician to peer in at the heart. In fact, because the ECG records the heart's electrical activity as sensed by electrodes on the patient's skin, the cardiac monitor produces only an indirect measurement on the electrical activity of the heart. The care provider must interpret the significance of these voltage changes and apply them to the clinical setting from the indirect surface recording.

In some instances the ECG's interpretation may be clear and unmistakable, even in a single lead. At other times, when it is difficult to make a definitive interpretation, additional leads provide supplementary information that may clarify the interpretation. In the case of myocardial infarction, multiple leads are absolutely necessary to recognize its presence and location. At present, the 12-lead ECG is the standard electrocardiogram used for the screening for infarction.

In the real world, sometimes even a 12-lead ECG does not always provide enough information to make a definitive interpretation. When this occurs, it is important to resist the notion that you must form an interpretation, any interpretation, and thus latch onto one without sufficient evidence. In those cases, the most intelligent and sophisticated answer may be "I don't know." Remember that "I don't know" can simply mean there is insufficient information to make a sound interpretation. Fortunately, the ECG provides a wealth of information and accurate interpretation is usually possible.

Overview of the 12-Lead ECG

FORMAT

At first glance there are a number of differences between a 12-lead ECG and a rhythm strip, the most obvious being an increased number of leads. Note the 3 row by 4 column format shown in Fig. 1-1. This example demonstrates the most common format for displaying the 12-lead ECG. An actual 12-lead is shown in Fig. 1-2 along with annotations describing various features of interest.

The 12-lead ECG only provides a 2.5-second view of each lead. When first introduced to the 12-lead ECG, these 2.5 seconds may seem prohibitively short. However, when looking for evidence of infarction, most of the information is obtained from analyzing a single, representative complex in each lead. It is assumed that 2.5 seconds is long enough to capture at least one representative complex. However, a 2.5-second view

1	AVR	V1	V4
2	AVL	V2	V5
3	AVF	V3	V6

FIG. 1-1 The most common format for displaying the 12-lead ECG.

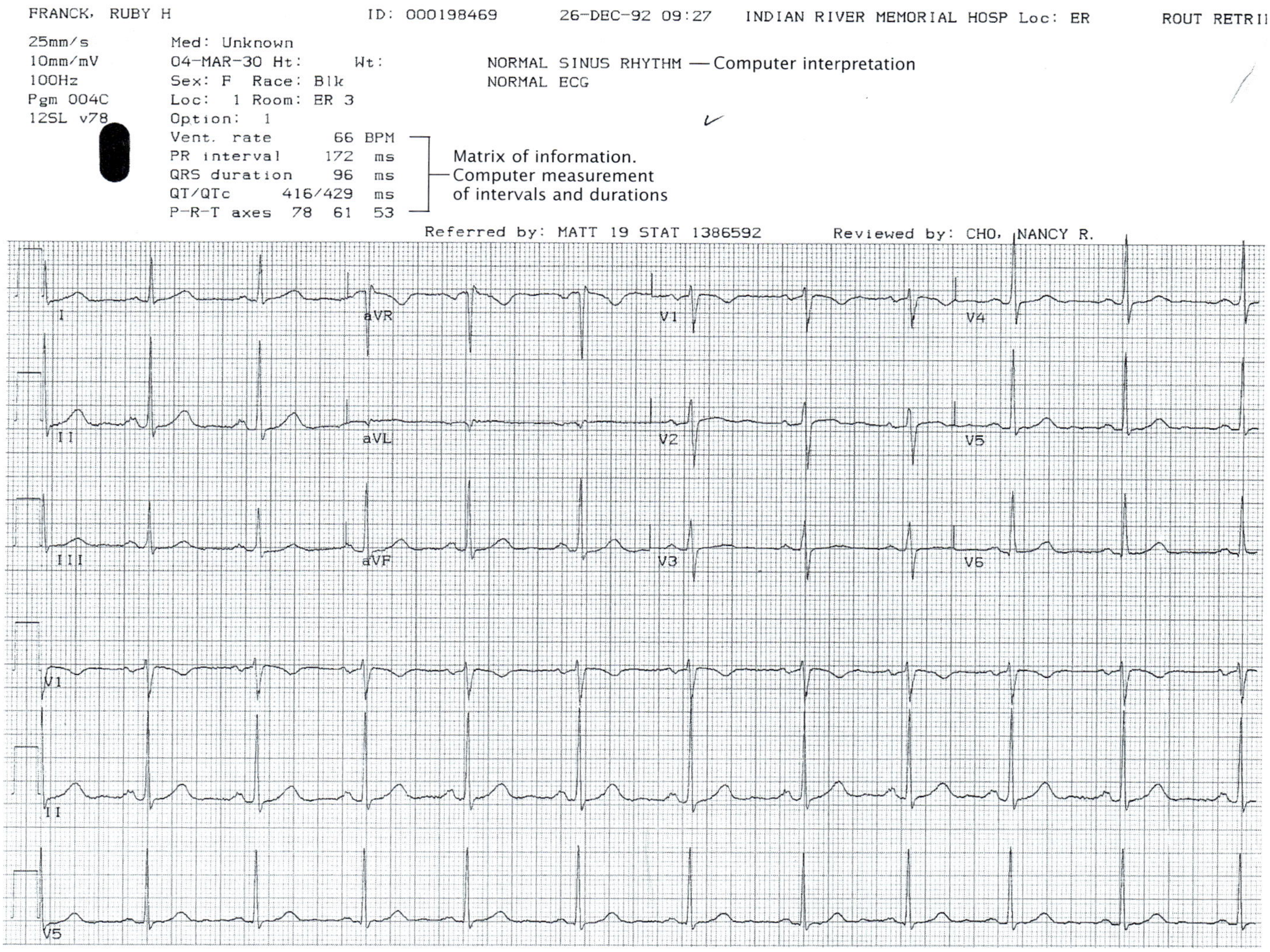

FIG. 1-2 An example 12-lead ECG.

is not long enough to properly assess rate and rhythm, so at least one continuous rhythm strip is usually included at the bottom of the tracing.

TIME

When intervals of the cardiac cycle are measured to determine rate and rhythm, time is most commonly expressed in seconds. If asked, "What is the maximum duration of the normal PR interval?", most emergency care providers would reply, "less than 0.20 seconds." The answer is correct, but in electrocardiography, intervals and duration are usually expressed in milliseconds. Fortunately, it is easy to convert seconds to milliseconds. Fig. 1-3 shows how

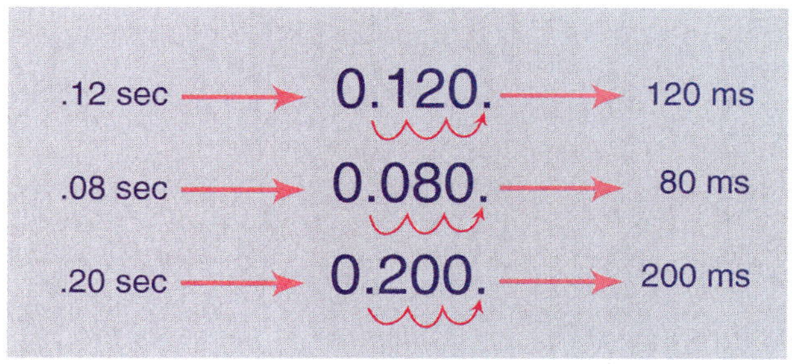

FIG. 1-3 Converting seconds to milliseconds.

the decimal point is moved three places to the right when converting from seconds to milliseconds.

Note that the information contained on the upper left corner of Fig. 1-2 includes measure-

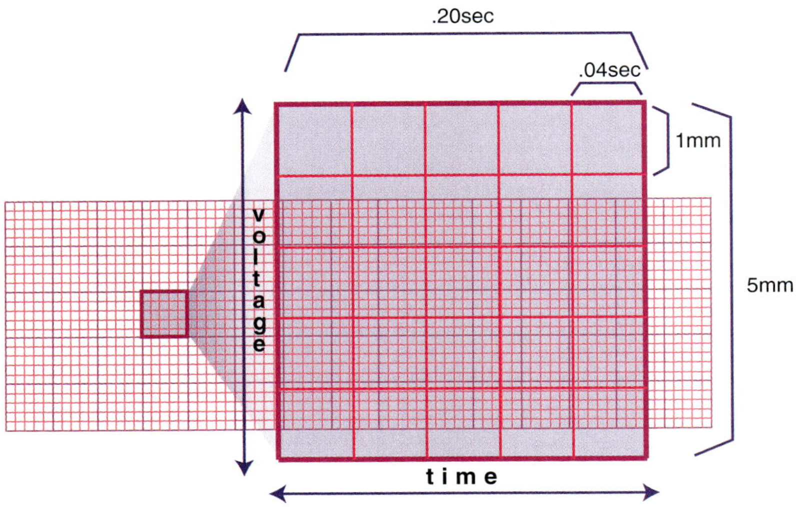

FIG. 1-4 This enlargement shows the relationship between time and voltage and the units used to measure them.

ments of the PR interval and the QRS duration. This information is provided by the computer's interpretive program, which is usually very accurate when measuring intervals and durations.

VOLTAGE

Voltage is expressed vertically on the ECG tracing, while time is expressed horizontally. As demonstrated in Fig. 1-4, each small box measures 1 millimeter (mm) in height and each large box measures 5 mm in height.

If the ECG monitor is set at standard calibration, a 1 millivolt (mV) impulse will produce a 10 mm deflection on the tracing. When a calibration pulse is produced, the monitor creates a 1 mV impulse that is sensed by the leads. If it is adjusted to standard calibration, the monitor will register a 10 mm deflection (two large boxes). Therefore, in standard calibration 1 mV = 10 mm.

If calibration is increased or decreased, the size of the deflection will change proportionately. Chapter 2 will provide more information on the significance of calibration as it relates to infarct recognition. At present, it is sufficient to know that voltage is measured vertically, and amplitude can be expressed in either millivolts or millimeters.

Lead Placement

Before discussion of the various lead placements, it is important to define three terms as they apply in this text: Electrode, lead, and cable. **Electrode** refers to the paper, plastic, or metal device that contains conductive media and is applied to the patient's skin. **Cable** refers to the wire that attaches to the electrode and conducts current back to the cardiac monitor. **Lead** is

Table 1-1 Comparison of Various Leads

I, II, III	Limb lead	Bipolar
AVR, AVL, AVF	Limb lead	Unipolar
V1-V6	Chest lead	Unipolar

used in a twofold manner: The term lead refers to the actual tracing obtained and the position of the electrode. For example, the term "V1 position" represents its proper location of the chest wall, while "lead V1" refers to the tracing obtained from that position.

The standard 12-lead is composed of six limb leads and six chest leads. These leads are referenced in Table 1-1. Leads I, II, III, AVR, AVL, and AVF are obtained from electrodes placed on the patient's arms and legs. As their names suggest, the six chest leads, V1-V6, are obtained from electrodes placed on the patient's chest. In viewing Fig. 1-5, it is noted that all 12 leads are obtained from only 10 electrodes. This is possible because the four limb electrodes are used for different purposes in different leads. For example, the left arm electrode is used as a negative electrode when lead III is obtained and is used as a positive electrode when lead AVL is obtained.

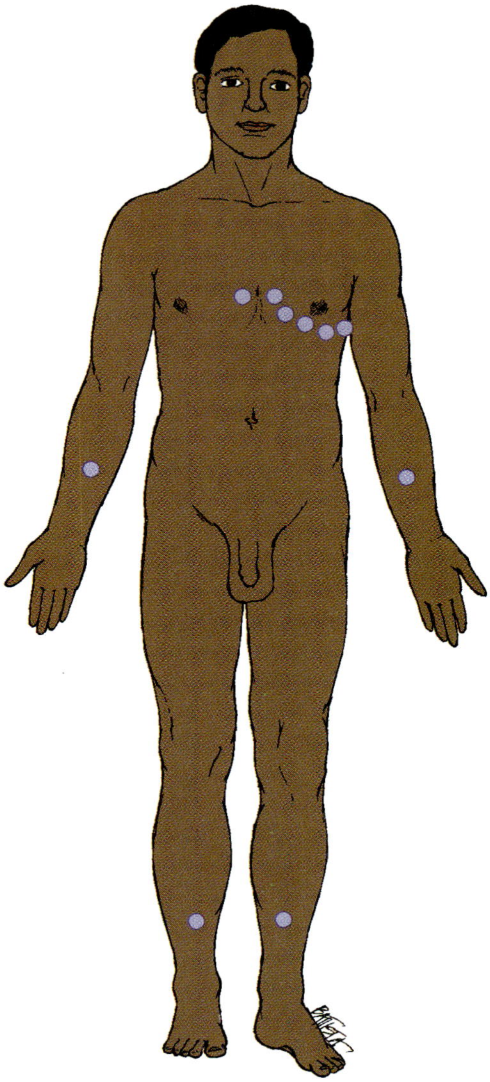

FIG. 1-5 The 12-lead ECG is obtained from ten electrodes positioned as shown here.

LIMB LEADS

Despite the common practice of attaching the electrodes for leads I, II, and III to the patient's trunk, these leads are properly positioned on the arms and legs. Why the switch? Over time, the placement of the limb leads seem to have crept up the extremities and onto the torso, probably in an effort to reduce artifact. However, proper position requires that these electrodes be placed somewhere on the limbs. It really doesn't matter where they are placed on the limbs as long as the bony prominences are avoided. The deltoid area is suitable for electrodes attached to the arms and is easily accessed. Either the thigh or the lower leg is suitable for the leg electrodes. Use the more convenient site.

Leads I, II, and III are the most familiar leads and were actually the first leads used when the electrocardiogram was developed around the beginning of this century. Since each of these three leads has a distinct negative pole and a distinct positive pole, they are considered **bipolar**. The positive electrode is located at the left wrist in lead I, while leads II and III both have their positive electrode located at the left foot. The difference in electrical potential between the positive pole and its corresponding negative pole is measured by each lead.

While leads AVR, AVL, and AVF have a distinct positive pole, they do not have a distinct negative pole. Since they have only one true pole, they are referred to as **unipolar leads**. In place of a single negative pole these leads have multiple negative poles, creating a negative field (central terminal), of which the heart is at the center. Theoretically, this makes the heart the negative electrode.

The positive pole in AVR is located on the right arm, AVL has a positive pole at the left arm, and AVF has a positive electrode positioned on the left leg. The position of the positive electrode corresponds to the last letter in each of these leads.

The letters "AV" were added because during the initial development of these leads, the size of the complexes were quite small and the researchers needed to "augment the voltage." So AVR represents Augmented Voltage Right arm. Likewise AVL indicates an Augmented Voltage lead at the Left arm, and AVF is an Augmented Voltage lead placed on the left Foot (actually the left leg). The augmented voltage leads are not the only unipolar leads in the standard 12-lead ECG.

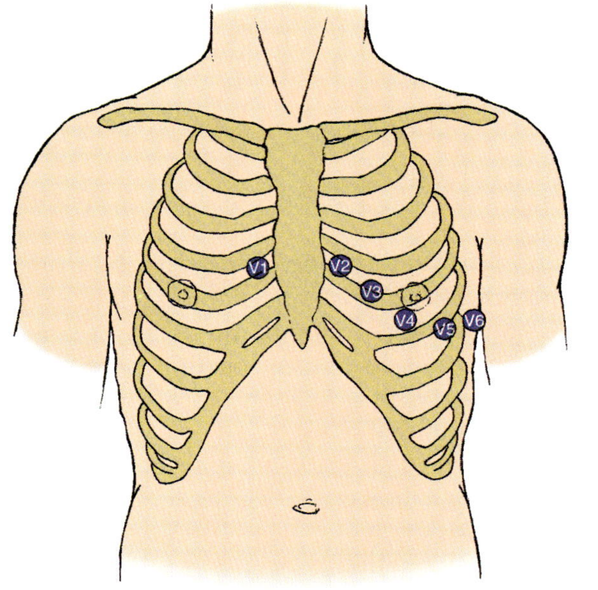

FIG. 1-6 The positions of the six chest leads, also known as precordial leads.

The chest leads, discussed in the next section, are also unipolar.

CHEST LEADS

Because the chest leads (also known as precordial leads) are unipolar, the positive electrode for each lead is placed at a specific location on the chest and the heart is the theoretical negative electrode. The location of each lead is displayed in Fig. 1-6. A method of locating each of these positions is described in Chapter 2.

What Each Lead "Sees"

Each positive electrode can be thought of as a camera or an eye looking in at the heart. The particular portion of the heart that each leads "sees" is determined by two factors. The first factor is the dominance of the left ventricle on the ECG and the second is the position of the positive electrode on the body. Both factors are discussed below, beginning with the dominance of the left ventricle on the ECG.

Because the ECG does not directly measure the heart's electrical activity, it does not "see" all of the current flowing through the heart. What the ECG does see from its vantage point on the body's surface is the net result of countless individual currents competing in a tug-of-war. For example, the QRS complex, which represents ventricular depolarization, is not a display of all the electrical activity occurring in the right and left ventricles. It is the net result of a tug-of-war produced by the numerous individual currents in both the right and left ventricles. Since the left ventricle is much more massive than the right, the left overpowers the right. What is seen in the QRS complex is the remaining electrical activity of the left ventricle, i.e., the portion not used to cancel out the right ventricle. Therefore, in a normally conducted beat, the **QRS complex represents the electrical activity occurring in the left ventricle.** It has been estimated that 80% of the cardiac electrical activity is canceled out by the tug–of–war leaving only 20% for the ECG to sense.

The second factor, position of the positive electrode on the body, determines which portion of the left ventricle is seen by each lead. The view of each lead can be committed to memory, or it can be reasoned easily by remembering where the positive electrode is located. The view of each lead is listed in Table 1-2, while Fig. 1-7 demonstrates the portion of the left ventricle that each lead views. Please note that AVR is not included in either Table 1-2 or Fig. 1-7. While AVR has several definite uses in electrocardiography, its use is limited in terms of infarct recognition. Therefore, AVR is not referenced throughout the remainder of this text.

Notice that certain limb leads share a common positioning of their positive electrode. For example, leads II, III, and AVF all have their positive electrode positioned on the left leg. However, while they all look at the same area of the heart, they all view it from a slightly different perspective. In keeping with the eye or camera analogy, imagine that the view of the eye or the angle of the camera lens is shifted towards the negative electrode. In the case of the inferior leads, while all three leads have their positive electrode in the same location, each lead sees the inferior wall in a slightly different perspective because each lead has a different position for its negative electrode.

Table 1.2 What Each Lead "Sees"

LEADS	VIEW
II, III, AVF	Inferior
V1, V2	Septal
V3, V4	Anterior
V5, V6, I, AVL	Lateral

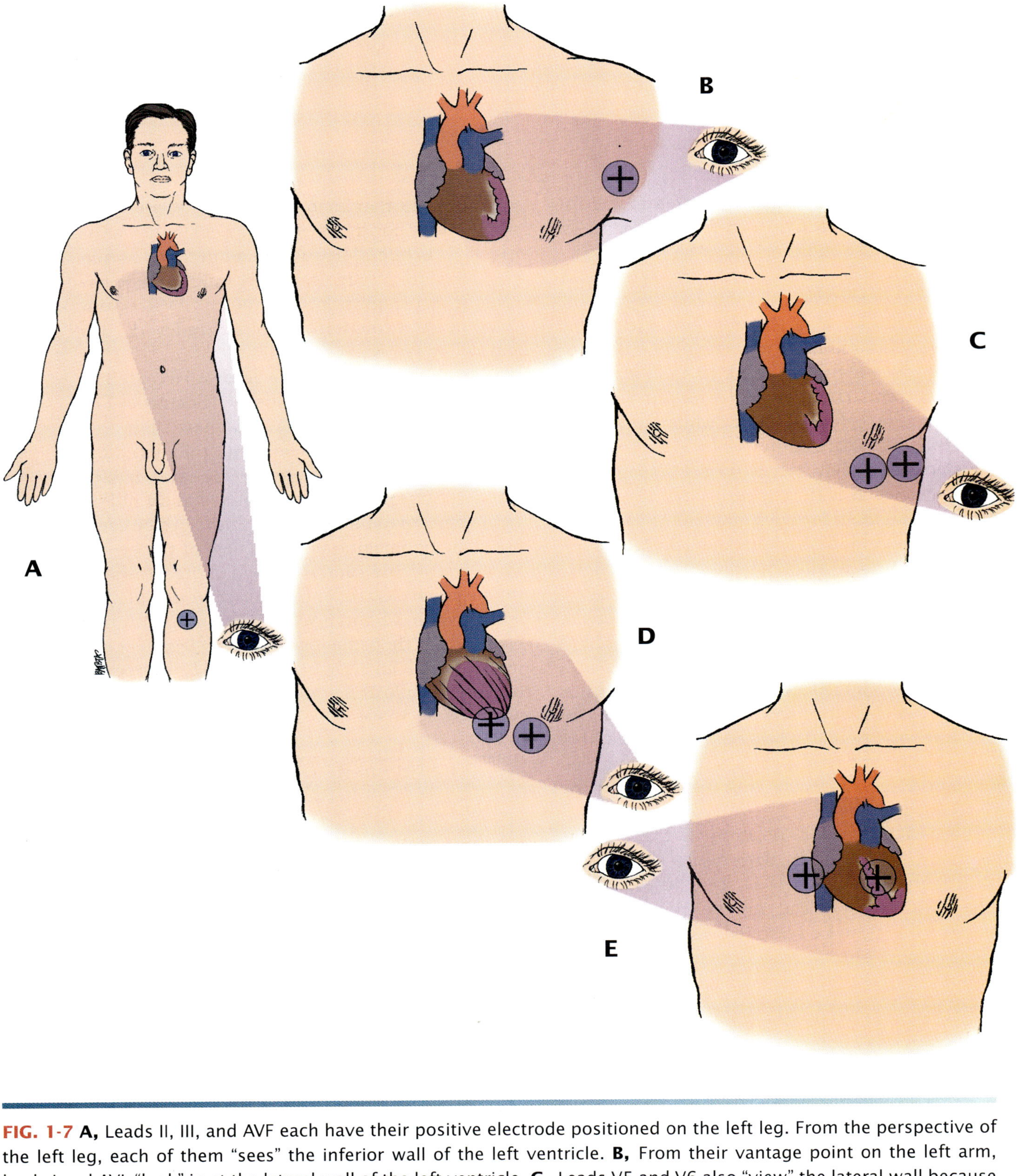

FIG. 1-7 **A,** Leads II, III, and AVF each have their positive electrode positioned on the left leg. From the perspective of the left leg, each of them "sees" the inferior wall of the left ventricle. **B,** From their vantage point on the left arm, leads I and AVL "look" in at the lateral wall of the left ventricle. **C,** Leads V5 and V6 also "view" the lateral wall because they are positioned on the axillary area of the left chest. **D,** Leads V3 and V4 are positioned in the area of the anterior chest. From this perspective, these leads "see" the anterior wall of the left ventricle. **E,** The septal wall is "seen" by leads V1 and V2, which are positioned next to the sternum.

Components of the QRS Complex

Though the term "QRS complex" refers collectively to the various forms of ventricular depolarization seen on the ECG, the QRS complex can be divided up into its component parts: the Q wave, the R wave, and the S wave. Definitions for all three of these waves are provided in this section. Before learning the definition of each component, it is helpful to know that not every QRS complex contains each of the three waves.

The **R wave** is defined as the first positive deflection of the QRS complex. The R wave begins as soon as the ECG leaves the isoelectric line in an upward direction, and continues until it returns to the isoelectric line. In Fig. 1-8, all of the QRS complex lying within the highlighted area is considered the R wave.

In addition to positive deflections, there may be negative deflections. When a negative deflection precedes an R wave, it is called a **Q wave**. The Q wave begins when the ECG leaves the isoelectric line in a downward direction and continues until it returns to the isoelectric line. The highlighted portion of Fig. 1-9 contains the Q wave.

Like the Q wave, the **S wave** is a negatively deflected complex. However, the S wave is a negative deflection that follows an R wave. The highlighted area of Fig. 1-10 signifies the S wave.

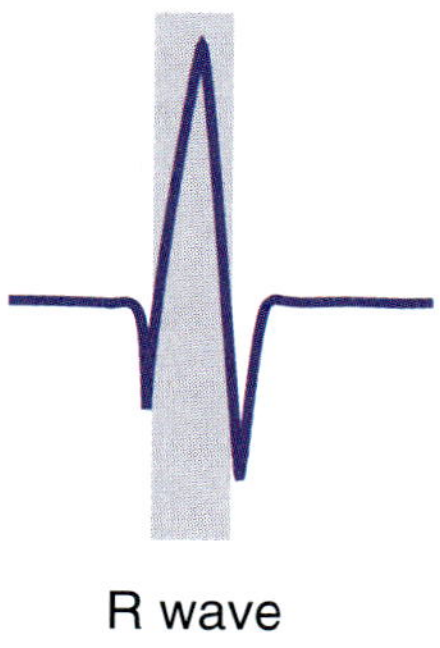

FIG. 1-8 The R wave is the first positive deflection.

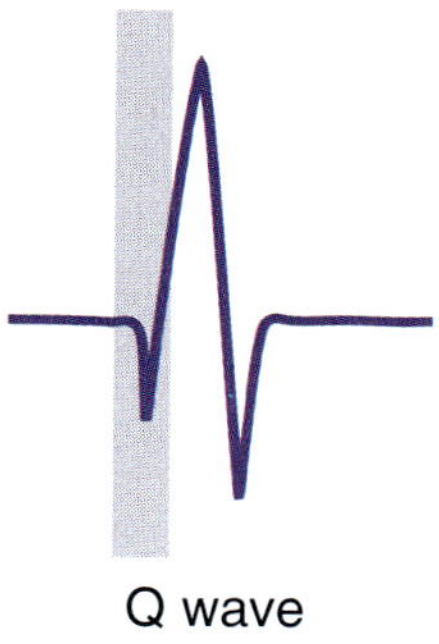

FIG. 1-9 The Q wave is a negative deflection preceding an R wave.

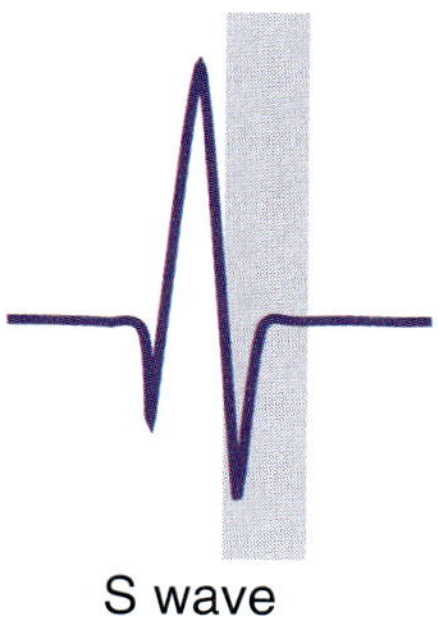

FIG. 1-10 The S wave is a negative deflection following an R wave.

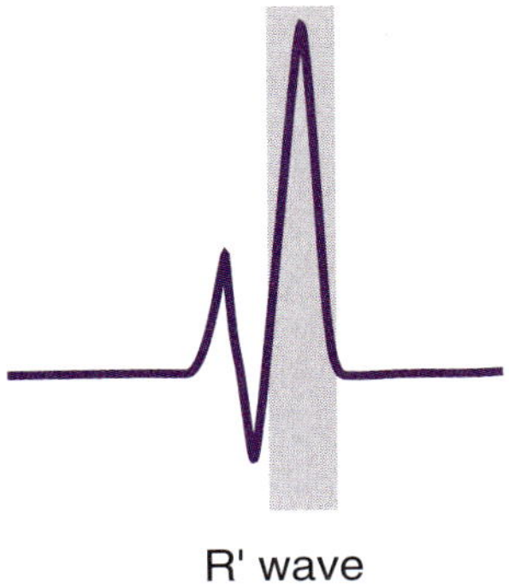

FIG. 1-11 The R primed wave is the second positive deflection occurring in a QRS complex.

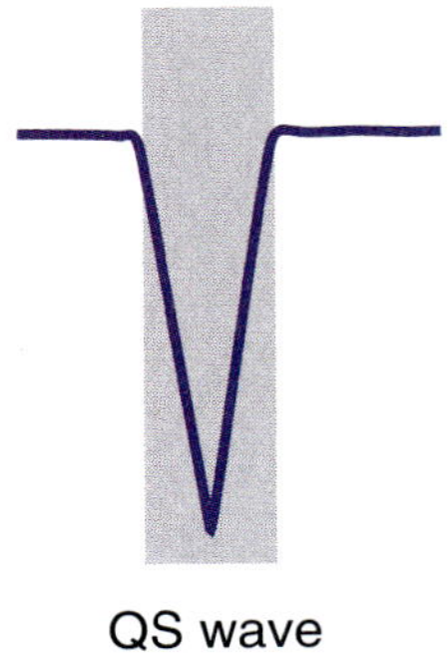

FIG. 1-12 QS complex is the name given to a QRS complex which is entirely negative.

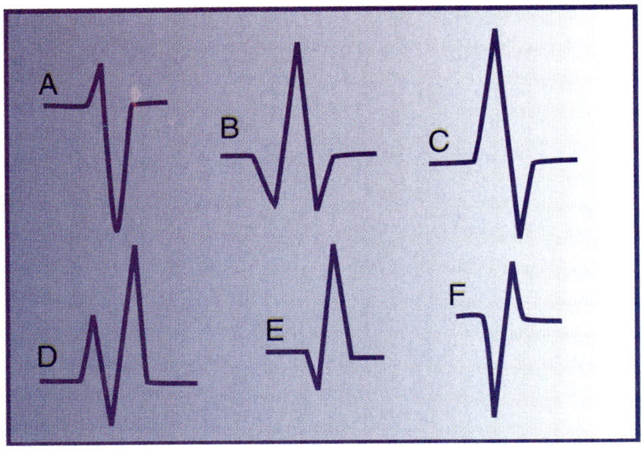

FIG. 1-13 Various QRS complex morphologies: A) rS B) qRs C) Rs D) RsR' E) qR F) Qr.

Occasionally there are some additional deflections in the QRS Complex. If there is a second positive deflection it is given the name **R primed** (R'). An example of an R' wave is demonstrated in Fig. 1-11.

Fig. 1-12 shows a QRS complex that is negatively deflected. In attempting to apply the rules mentioned above, the negative deflection should be referred to as either a Q wave or an S wave, depending upon whether it precedes or follows the R wave. However, in this case there is no R wave to help identify the complex as a Q or an S wave. In such instances, when the entire QRS complex is a negative deflection it is referred to as a **QS complex**.

Examples of various QRS complex morphologies are shown in Fig. 1-13 along with the appropriate nomenclature for each. Note how uppercase and lowercase letters are used to designate the relative size of each component.

Q Waves

Q waves are often present as part of the QRS complex and may be a completely normal finding. However, Q waves can signify the presence of myocardial infarction. It is sometimes a challenge to differentiate normal Q waves (**physiologic Q waves**) from those present as the result of infarction (**pathologic Q waves** or **significant Q waves**). Generally, it is the depth and width of a Q wave that is used to distinguish between the two cases.

When a Q wave is physiologic (present as a normal part of the QRS) it is usually less than 40 ms (less than .04 seconds, or one small box) and its amplitude is less than one-third the amplitude of the R wave. Conversely, when Q waves are pathologic (for example, the result of infarction), they are generally 40 ms or more in duration and may exceed one-third the amplitude of the R wave.

Since infarction is a possible cause of Q waves, the duration and amplitude of every Q wave noted on the ECG should be examined. Fig. 1-14 shows examples of physiologic and pathologic Q waves.

In the early hours of infarction, a pathologic Q wave may not have developed to its full width or amplitude. Therefore, a single ECG may not properly identify a Q wave as pathologic. However, even when Q waves do not meet the objective criteria of 40 ms in duration or one-third the amplitude of the QRS complex, pathology must be considered if the Q waves become wider or deeper in each subsequent tracing.

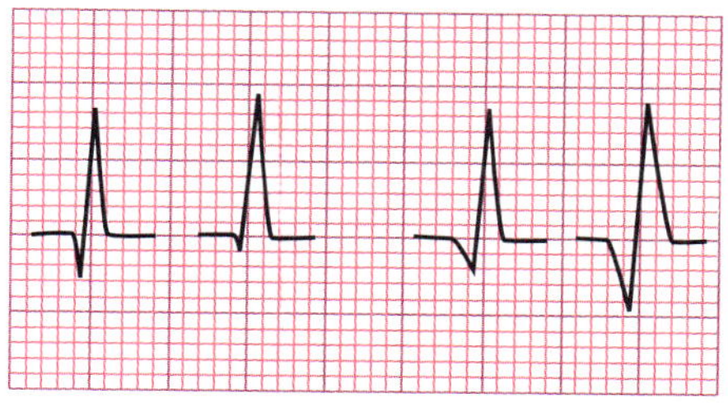

FIG. 1-14 Physiologic and pathologic Q waves.

ST Segment

The **ST segment** marks the beginning of ventricular repolarization. The ST segment begins exactly where the QRS complex ends. The junction between the QRS complex and the ST segment is referred to as the junction point or **J Point** (Fig. 1-15).

The ST segment is normally isoelectric but a number of conditions may cause it to be elevated or depressed. When assessing for ST segment deviation, first locate the J Point which identifies the beginning of the ST segment. Next use the TP segment and the PR segment to estimate the position of the isoelectric line. Then compare the level of the ST segment to the isoelectric line. While some deviation of the ST segment from the isoelectric line can be a normal finding, ST segment deviation of 1 mm or more from the isoelectric line is considered significant.

Myocardial ischemia, injury, and infarction are among the causes of ST deviation. In the following chapters, much attention will be focused on determining if ST segment elevation is present.

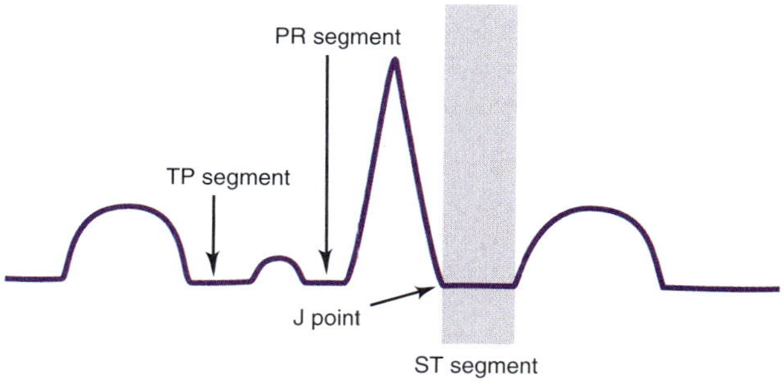

FIG. 1-15 The ST segment begins at the point where the QRS complex ends. The junction point between the QRS and the ST segment is known as the J Point.

QRS Duration

The QRS duration is a measurement of the time required for ventricular activation. It normally requires about 80–100 ms for an electrical impulse to travel down the electrical conduction system of the ventricle and to depolarize the myocardium. If the electrical impulse is diverted and not allowed to follow the normal ventricular conduction pathway it will take longer to depolarize the myocardium. Of course, this delay in conduction through the ventricle produces a wider QRS complex.

Emergency care providers are accustomed to measuring QRS complex width as a means of differentiating a premature ventricular contraction (PVC) from a premature atrial contraction (PAC). Chapters 6-9 measure QRS complex duration to detect the presence of bundle branch block.

The same criteria are used for measuring QRS duration regardless of the reason. Remember, a QRS complex that is 120 ms or more in duration (three small boxes wide) is considered abnormal.

R Wave Progression

The morphologies of the QRS complexes seen in the chest leads usually follow a predictable pattern as they progress from V1 to V6. In V1 the QRS complex is primarily negative with a very small R wave and a predominant S wave (rS complex). As the leads progress towards the left, the QRS complexes become more positively deflected as the R wave increases in height and the S wave decreases in depth. This progression continues and by the time V6 is reached, the complex is predominantly upright.

The pattern observed in the V-leads in which the QRS complex changes from a primarily negative complex to a primarily positive complex in V6 is called **R wave progression.** The area in which this occurs is called the **transition zone.** Transition usually occurs either at V3 or between V3 and V4, as is demonstrated in Fig. 1-16.

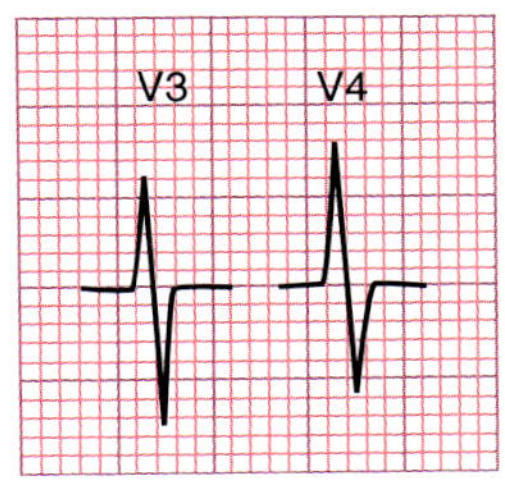

FIG. 1-16 In normal R wave progression, the QRS complex is negative in V1, positive in V6 and switches from negative to positive in the V3-V4 transition zone.

Many conditions can affect R wave progression, infarction being only one of them. While changes in R wave progression alone is not strong enough evidence to diagnose infarction, patterns of altered R wave progression will be seen in association with many infarctions.

SUMMARY

- **The ECG operates like a voltmeter and senses change in electrical potential across the skin.**
- **Milliseconds are used to express time on the 12-lead ECG.**
- **The 12-lead ECG is obtained through four limb electrodes and six chest electrodes.**
- **Each lead "views" the left ventricle from the position of its positive electrode.**
- **The term QRS complex refers to ventricular depolarization but not every QRS complex has a Q wave, an R wave, and an S wave.**
- **The R wave is the first positive deflection in the QRS complex.**
- **Both the Q wave and the S wave are negative deflections. The Q wave precedes the R wave while the S wave follows it.**
- **Q Waves may be a normal, physiologic finding or an abnormal, pathologic one.**
- **Q waves that equal or exceed 40 ms, or are more then one-third the amplitude of the R wave, tend to be pathologic.**
- **The J point is the junction between the QRS complex and the ST segment.**
- **The ST segment is normally level with the isoelectric line. Use both the TP segment and the PR segment to establish the position of the isoelectric line.**
- **The normal duration of a QRS complex is 80–100 ms. A QRS complex 120 ms or more in duration is abnormal.**
- **The QRS complex is primarily negative in V1, primarily positive in V6, and normal transition can occur at V3, at V4, or between the two.**

2

Acquiring the 12-Lead ECG

CHAPTER

OBJECTIVES

- Develop a reliable approach to locating the proper positions of the six chest leads.
- Describe a method for obtaining a multi-lead ECG using a standard "3-lead" monitor.
- Understand the significance of frequency response in producing a reliable tracing.
- Identify normal calibration and instances when it should be changed.
- Recognize the importance of skin preparation before obtaining the ECG.

Lead Placement

CHEST LEADS

Proper placement of the chest leads requires the ability to pinpoint specific anatomic locations, particularly certain intercostal spaces (Fig. 2-1). Various landmarks can be used to ascertain the correct location of these intercostal spaces and the particular method used is of little consequence, as long as the leads are properly located. One method of locating the appropriate intercostal spaces is described here and illustrated in Fig. 2-2.

Begin by locating the jugular notch. Move inferiorly until the articulation between the manubrium and the sternum (sternal angle or angle of Louis) is found. Following that articulation to the right sternal border will lead to the second rib. Immediately below the second rib is the second intercostal space. Move down two intercostal spaces and position the V1 electrode in the fourth intercostal space, just right of the sternum.

Next, move across the sternum to the corresponding intercostal space and position the V2 electrode in the fourth intercostal space, just to the left of the sternum. From the V2 position, palpate down one intercostal space and follow the fifth intercostal space to the midclavicular line. The fifth intercostal space, at the midclavicular line, marks the position for the V4 electrode.

The remaining three chest electrodes do not have specific intercostal landmarks, but are positioned in relation to the V2 and V4 positions. The position of lead V3 is the midpoint between V2 and V4. From the V4 position, if an imaginary horizontal line is drawn level with the V4 position, V5 and V6 will fall on that line. The position of V5 is in the anterior axillary line (where the arm joins the chest), level with V4. Lead V6 is positioned in the midaxillary line, level with V4 and V5. In the female patient, chest leads must be positioned under the breast.

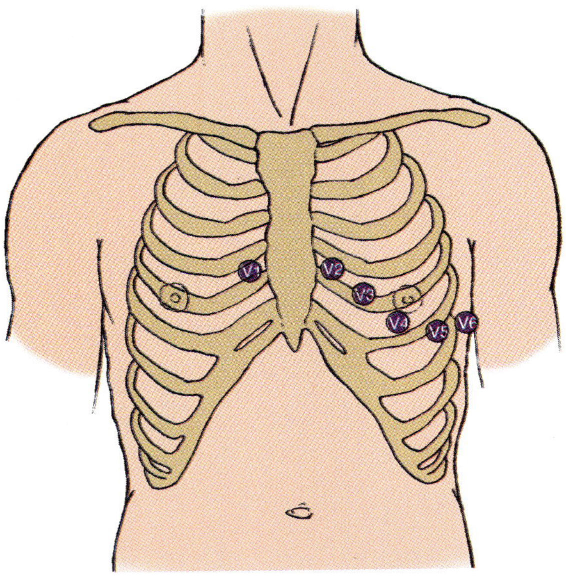

FIG. 2-1 Proper chest lead placement.

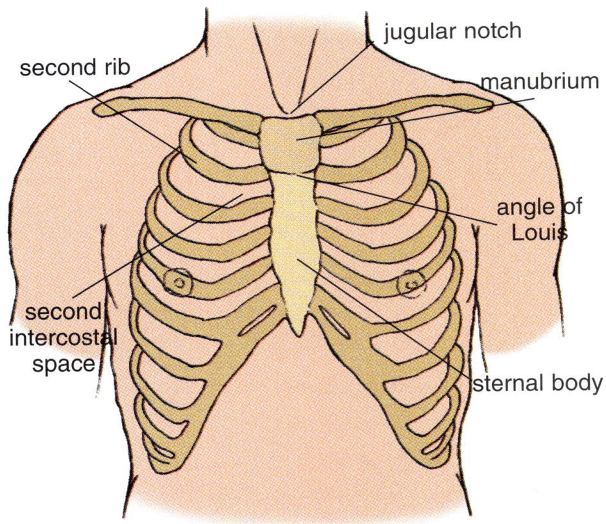

FIG. 2-2 A, The relationship between the jugular notch (sternal notch), manubrium, the angle of Louis, the sternal body and the intercostal spaces.

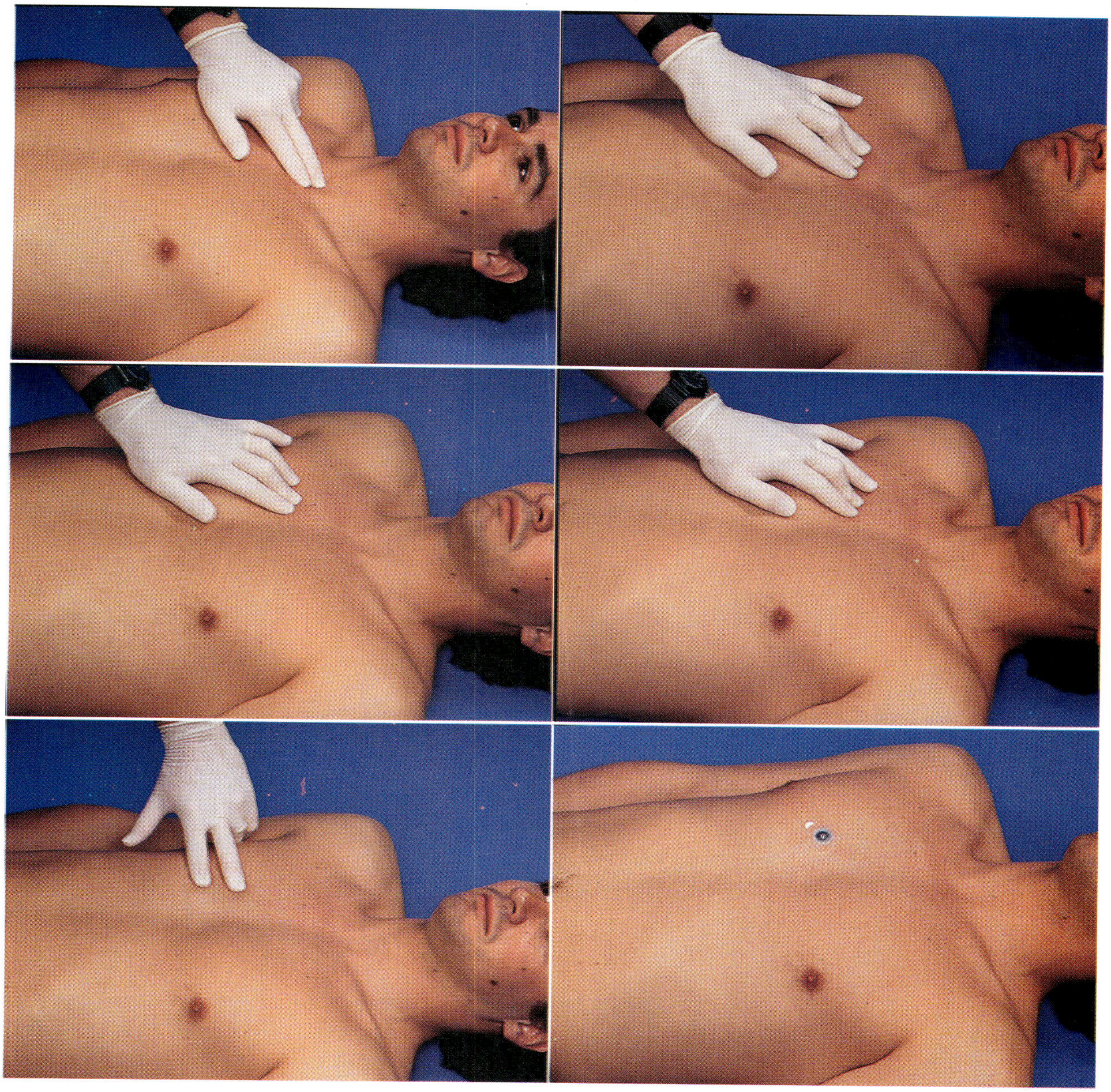

B C D E F G

FIG. 2-2, continued. **B,** Locate the jugular notch. **C,** Palpate for the angle of Louis. **D,** Follow the angle of Louis to the patient's right until it articulates with the second rib. **E,** Locate the second intercostal space (immediately below the second rib). **F,** From the second intercostal space the third and fourth intercostal spaces can be found. **G,** V1 is positioned in the fourth intercostal space just to the right of the sternum.

Continued.

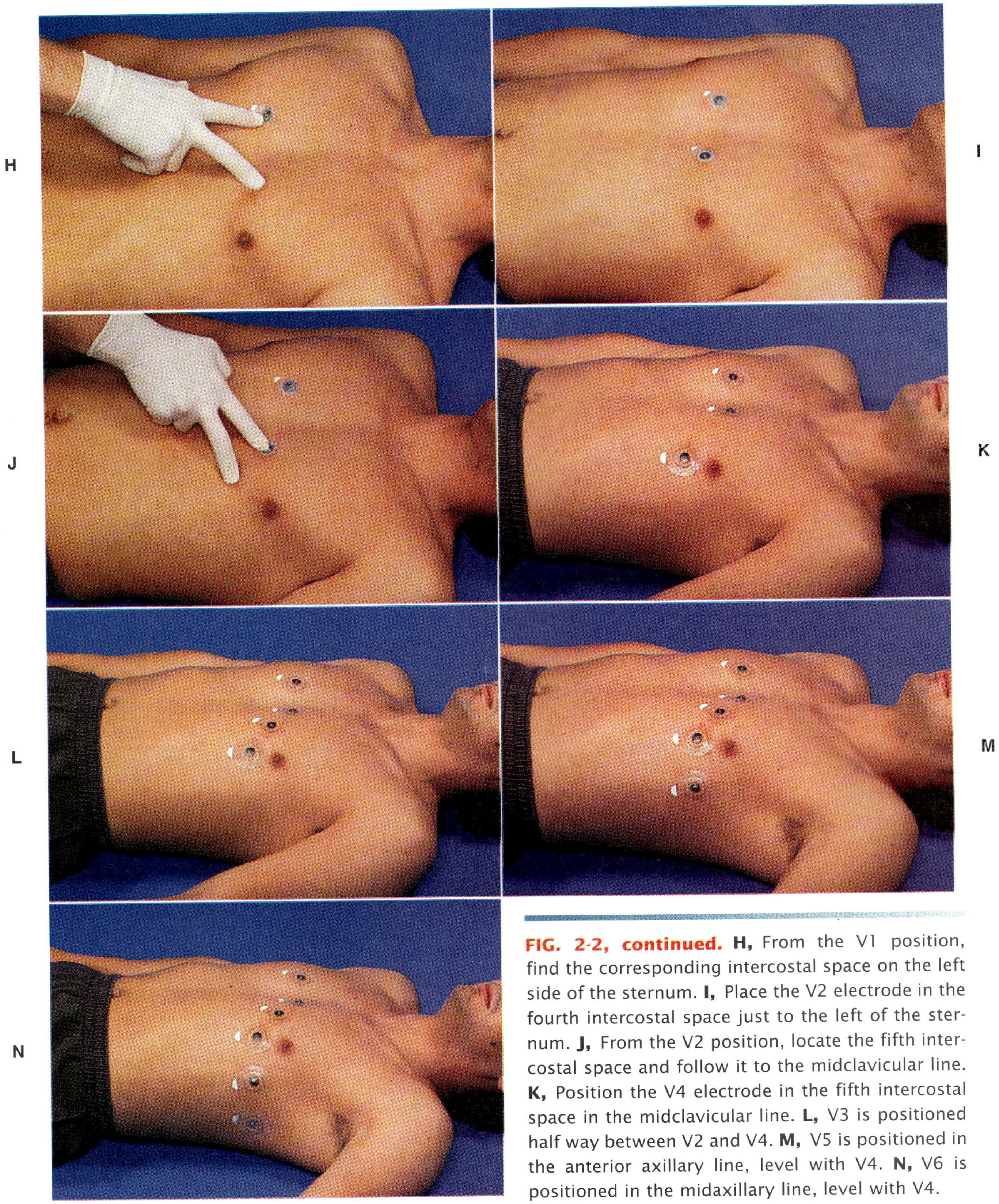

FIG. 2-2, continued. H, From the V1 position, find the corresponding intercostal space on the left side of the sternum. **I,** Place the V2 electrode in the fourth intercostal space just to the left of the sternum. **J,** From the V2 position, locate the fifth intercostal space and follow it to the midclavicular line. **K,** Position the V4 electrode in the fifth intercostal space in the midclavicular line. **L,** V3 is positioned half way between V2 and V4. **M,** V5 is positioned in the anterior axillary line, level with V4. **N,** V6 is positioned in the midaxillary line, level with V4.

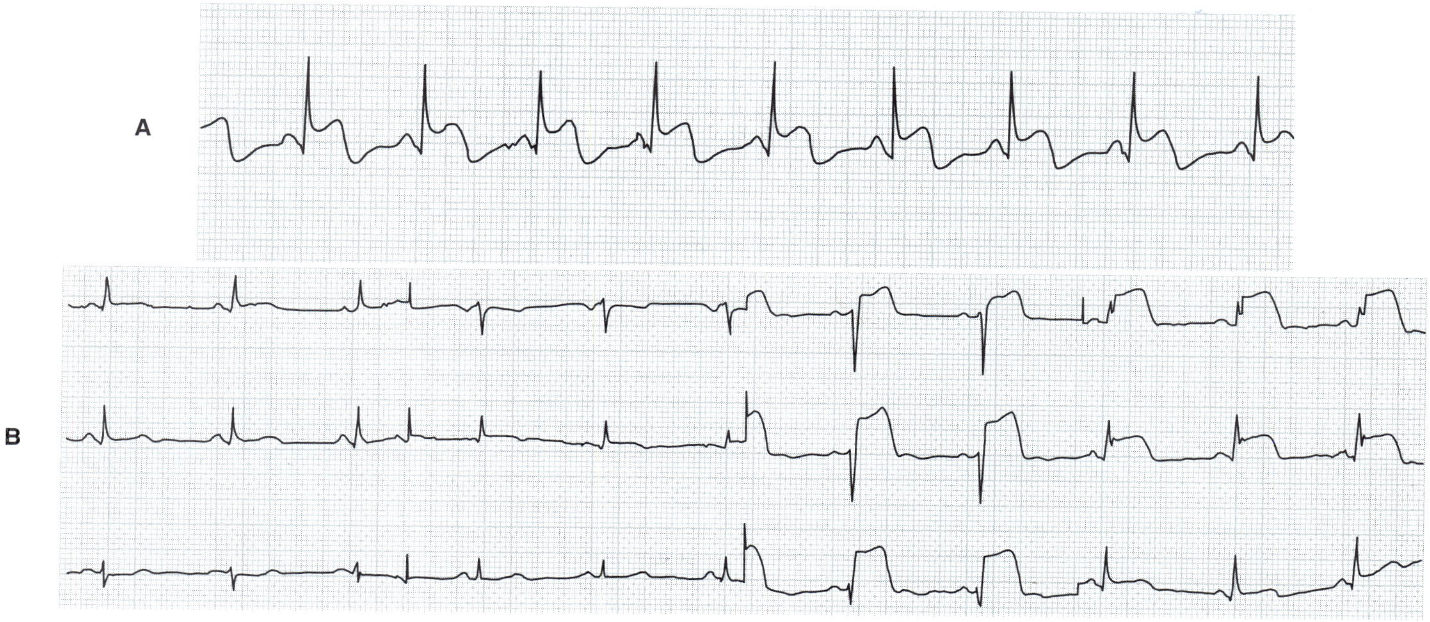

FIG. 2-3 **A,** This tracing shows ST segment elevation in what was labeled as "lead II" but, it was actually obtained from the upper abdomen. **B,** The 12-lead from the same patient with proper lead placement. No ST segment elevation is seen in lead II. It is correctly shown in the V leads.

Later chapters discuss the use of some right-sided chest leads. Right-sided chest leads are positioned symmetrically, on the contralateral side. Therefore, V4R is positioned in the fourth intercostal space, midclavicular line, on the right side of the chest. The positions of V5R and V6R are in a horizontal line with V4R, placed respectively in the anterior axillary line and the mid-clavicular line on the right chest.

LIMB LEADS

As previously mentioned, limb leads can be placed anywhere on the appropriate limb, as long as bony prominences are avoided. Leads I, II, and III are routinely obtained and very familiar to the cardiac care provider. However, many position them on the trunk rather than positioning them on the appropriate limb. Fig. 2-3A demonstrates ST segment elevation in a tracing labeled as lead II. Fig. 2-3B shows no similar ST segment elevation in a 12-lead from the same patient. Interestingly, the electrode used to obtain this lead II rhythm strip was not positioned on the left leg, but on the trunk, near the V5 position. Note how similar the "lead II" tracing is to the V5 tracing. In this instance, improper limb lead placement resulted in an ECG more closely resembling a chest lead than a limb lead. As a rule, place limb leads on the appropriate limbs. If this is not feasible, place them on the trunk as close to the appropriate limb as possible.

Equipment

The maximum number of leads that a cardiac montior can obtain is not limited by the number of cables attached to the monitor. In fact, any number of leads can be produced from a "3–lead" monitor. This chapter describes two methods for acquiring a 12–lead ECG and discusses a method of producing a 9-lead ECG from a "3–lead" monitor.

Why is it helpful to understand how to obtain a 12-lead ECG from a standard monitor when monitors capable of producing 12-lead electrocardiograms are readily available in most settings? Occasionally, situations present when the availability of a stat 12-lead ECG is desirable, but a 12-lead machine is not available. When this occurs, the emergency cardiac care provider may opt to obtain the 12-lead ECG using a standard monitor. In the prehospital setting, monitors capable of providing a 12-lead ECG were only recently introduced. Therefore, the ability to produce a multilead ECG from a "3-lead" monitor may have greater significance to the prehospital cardiac care provider.

Those emergency cardiac care providers interested in multilead acquisition from a standard monitor must be certain to read the sections discussing frequency response and calibration, because these topics, to a great extent, determine the fidelity and accuracy of the ECG produced.

12-Lead Acquisition

12-LEAD MONITOR

Once the electrodes have been properly positioned, the cables can be attached. With a 12-lead monitor it is simply a matter of following the manufacturer's instructions and pushing the right button(s) to record the tracing (Fig. 2-4). Most modern 12-lead monitors record all 12 leads simultaneously but display them in the conventional 3 row by 4 column format. Therefore, all of the QRS complexes in a row are consecutive while QRS complexes that are aligned vertically represent a simultaneous recording of the same beat (Fig. 2-5).

The primary advantages of using a 12-lead machine are speed and accuracy. Because the leads are obtained simultaneously, only 10 seconds of sampling time is required to record all twelve leads. The 12-lead monitor is the gold standard to which other means of acquisition are compared. Additional benefits include the interpretive program and the information matrix measuring intervals and durations.

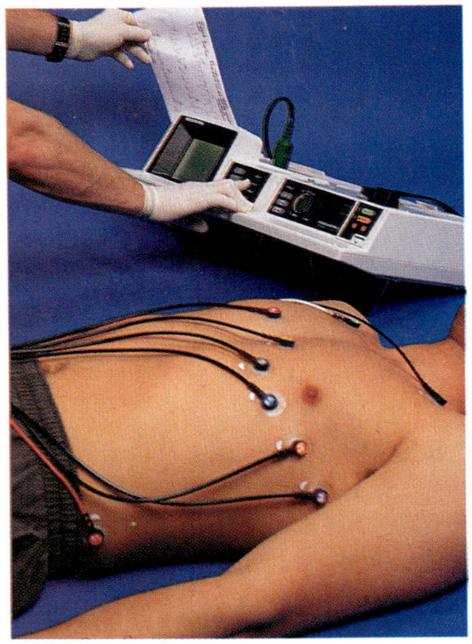

FIG. 2-4 To obtain a 12-lead ECG when using a 12-lead monitor or machine, simply attach the cables to the electrodes, ask the patient to be still, and push the record button. Acquisition requires only 10 seconds.

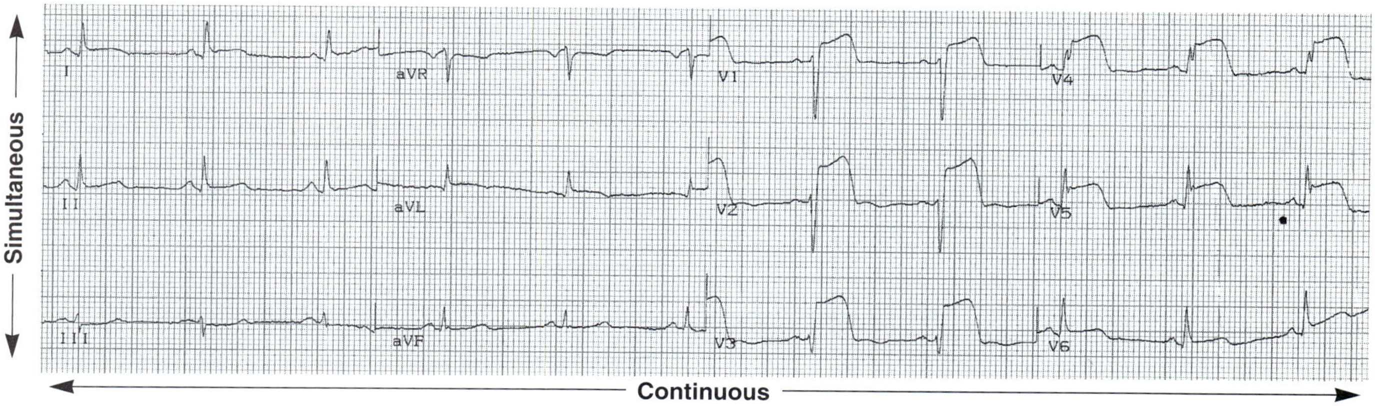

FIG. 2-5 In a simultaneous tracing, the beats in a vertical column are all the product of the same ventricular contraction. Likewise, beats in a horizontal row are continuous, even as the leads change.

From the prehospital perspective, a 12-lead monitor allows for transmission of the 12-lead ECG to the receiving facility. The technology for ECG transmission has improved considerably over the past few years and it is now possible to produce a copy at the receiving facility that is identical to the original obtained in the field.

12-LEAD ADAPTER

Some manufacturers offer a 12-lead adapter for use with standard monitors, as shown in Fig. 2-6A. The 12-lead adapter plugs into the monitor's cable port and consists of selector box and 10 ECG cables. The 10 cables are then attached to the electrodes, just as they are for a true 12-lead monitor. The monitor is placed in lead II, and the lead selector is set to lead I.

Once an adequate sample of lead I has been obtained (two or three similar complexes with a steady baseline), the selector can be moved to lead II. This procedure is repeated until all six limb leads have been obtained. The last stop on the first dial is marked "V LEADS." When the first dial is set to "V leads," the second dial determines which chest lead is being acquired. Leads V1-V6 may be obtained by changing the position

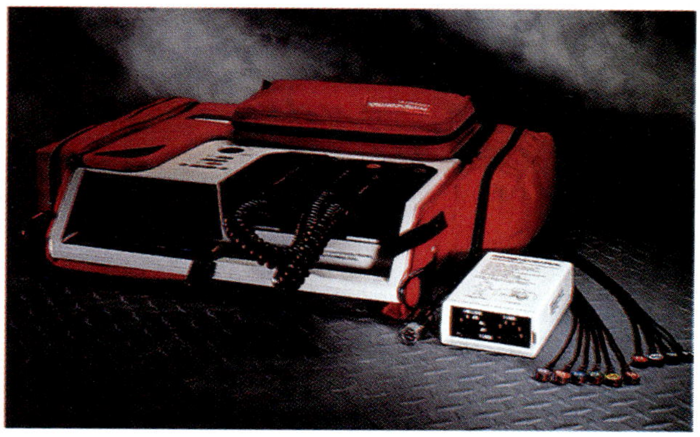

A

FIG. 2-6 A, The LIFEPAK® 10 defibrillator/monitor/pacemaker with the 12-lead adapter. (*Courtesy of Physio-Control Corporation, Redmond, WA.*)

Continued.

B

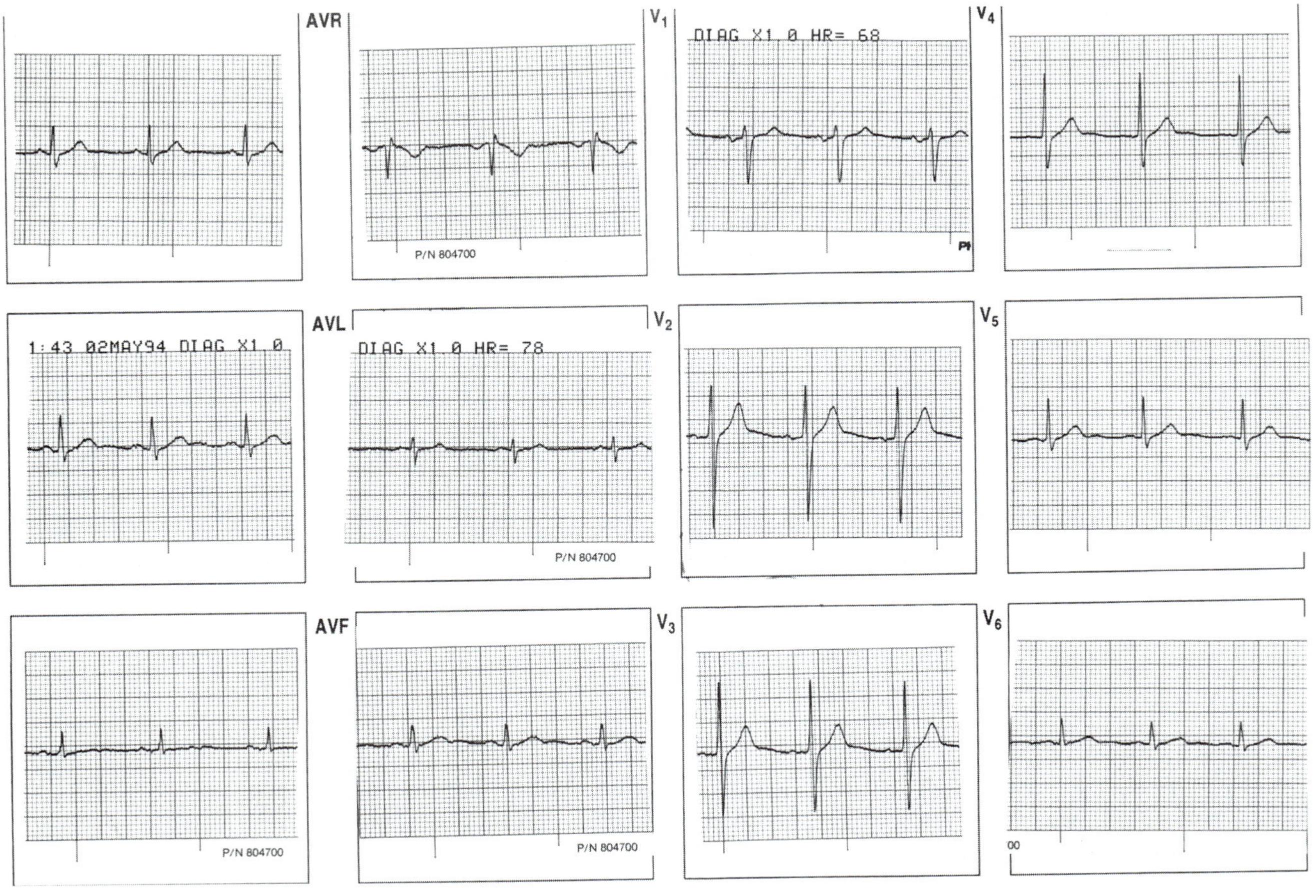

FIG. 2-6, continued. B, The tracing mounted in the standard 12-lead format.

of the dial, after collecting a representative sample of each lead. The result is a serial 12-lead ECG, which obtains true unipolar leads.

The chief disadvantage of this method is time requirement. Every time a new lead is selected the tracing usually goes off the screen. One must, therefore, wait for the tracing to center itself, then gather two or three complexes of similiar morphology before switching to the next lead. This process may take 10–20 seconds per lead, requiring 2–4 minutes for acquiring all twelve leads. The other disadvantage of this method is the format of the tracing.

When a serial 12-lead is obtained by this method the tracing is printed out over many feet of paper. The resulting output, however accurate it may be, does not look like a 12-lead. This could raise eyebrows and make some hesitant to form any treatment decision based on these tracings.

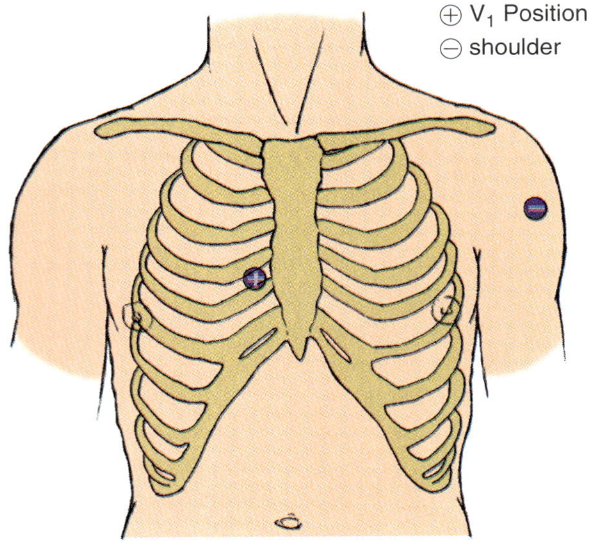

FIG. 2-7 Obtaining a MCL1 lead.

STANDARD "3-LEAD" MONITOR

If a 12-lead monitor or adapter is not available, but a "3-lead" monitor is available, then a multi-lead ECG may be the only alternative. With the multi-lead ECG, bipolar versions of the chest leads are used rather than the true unipolar versions. Most emergency cardiac care givers are already familiar with at least one bipolar version of a chest lead, MCL1.

To obtain MCL1 the negative electrode is placed at the left shoulder — the "L" of MCL — and the positive electrode is placed at the V1 position (Fig. 2-7). To obtain any other V lead, the negative electrode remains at the left shoulder while the positive electrode is moved to the corresponding V lead position. For example, MCL4 is obtained by placing the negative electrode at the left shoulder and the right electrode at the fifth intercostal space in the midclavicular line. Each of the V leads may be approximated in this way. Therefore, the MCL system accounts for six of the twelve leads.

To obtain a 9-lead ECG, place an electrode on the left arm, the right arm, and the left leg. The three cables are then attached to the appropriate

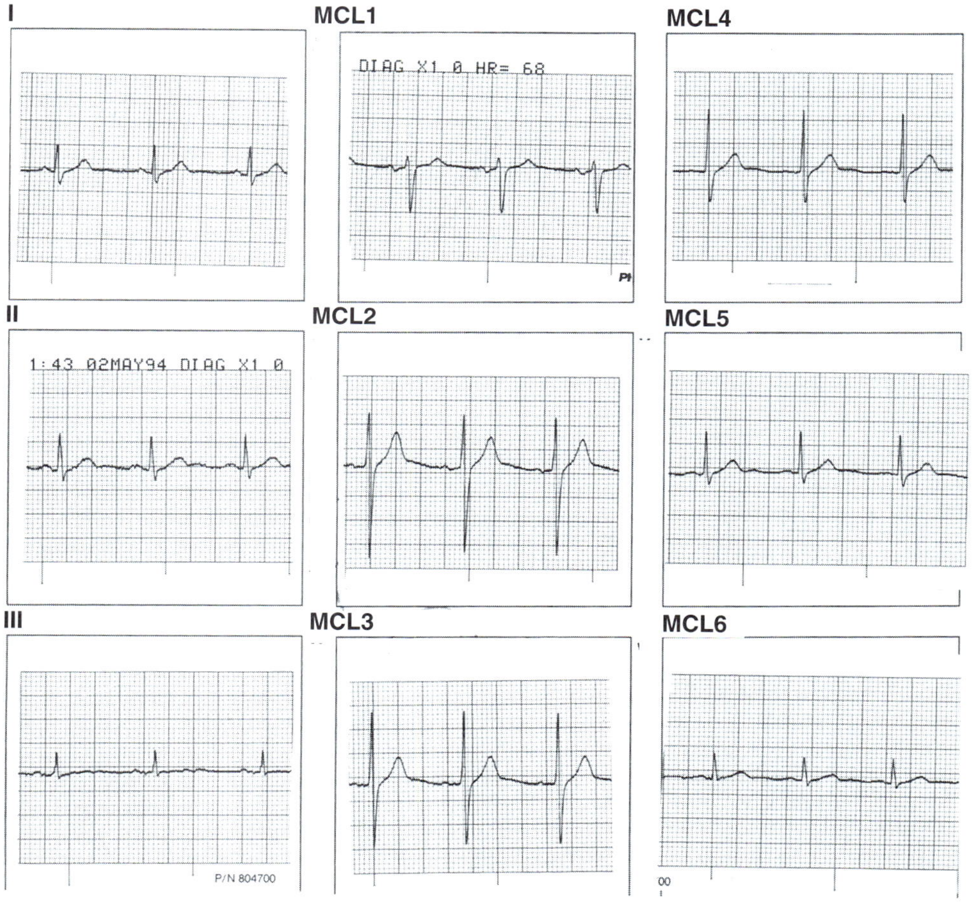

FIG. 2-8 Nine leads are obtained: I, II, III, and MCL1–MCL6.

limbs and the monitor is used to assess cardiac rate and rhythm. When ready to search for evidence of infarction, place an electrode at each of the six chest lead positions. Then record a representative sampling of leads I, II, and III. Leave the monitor in lead III — this places the negative electrode at the left shoulder — and move the left leg cable to the V1 position and record MCL1. When an adequate sample of MCL1 has been obtained, repeat this procedure for MCL2-MCL6. An ECG obtained by using a 3-lead monitor is shown in Fig. 2-8.

The remaining three limb leads, AVR, AVL, and AVF, may also be obtained in a modified bipolar version. However, since AVR is not used for infarct recognition it may be omitted. In fact, one may opt to omit leads AVL and AVF and produce a 9-lead ECG instead of a full 12-lead ECG.

While a 9-lead ECG does not include AVR, AVL, and AVF, remember that leads I, MCL5, and MCL6 are still available to provide information about the lateral wall, and leads II and III can provide a view of the inferior wall. The assumption is that with these nine leads, the interpreter would arrive at the same conclusions as if he or she had used a full 12-lead. However, this has yet to be proven in the setting of infarct recognition.

As of the writing of this text, a study is underway that investigates multilead ECGs and their use in the setting of infarction. The validity of modified leads for infarct recognition and the minimum number of leads required to recognize infarction are concerns specifically addressed in the study. Results may affect the clinical application of this method.

Frequency Response

The heart is not the only source of electrical activity that is detected by the ECG. Competing with the heart are such things as muscle tremor, movement artifact, 60-cycle interference, and other types of background "noise." Therefore, engineers work to produce a situation in which the monitor clearly sees the signal produced by the heart but ignores those signals that produce artifact.

To better understand this concept, once again think of the ECG monitor as a voltmeter. Like any other voltmeter, it functions within a certain range or spectrum. If electrical activity occurs within that spectrum the monitor senses it; if it occurs outside of the spectrum the monitor does not sense it. The spectrum in which an ECG can accurately reproduce the signals it is sensing is referred to as the **frequency response**. Monitors may be designed with either a narrow or wide frequency response. Each has its own set of advantages and disadvantages.

Frequency response can be considered the window through which the ECG looks. If the window is large, the ECG sees a lot; if the window is smaller the ECG sees less. Which is better? The answer depends upon the purpose for which the ECG monitor is being used. If rate and rhythm are the primary objective, a narrow frequency response is desirable. The narrow frequency response does not let the monitor see much of the artifact and noise that can produce an unclear tracing. This simplifies the process of locating P waves, measuring intervals, and all the other aspects of rhythm assessment. However, as helpful as a narrow frequency response can be when determining rate and rhythm, infarct recognition requires a wide frequency response. Figs. 2-9A and 2-9B graphically demonstrate how changes in frequency response affect what the monitor can and can't see.

The range in which ST segment elevation can be detected is in the lower end of the frequency

A

B

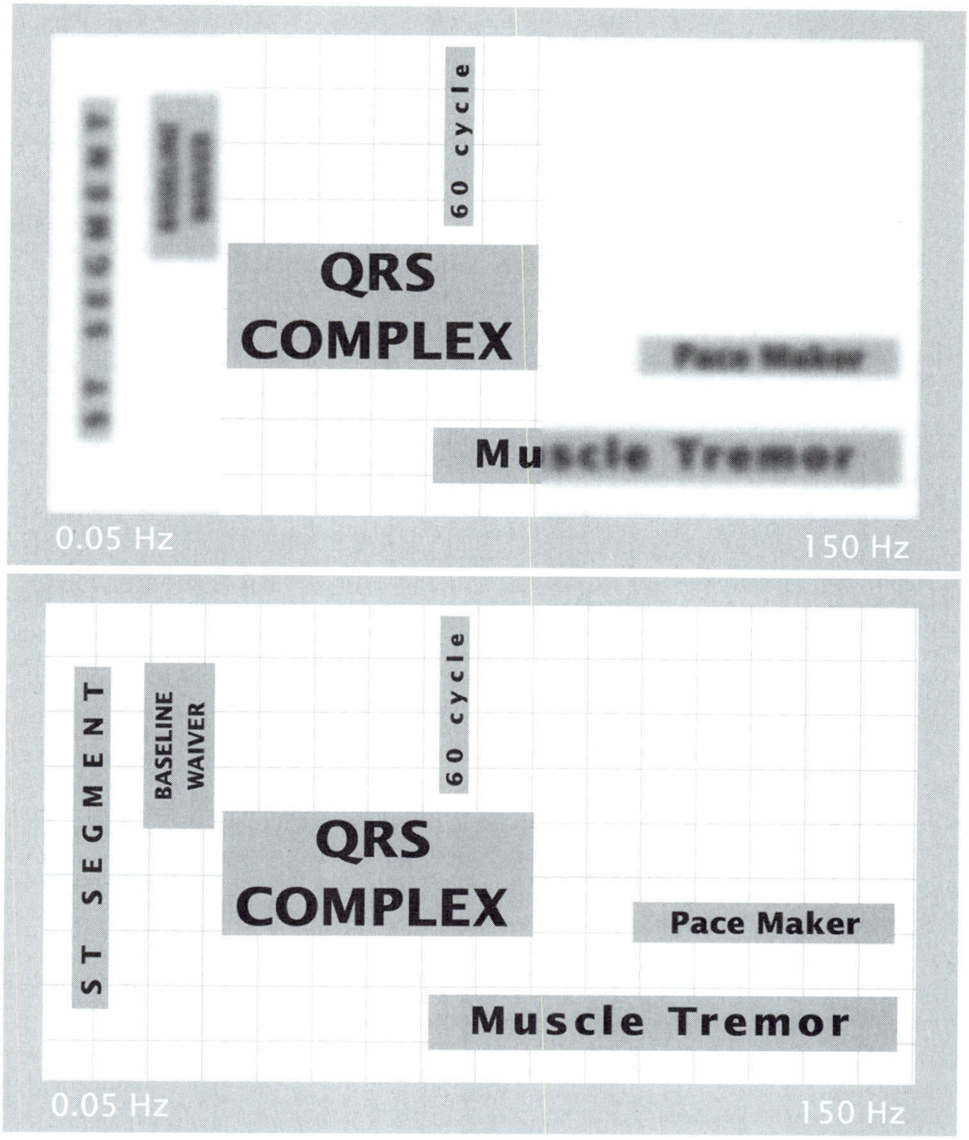

FIG. 2-9 **A,** With a limited frequency response the monitor can clearly "see" the QRS complex but cannot see the other features as clearly. **B,** With a wider frequency response, the monitor can not only see the QRS complex but also the ST segment as well.

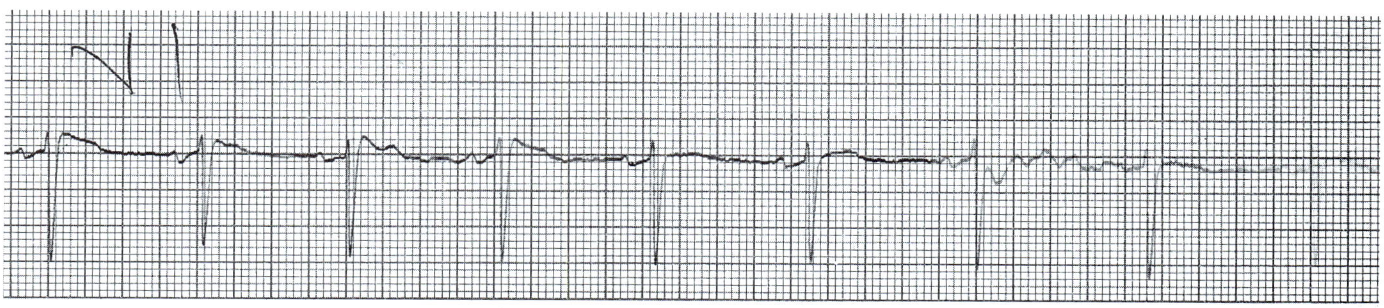

FIG. 2-10 The first four beats were obtained in monitor quality and demonstrate 2 mm of ST segment elevation. The fifth beat was obtained in diagnostic quality and shows no ST segment elevation.

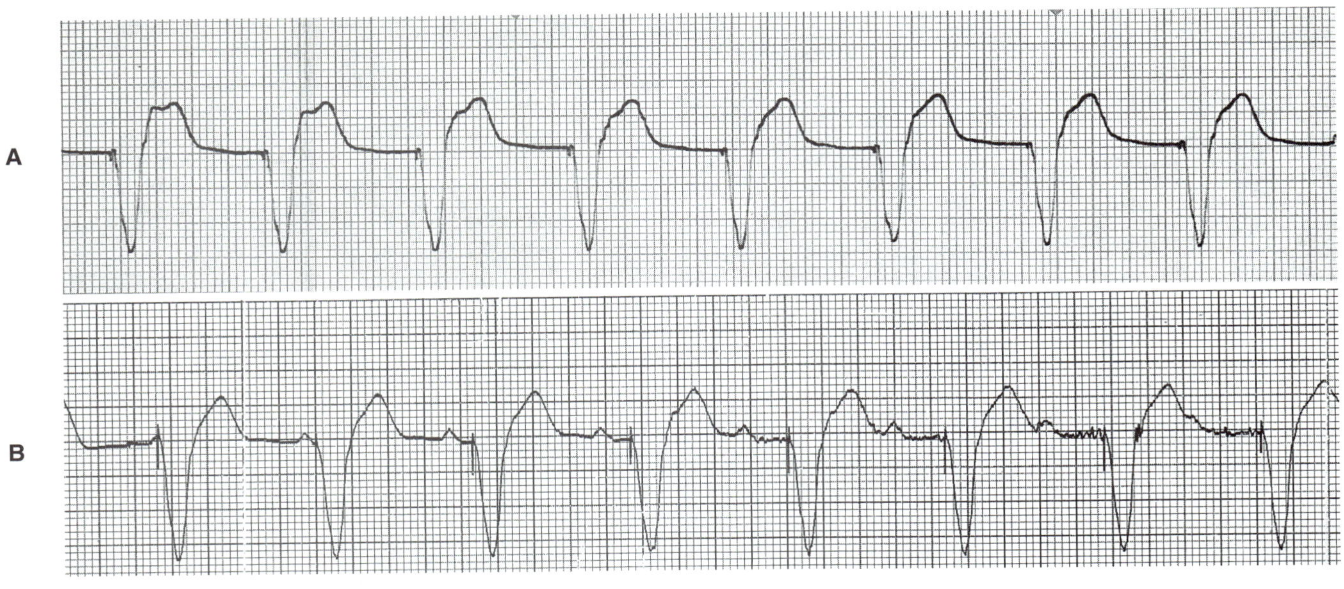

FIG. 2-11 **A,** Tracing obtained in monitor quality. The patient's pacemaker was firing, but no pacemaker spikes are visible. The ST segment elevation is prominent. **B,** The same patient, tracing obtained in diagnostic quality. The pacemaker spikes are now visible.

spectrum. A narrow frequency response can distort readings in the lower end of the spectrum and may not accurately reproduce all of the electrical activity occurring while the ST segment is recorded. This lack of sensitivity in the lower end of the frequency spectrum can alter the position of the ST segment. Therefore, a wide frequency response is needed for accurate ST segment analysis.

A narrow frequency response can be referred to as "monitor quality" and a wide frequency response can be referred to as "diagnostic quality." The ECG in Fig. 2-10 was obtained from a healthy 30-year-old emergency care provider. The ST segment is elevated by approximately 2 mm in VI when recorded in monitor quality. While this tracing was being recorded the monitor was switched from monitor quality into diagnostic quality. The fifth beat was the first to be captured in diagnostic quality. Notice that the ST segment is no longer elevated. ECG tracings obtained in monitor quality frequency response display ST segment elevation which is not present in diagnostic quality. This could lead to misidentification of infarct patients. Furthermore, the ST segment may appear normal in monitor quality but show ST segment elevation when obtained in diagnostic quality. Also note there is more artifact in the later portion of the tracing. This demonstrates the tradeoff: Increased fidelity often results in greater artifact.

Another example of how frequency response can change the ECG is demonstrated in Fig. 2-11. These strips were obtained within seconds of each other, first using monitor quality, then using diagnostic quality. Once again a monitor quality recording has produced ST segment elevation beyond the amount present in a diagnostic quality tracing. In addition, the pacemaker spike is not visible in the fist tracing (monitor quality), but is very prominent in the second tracing (diagnostic quality).

Again, the more appropriate frequency response depends on the intended use. Monitor quality aids in rhythm analysis, while diagnostic quality is necessary for accurate ST segment analysis. Fortunately, many newer monitors are designed to allow the user to instantly switch between monitor quality and diagnostic quality. This allows emergency cardiac care providers to use monitor quality when determining rate and rhythm and to later switch to diagnostic quality for ST segment analysis. Fig. 2-12 shows the

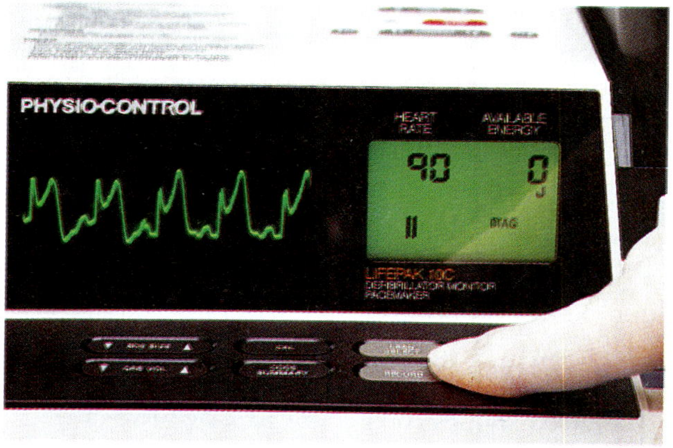

FIG. 2-12 Press the record button, and hold it. After a few seconds, the letters "DIAG" will appear in the information window. At this point the monitor has changed frequency response. It is not necessary to continue to hold the record button. However, once the record is turned off the machine reverts back to diagnostic quality.

method by which one monitor allows the user to enable the diagnostic quality in a common ECG monitor.

The method of accessing diagnostic-quality varies among different brands and models of ECG equipment. Always check the monitor's technical manual for specific information regarding diagnostic quality before using it in the clinical setting. Current recommendations suggest a low end of 0.05 MHz and a high end of 150 MHz. Be certain to check the low end carefully. Some monitors' lower frequency response is 0.5 MHz, which is still considered monitor quality.

Calibration

The significance of standard calibration is moot when the monitor is used only to determine rate and rhythm. However, proper calibration is critical when analyzing ST segments.

The cardiac monitor's sensitivity to electrical current is variable. When the sensitivity is increased, a larger complex is produced. Likewise, a smaller complex is the result of decreased sensitivity. The button or control which adjusts the monitor's sensitivity can be labeled with a variety of names, some of which are ECG size, sensitivity, gain, and calibration. While the adjustment of sensitivity allows for an almost infinite number of possible settings, one setting is considered the standard for ECG recording: 1 mV = 10 mm. This means that when an ECG monitor is in standard calibration, a 10 mm (two big boxes) deflection is produced for every millivolt that is sensed.

In Chapter 3, ST segment elevation is used to spot possible myocardial infarction. However, the amount of ST segment elevation varies depending upon the calibration. For example, 1 mm of ST segment is significant when seen in standard calibration. However, 1 mm of ST segment elevation is not significant when noted in a complex printed at two times its normal size. Once the complex is reduced to its proper size, the amount of ST segment elevation would also be proportionately reduced and would be well below 1 mm. Therefore, all tracings should be recorded in standard calibration and the calibration pulse should be included in the tracing.

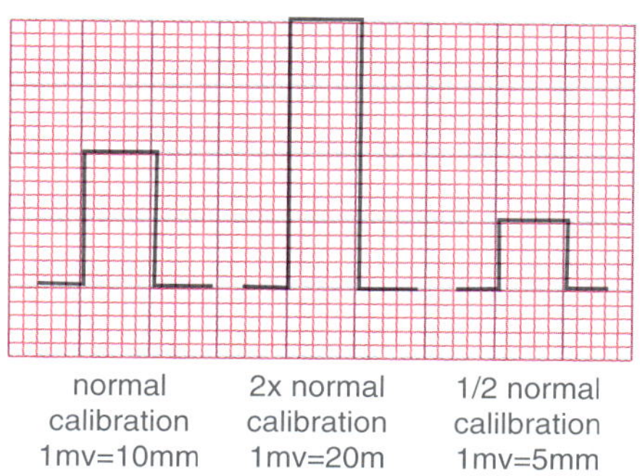

FIG. 2-13 The size of the ECG may be adjusted as needed. However, ST segment analysis must be adjusted accordingly whenever non-standard calibration is used.

Certain instances may warrant the use of a non-standard calibration. If the complexes are too large to fit the page, the calibration should be reduced. Likewise, if the complexes produced are too small to read, then the calibration should be increased. When changes in calibration are necessary, choose a calibration which will make interpretation easier. Therefore, if an increase in QRS size is needed, double the calibration. Likewise, if a reduction in ECG size in necessary, halve the calibration. Always include a calibration pulse and note the change in calibration on the ECG (Fig. 2-13).

Wandering Baseline

When the position of the baseline is in a state of flux, ST segment analysis is very difficult. As the baseline wanders, the isoelectric point changes from moment to moment. In this situation, the J point, though it may have been isoelectric when inscribed, can appear elevated above the PR and TP segments as shown in Fig. 2-14.

This ST segment elevation may not be the result of infarction, but just an expected finding which occurs as the monitor centers the isoelectric line in the screen. Therefore, be very cautious about analyzing ST segment elevation in leads with a wandering baseline. If an ECG is being obtained via a standard monitor, the care giver should wait until the tracing is centered for several beats before moving to the next lead.

A common cause of a wandering baseline is patient movement, often due simply to the patient's respirations. When the tracing quality precludes a good interpretation the tracing should be repeated. Efforts made to reduce the source of patient movement can improve the tracing quality, as can good skin preparation technique.

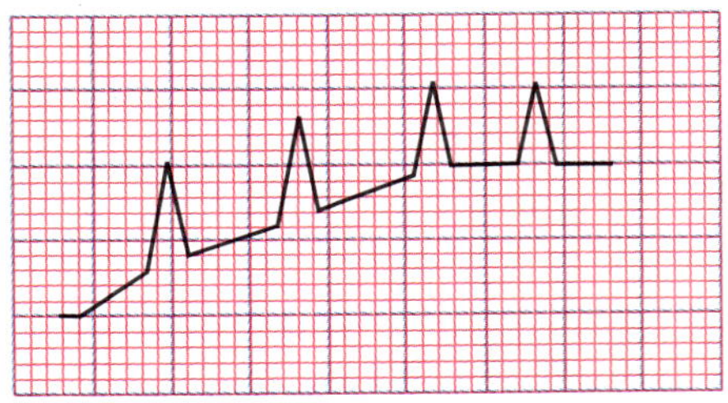

FIG. 2-14 The J Point is isoelectric, but when compared to the TP and PR segments it appears elevated. Note that when the baseline returns to the centered position, the ST segment no longer appears elevated. Do not perform ST segment analysis in this situation.

Skin Preparation

An often neglected component of ECG acquisition is skin preparation. For the monitor to properly detect current flow on the patient's skin, it must be able to penetrate through the dead skin and oil. A simple wipe of the skin with water or alcohol, followed by a brisk rub, may greatly improve the tracing quality. Many electrode manufacturers include an abrasive area on the disposable backing of the electrode for this purpose, but a gauze sponge works well too.

In the emergency setting, skin preparation techniques may take a back seat to the many other tasks being accomplished. However, if a "noisy" tracing has been produced and the artifact makes the tracing difficult to interpret, the skin should be quickly prepped and another ECG obtained. In the final analysis, it may be more efficient to routinely prep the skin before the first tracing.

Patient Position

While it may not be immediately obvious, the position of the patient can have an effect on the ECG. One reason for differences between tracings obtained in various positions is that while the electrode does not move when the patient changes position, the position of the heart does move relative to that electrode. Strictly speaking, a patient should be supine when the ECG is acquired. This makes comparison of serial ECGs more meaningful. However, this is not always possible or desirable in the chest-pain patient. If the patient is not supine when the tracing is obtained, simply note the patient's position on the 12-lead.

Electrodes

Two primary types of electrodes are available. One is used with cables that snap into place, the other is intended for cables using alligator clips instead of snaps. Often the former is used in the prehospital setting and the latter is most often seen in the hospital. When an EMS provider obtains a 12-lead and leaves the snap-on electrodes in place, they need not be removed before acquiring a follow-up 12-lead with the alligator–type clip cable. To accomplish this, simply attach the alligator clips of the hospital monitor to the metal posts of the snap-on electrode. Aside from the saving time, this method allows for better comparison of the field versus the hospital 12-lead, since lead position is unchanged.

When the snap-on type electrodes are used, some overlap in the chest leads is likely. In smaller framed patients, the use of pediatric electrodes may eliminate this situation.

SUMMARY

- Limb leads should be attached to the limbs and not to the chest.
- Proper positioning of V1, V2, and V4 requires the location of specific intercostal spaces.
- Leads V3, V5, and V6 do not have specific intercostal sites but are positioned relative to the other three chest leads.
- A standard monitor can produce a 9-lead or 12-lead ECG, but it must be capable of recording in diagnostic quality.
- To use ST segment elevation as an indicator of infarction, the monitor must be set to standard calibration, and in diagnostic quality.
- When the baseline wanders, ST segments may appear elevated when in fact they are not.
- Neglecting proper skin preparation can lead to a poor quality tracing.

3

OBJECTIVES

Myocardial Infarction: Recognition and Localization

CHAPTER 3

- Recognize the progressive ECG changes produced by myocardial infarction.
- Localize the area of myocardial infarction.
- Appreciate the great variance in normal coronary artery distribution.
- Predict which coronary artery is occluded.
- Assess the extent of infarction.
- Identify the clinical and ECG features of right ventricular infarction.

The Process of Infarction

In the strictest sense, the term myocardial infarction relates to necrosed myocardial tissue. In a practical sense, the term myocardial infarction is applied to the process which results in the death of myocardial tissue. Consider the entire "process" of myocardial infarction as a continuum rather than the presence of dead heart tissue. If efforts are made to recognize the process of myocardial infarction, patients may be identified earlier and, if promptly treated, may altogether avoid the loss of myocardial tissue. The American Heart Association has introduced the phrase "myocardially infarcting" and recommends its use to highlight the fact that an acute process is under way.

The process of myocardial infarction occurs when a coronary artery is unable to sufficiently supply myocardial tissue. The process usually begins when a blood clot forms in a coronary artery and occludes blood flow. Immediately after the onset of occlusion, myocardial cells begin to experience ischemia and then injury. This clot may spontaneously dissolve or may continue to occlude the coronary artery. If the occlusion persists, then loss of myocardial tissue will occur, beginning even within the first hour. It is important to understand the mechanisms of ischemia, injury, and infarction before discussing the changes produced on the ECG.

Ischemia refers to a temporary shortage of oxygen at the cellular level. This shortage is most often due to an increase in oxygen demand in the presence of a narrowed coronary artery. The narrowing will not allow for additional blood to be supplied and this mismatch in supply and demand results in ischemia. The pain produced by myocardial infarction is resolved when the demand for oxygen is reduced (the patient rests) to a level which can be supplied by the narrowed coronary artery.

Injury, like ischemia, also occurs when the supply of oxygen falls short of its demand. In the case of injury, this imbalance is not necessarily due to an increased demand. More commonly, the imbalabnce results from a diminishing supply of oxygen. The cells experiencing injury are still alive but cannot indefinitely survive in this condition, and will die if the hypoxia is not corrected. The injury can be extensive enough to produce a decrease in pump function or electrical conductivity in the affected cells.

As injury continues, some of the cells will begin to **infarct** (die) from the anoxia. As time progresses all of the cells experiencing injury will ultimately die unless the occlusion is corrected. Of course, infarcted cells are without function and cannot respond to electrical stimulus or provide any mechanical function.

In the ECG there are certain clues which serve to indicate the presence of ischemia, injury, and infarction. Familiarity with these clues may help to establish the presence, location, extent, and duration of the infarct.

ECG Changes Due to Infarction

The most fundamental use of the ECG is to identify the underlying cardiac rate and rhythm. When the ECG is used for this purpose, the clinician calculates the number of beats per minute and inspects for the presence of a dysrhythmia. However, a new set of criteria is needed in order to recognize the presence of myocardial infarction. While infarction can produce changes in rate and rhythm, infarct recognition in the ECG relies on the detection of morphologic changes (i.e., changes in shape) of the QRS complex, the T wave, and the ST segment. These changes occur in relation to certain events during the infarction. Therefore, as shown in Fig. 3-1A, they often occur in a predictable pattern which is recognizable on the ECG. The changes described below are not seen in every lead. They appear only in leads looking at the infarct site.

The first change that one might detect in the ECG is the development of a **tall T wave**. In addition to an increase in height, the T wave becomes more symmetric and may also become pointed (Fig. 3-1B). These T wave changes may occur within the first few minutes of infarction, during what has been described as the hyperacute phase of infarction.

As time progresses, signs of myocardial injury may develop. **ST segment elevation** (Fig. 3-1C) provides the primary indication of myocardial injury in progress. ST segment elevation may occur within the first hour or first few hours of infarction, and is considered to occur in the acute phase of infarction. Also in the acute phase of the infarction, one may see the presence of **T wave inversion,** suggesting the presence of ischemia (Fig. 3-1D). In fact, T wave inversion may precede the development of ST segment elevation, or they may occur simultaneously.

A few hours later, although still within the acute phase, the ECG may give its first evidence that tissue death has occurred. That evidence comes with the development of a **pathologic Q wave** (Fig. 3-1E) and is often seen in the first few hours to the first several hours. As mentioned in the Chapter 1, Q waves may occur normally, but a Q wave which is 40 ms or more wide (one small box or more wide) is suggestive of infarction.

In time, the T wave regains its normal contour and the ST segment returns to the isoelectric line. The Q wave, however, remains as evidence that an infarct has occurred (Fig. 3-1F). When this pattern is seen, establishing the time of the infarct is impossible. It is only possible to recognize the presence of a previous MI.

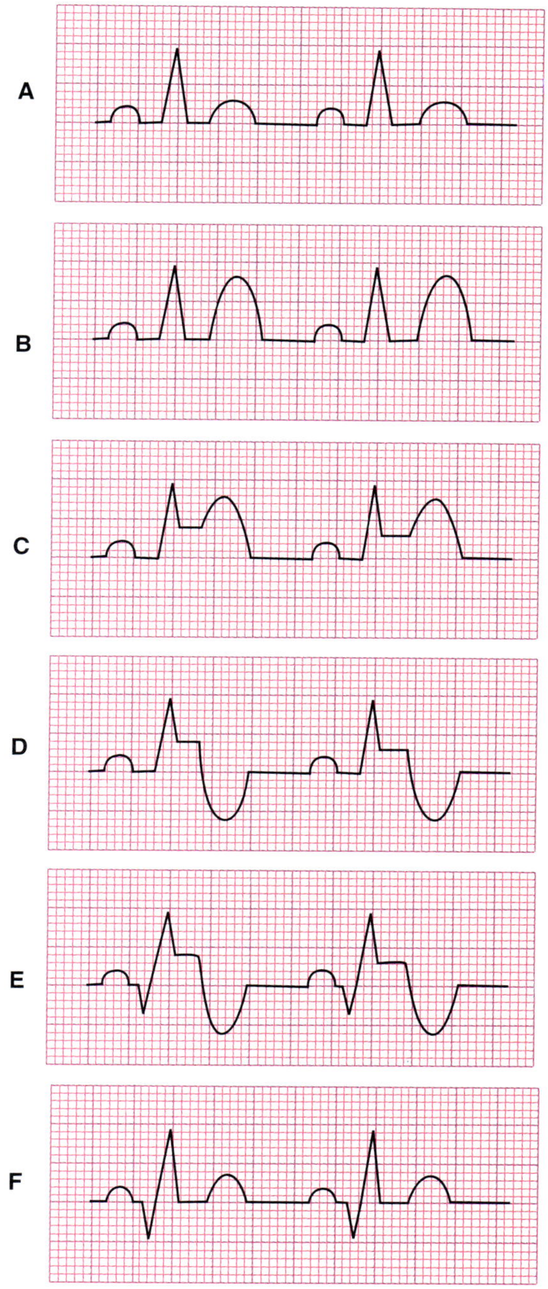

FIG. 3-1 A-F, The evolving pattern of myocardial infarction on the ECG.

The changes just described can be referred to as the **indicative changes** of myocardial infarction. Of the indicative changes, ST segment elevation is especially well-suited for the detection of MI in the early hours. A tall T wave alone is

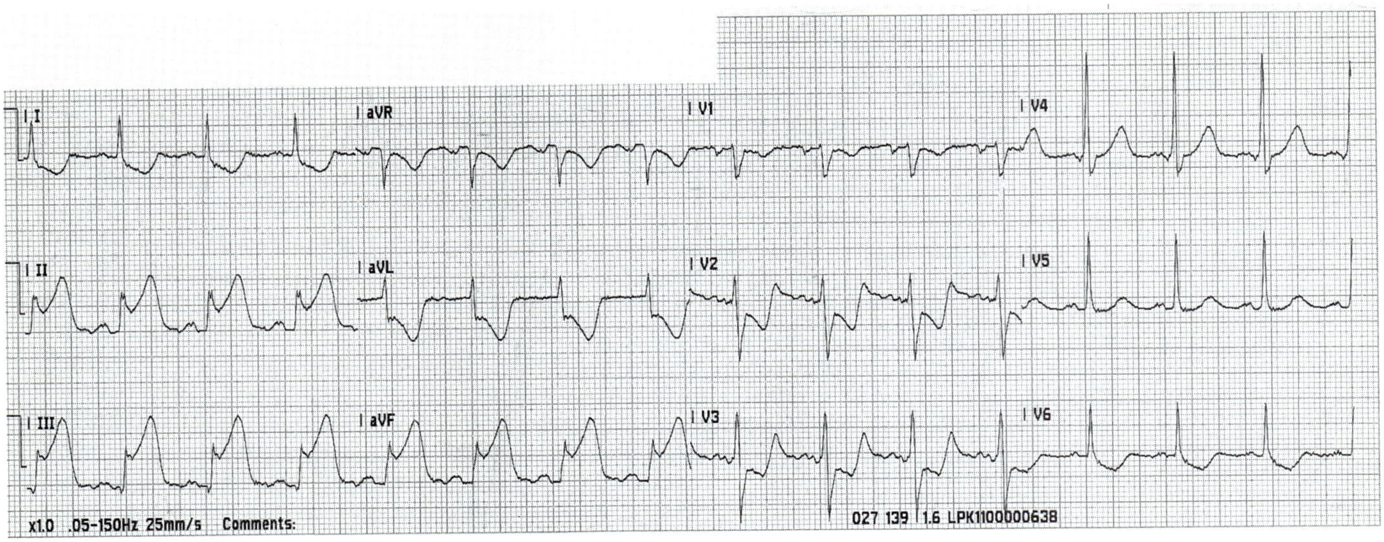

FIG. 3-2 ST segment elevation in leads II, III and AVF.

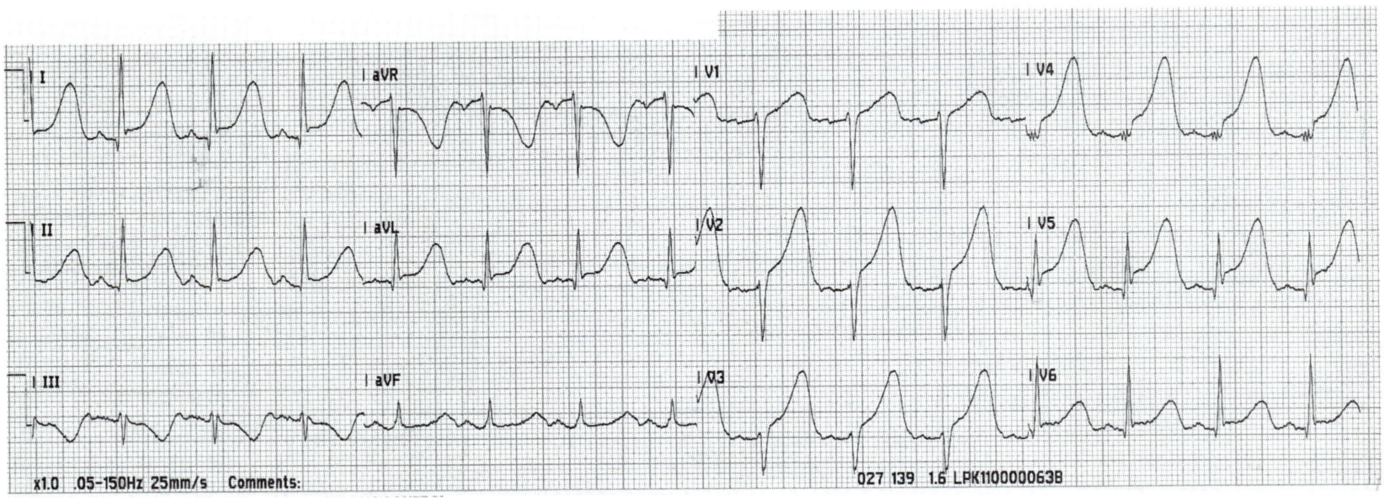

FIG. 3-3 ST segment elvation in leads I, AVL, and V1-V6 suggests a large infarct affecting the septum, anterior, and lateral walls.

not specific enough to diagnose MI, and T wave inversion may occur in simple angina. The development of a pathologic Q wave is the most accurate method of recognizing infarction, but, it may not be present in the first hours when patients are encouraged to seek treatment. ST segment elevation, however, is reasonably specific to infarction, and is often present in the early hours of infarction. Therefore, **ST segment elevation provides the strongest ECG evidence for the early recognition of myocardial infarction.**

When indicative changes of myocardial infarction occur, they are not found in every lead of the ECG. In fact, they are only present in the leads "looking" directly at the infarct site. When indicative changes are seen in two or more leads which "look" at the same portion of the heart (**anatomically contiguous leads**), enough evidence exists to suspect a myocardial infarction. Fig. 3-2 shows ST segment elevation in leads II, III, and AVF. These three leads are anatomically contiguous because they all look at adjoining tis-

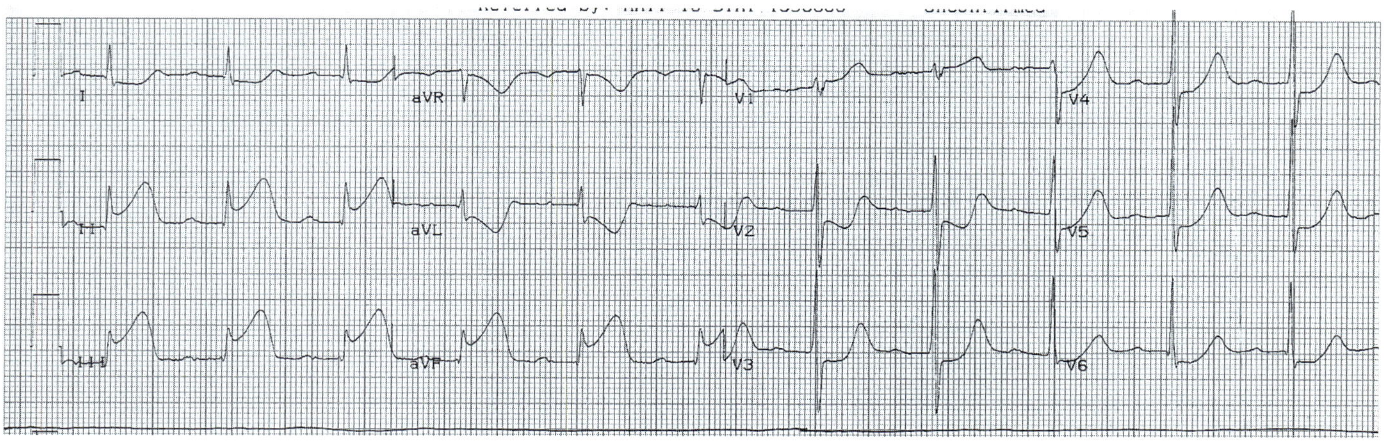

FIG. 3-4 **Inferior infarction.**

sue in the inferior region of the left ventricle. Therefore, an inferior wall infarction is suspected to be the cause of the ST segment elevation.

However, when ST segment elevation is seen in two or more leads that are not anatomically contiguous, infarction is not the suspected cause. For example, if ST segment elevation is noted in leads II and V2, one would not suspect myocardial infarction since leads II and V2 are not anatomically contiguous (lead II looks at the inferior wall while V2 looks at the septum). This fact demonstrates how infarct recognition and infarct localization are closely tied together: To recognize infarction, it is necessary to know which portion of the heart each lead is viewing. To localize the infarct, simply note which leads are displaying that evidence and consider which part of the heart that those leads "see."

Fig. 3-2 shows ST segment elevation and tall T waves in leads II, III, and AVF. These leads are anatomically contiguous because they look at the same general area of the heart. And since they "look" at the inferior wall of the left ventricle, an inferior wall MI is suspected. Fig. 3-3 shows an ECG with indicative changes in the V leads, lead I, and AVL. Since these leads view the septum, the anterior wall, and the lateral wall, an infarct in these areas is suspected.

Is that all there is to it? Yes, at least for now. Recognizing and localizing infarction is simply a matter of knowing what ECG changes to look for and knowing which portion of the heart each lead "looks" at.

Use Table 3-1 as a guide to localize the site of infarction in the following ECGs. Figures 3–4 through 3-7 are practice ECGs.

Looking at Figs. 3–5 and 3–7, it becomes apparent that indicative changes may be present in some of the V leads but not necessarily all of the V leads. Likewise, leads I and AVL may or may not show indicative changes when these same changes are present in the V leads. This situation may initially generate confusion when trying to localize the infarction. For example, if indicative changes are noted in V2 and V3, would the infarction be most appropriately referred to as a septal infarction or as an anterior infarct? It is more important that emergency cardiac care providers have an understanding of which area is infarcting rather than applying just the right name to it. To have a better understanding of infarct localization, an appreciation of coronary artery anatomy is necessary, which is the subject of the next section.

Table 3.1

LEADS DISPLAYING INDICATIVE CHANGES	LOCATION OF THE INFARCT SITE
II, III, and AVF	Inferior
V1 and V2	Septal
V3 and V4	Anterior
V5, V6, I, and AVL	Lateral

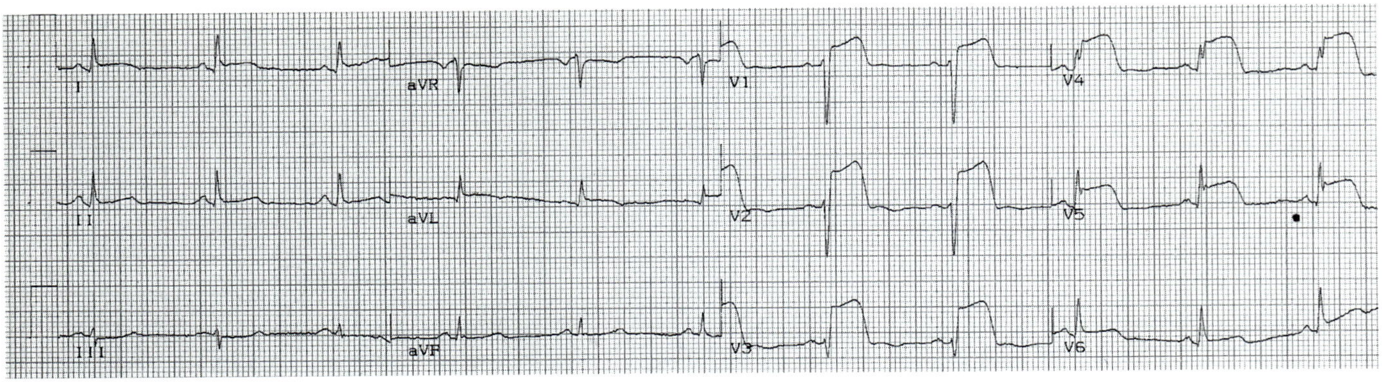

FIG. 3-5 Anteroseptal infarct with lateral extension.

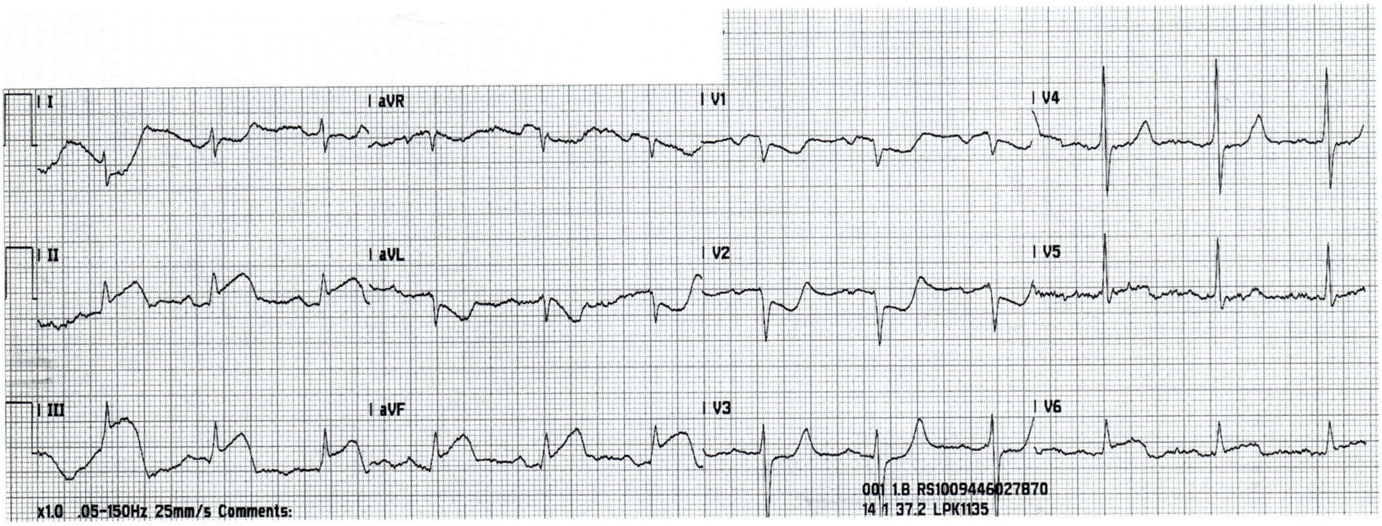

FIG. 3-6 Inferior infarct.

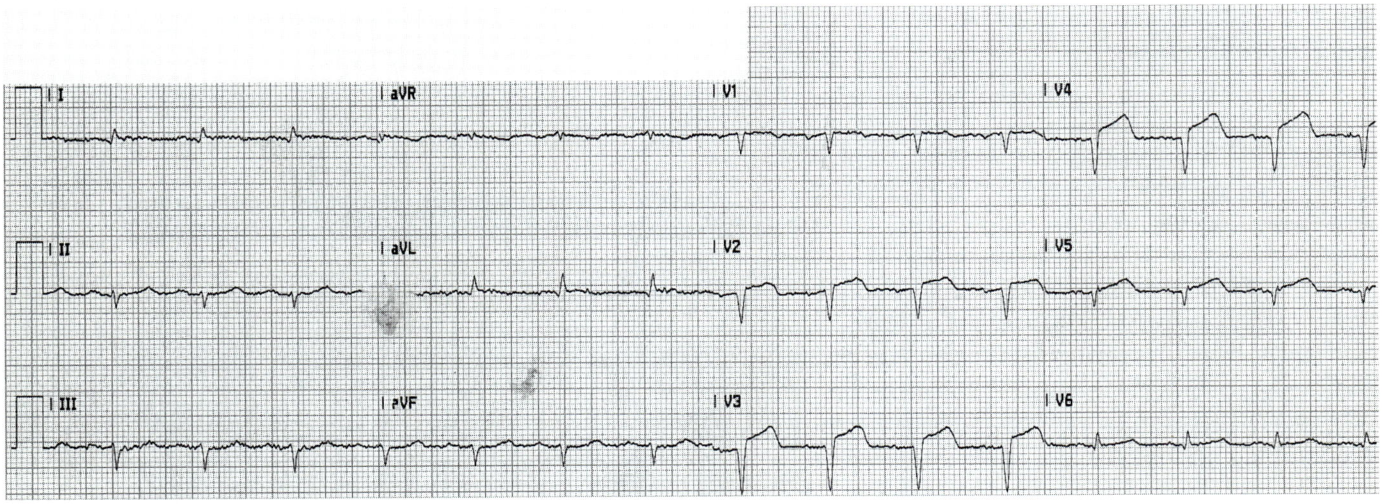

FIG. 3-7 Anteroseptal infarct with lateral extension.

Coronary Artery Anatomy

Since myocardial infarction is the result of an occluded coronary artery, it is worthwhile to develop a familiarity with the coronary arteries that supply the heart. Once the infarction has been recognized and localized, even a basic understanding of coronary artery anatomy makes it possible to predict which coronary artery is occluded. Chapter 4 discusses how determining the site of coronary artery occlusion can allow for complications to be anticipated in advance, and help emergency care providers develop a more effective treatment plan. This section focuses on how a knowledge of the coronary artery anatomy helps to localize the infarction and gauge the extent of the infarct.

Fig. 3-8 shows which coronary artery supplies blood to each portion of the heart. Note where

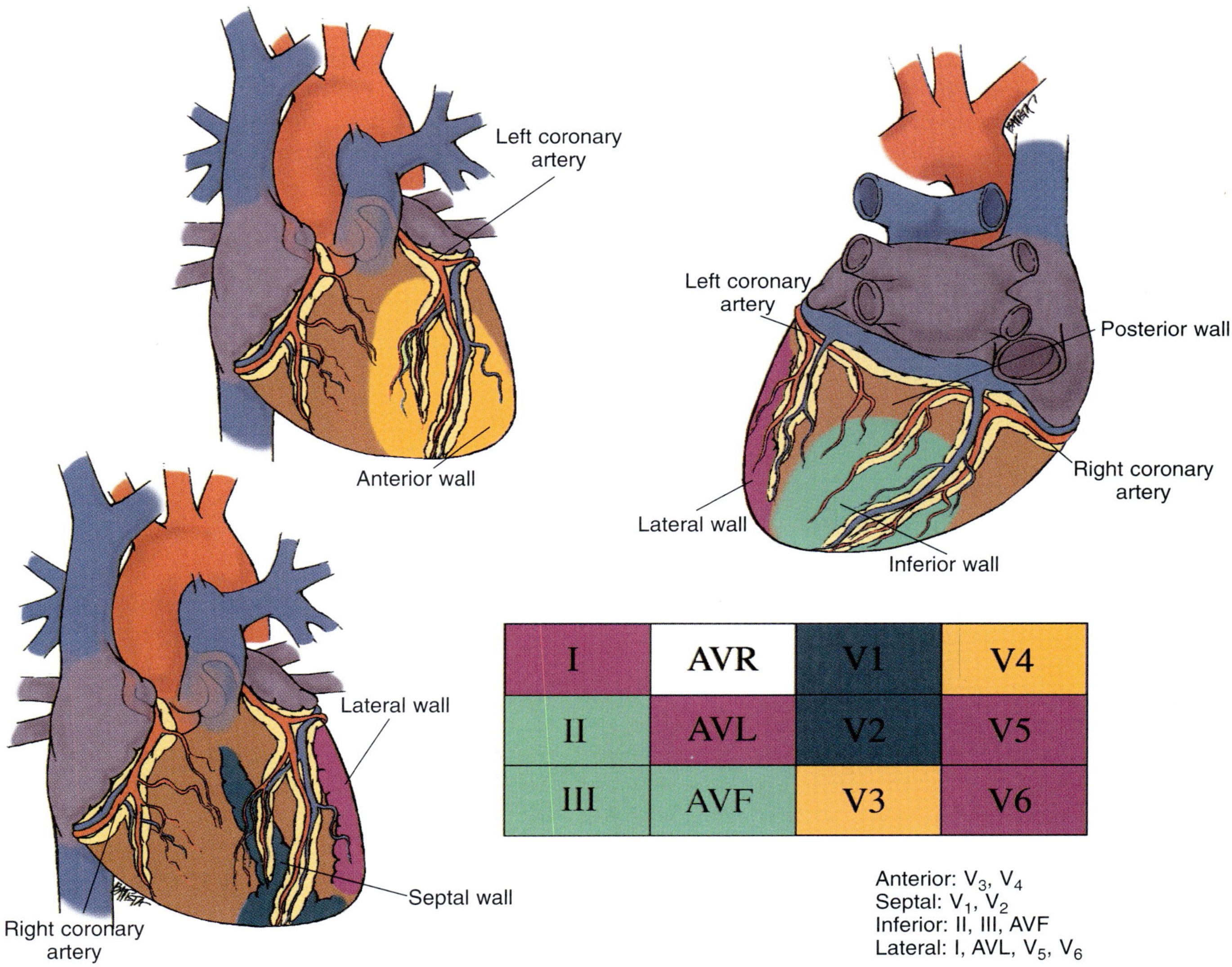

I	AVR	V1	V4
II	AVL	V2	V5
III	AVF	V3	V6

FIG. 3-8 Coronary artery anatomy.

Table 3.2 Coronary Artery Distribution

RIGHT CORONARY ARTERY	LEFT CORONARY ARTERY
Right ventricle	Septal wall of left ventricle
Inferior wall of left ventricle	Anterior wall of left ventricle
Posterior wall of left ventricle	Lateral wall of left ventricle Posterior wall of left ventricle

the two coronary arteries branch off from the aorta. It seems that the heart makes sure to feed itself first because the right and left coronary arteries branch out from the most proximal portion of the aorta. As the illustrations indicate, the right and left coronary artery have separate origins. However, from that point on there is great individual variance in the normal coronary artery distribution. These illustrations represent an average pattern of coronary artery anatomy. A brief description of the average or "normal" coronary artery anatomy is provided below.

Once the **left coronary artery** leaves the aorta it quickly divides into the left anterior descending artery and the circumflex artery. Both of these arteries have numerous branches that form a network. That network supplies the septal wall, the anterior wall, and the lateral wall of the left ventricle. The **right coronary artery** supplies the right ventricle with its more proximal branches and continues around the right ventricle into the posterior region of the left ventricle.

It is in the posterior portion of the heart, also referred to as the crux, that the right coronary artery and the left coronary artery meet head-on. One of these arteries will go on to form the posterior descending artery and supply the inferior wall of the left ventricle. In approximately 90% of the population, the right coronary artery forms the posterior descending branch and supplies the inferior wall of the left ventricle. In the remaining 10% of the population, the left coronary artery forms the posterior descending artery. Table 3-2 summarizes the pattern in which coronary arteries most commonly supply the myocardium.

Predicting the Site of Coronary Artery Occlusion

Armed with this basic understanding of coronary anatomy, it is now possible to predict which coronary artery is occluded. The approach used throughout this text is to predict whether the occlusion is located within the left coronary artery or within the right coronary artery. There are two reasons for this dichotomy. The first is the tremendous variation in the "normal" distribution of coronary arteries. For example, the extent to which the lateral wall is supplied by the left anterior descending artery versus the circumflex artery may vary greatly from individual to individual, but in most of the population the lateral wall is supplied by some division of the left coronary artery. Therefore, by limiting our prediction to either a right coronary artery occlusion or a left coronary artery occlusion, we recognize the great diversity in coronary artery distribution. The second reason for placing the occlusion in either the right or left coronary artery is clinical practicality. This approach puts an infarction into one of two categories, each very clinically distinct from the other. Any further subdivision would only create additional categories, none of which are completely distinct from each other. Therefore, infarctions will be identified as resulting from either a left coronary artery occlusion or from a right coronary artery occlusion.

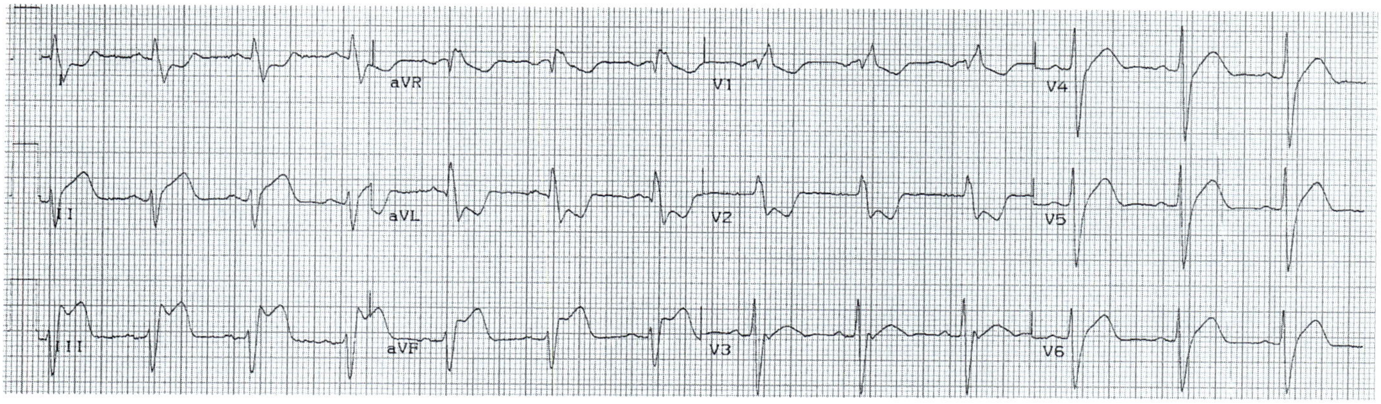

FIG. 3-9 **Inferior wall infarction, lateral extension (V5 and V6). Right coronary artery occlusion.**

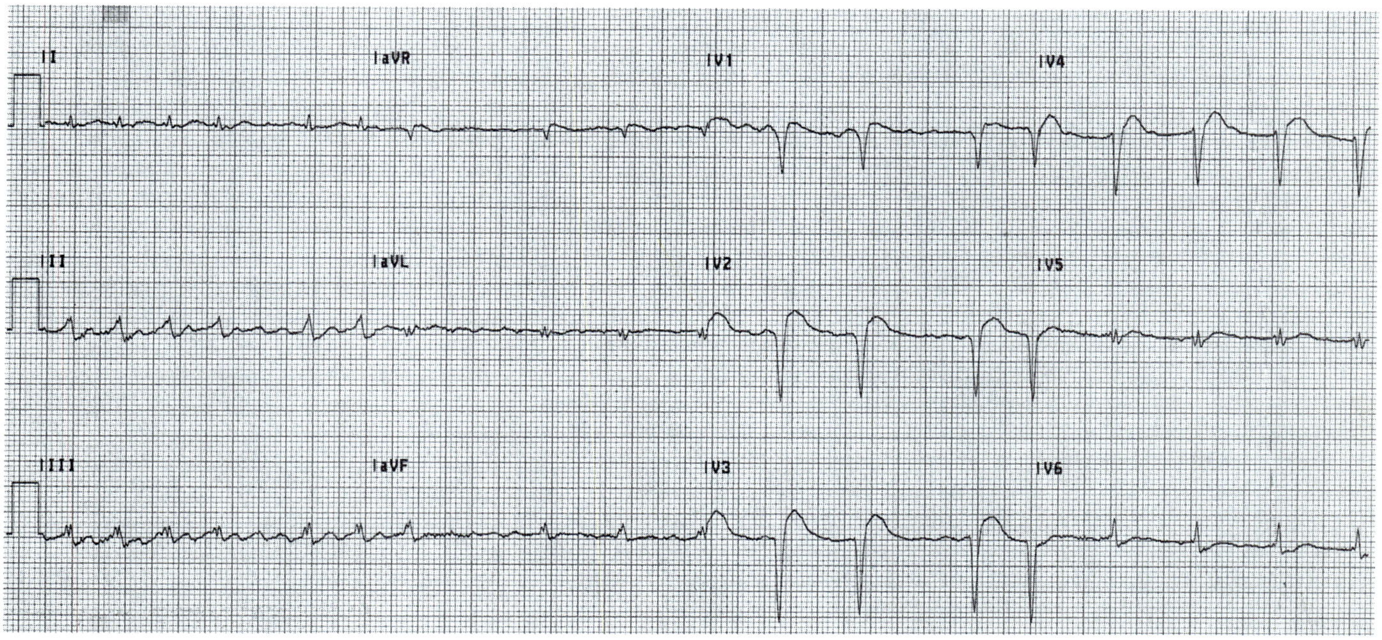

FIG. 3-10 **Anteroseptal. Left coronary artery occlusion.**

To identify the site of occlusion, one only needs to compare the infarct location with the coronary anatomy. An ECG showing indicative changes in leads II, III, and AVF directs one to suspect an inferior wall infarction. Since the inferior wall of the left ventricle is supplied by the right coronary artery in 90% of the population, it is reasonable to suppose that this infarct is due to a right coronary artery occlusion. When indicative changes are seen in the leads viewing the septal, anterior, and/or lateral walls of the left ventricle (V1-V6, I, and AVL), it is then reasonable to suspect a left coronary artery occlusion . Look at the following practice ECGs (Figs. 3-9 through 3-12) and determine which coronary artery is most likely occluded. To save time, assume that the occlusion is located in the left coronary artery unless indicative changes are noted in leads II, III, and AVF.

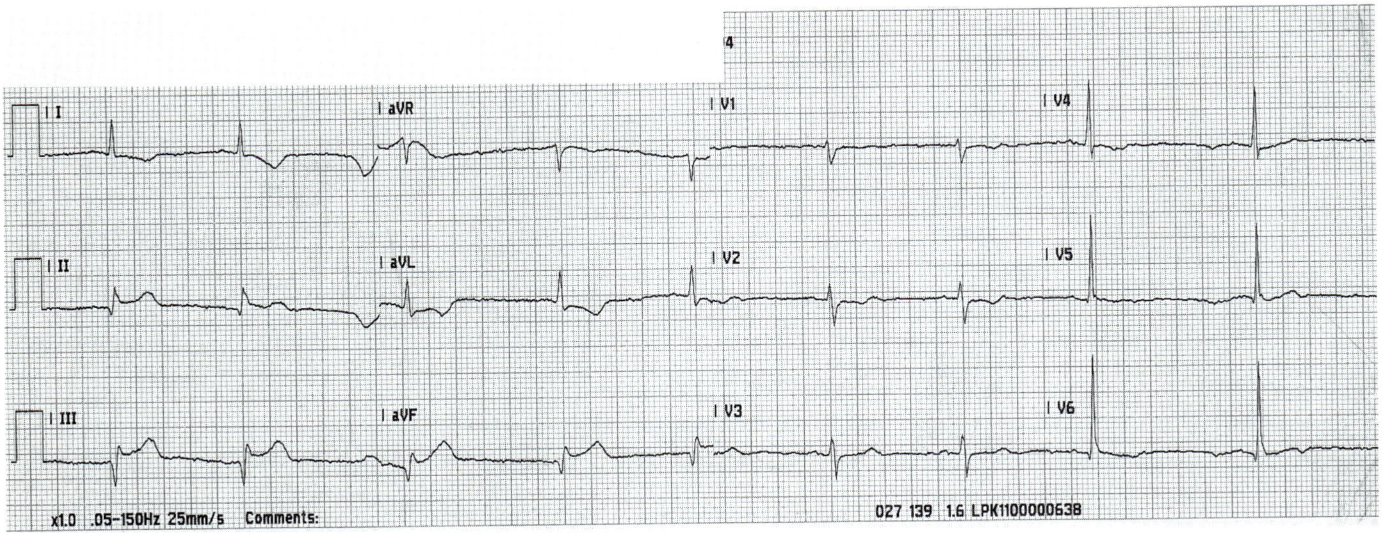

FIG. 3-11 **Inferior wall infarction. Right coronary artery occlusion.**

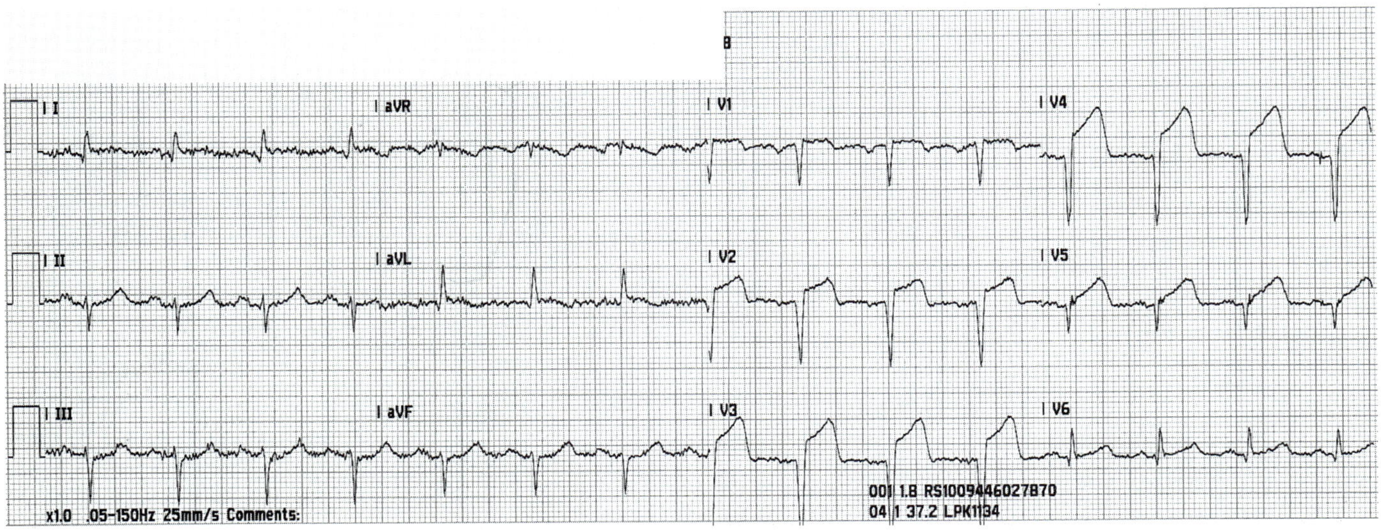

FIG. 3-12 **Anteroseptal infarction with lateral extension. Left coronary artery occlusion.**

Assessing the Extent of Infarction

One way to gauge the relative extent or size of an infarction is to evaluate how many leads are showing indicative changes. As one might expect, an ECG showing changes in only a few leads suggests a smaller infarction than one which produces changes in many leads. Discussed below are methods used to estimate the size of an infarct.

Four specific locations along the left coronary artery are identified in Fig. 3-13, marked A-D. Consider which tissues would be affected by an occlusion at each of these sites, then imagine

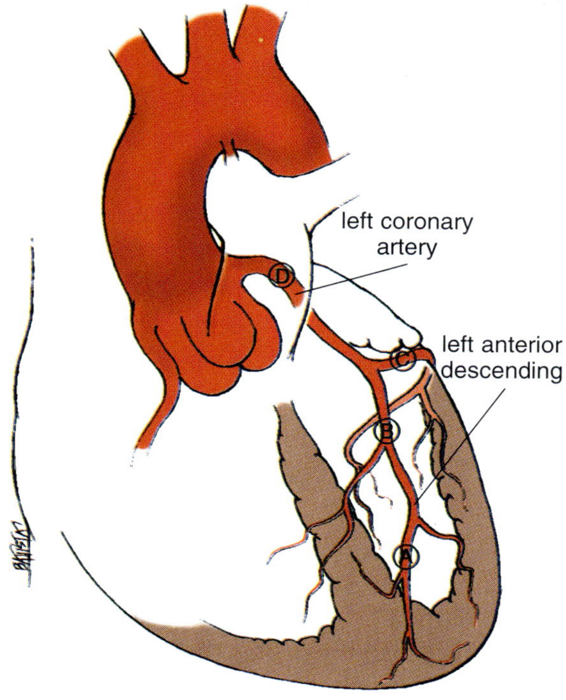

FIG. 3-13 Extent of infarct as related to various occlusion sites in the left coronary artery.

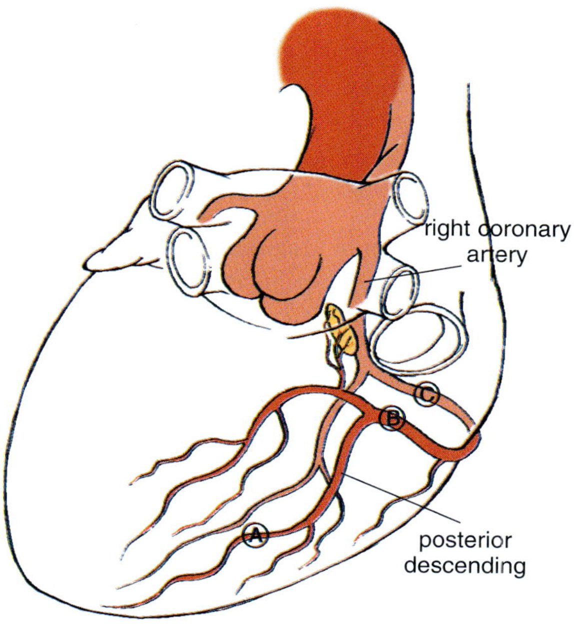

FIG. 3-14 Extent of infarct as related to various locations of right coronary artery occlusion.

which leads might show ECG changes resulting from an occlusion at each site. If an occlusion were to occur at site *A*, then a portion of the anterior wall would be affected, and leads V3 and V4 may show changes as a result. If the occlusion were at site *B*, then the septum would be affected by the infarction and leads V1 and V2 would also be expected to display indicative changes. If the circumflex were to occlude at site *C*, then a lateral wall infarction would be the concern, and leads V5, V6, I, and AVL might reveal indicative changes. A more proximal occlusion, such as one at site *D*, would affect a large portion of the left ventricle and could produce an ECG variation in most or all of leads V1-V6, I , and AVL.

This exercise clarifies how the location of the occlusion affects the amount of tissue at risk, and the number of leads showing indicative changes. In general, the more proximal the occlusion, the larger the infarction, and the greater the number of leads showing indicative changes. In the standard 12-lead, eight leads "look" at tissue supplied by the left coronary artery (I, AVL, V1-V6). When assessing the extent of an infarct produced by a left coronary artery occlusion, count how many of those eight leads are showing indicative changes. The more of these eight leads demonstrating indicative changes, the larger infarct is assumed to be. When evaluating the extent of an infarct due to a right coronary occlusion the same concept applies. However, a new problem arises.

While the standard 12-lead ECG provides a full view of tissue supplied by the left coronary artery, it gives only an incomplete view of tissue supplied by the right coronary artery. In Fig. 3-14, three potential sites of a right coronary artery occlusion are marked A-C. An occlusion at site *A* would only involve the distal-most portion of the right coronary artery, and would be expected to produce an inferior wall infarction with changes visible in leads II, III, and AVF. An occlusion at site *B* would involve a larger amount of tissue and probably produce a larger infarction. However, there are no leads in the standard 12-lead ECG which "look" at the posterior wall, so indicative changes would only be seen in leads II, III, and AVF. A more proximal occlusion, such as one at site *C*, would not only involve a much larger portion of the myocardium, but would also produce an infarction in both ventricles. Once again though, the ECG would only display changes in leads II, III, and AVF. This example illustrates the difficulty in assessing the extent of an infarction in the setting of a right coronary artery occlusion. Fortunately, there are a few ways to obtain that important information.

Right Ventricular Infarction

The topic of right ventricular infarctions (RVI) is not new, yet it is new to many emergency cardiac care providers. Until a few decades ago, there was a general consensus that infarctions of the right ventricle occurred infrequently and that when they did occur, they were of little consequence. To compound the problem, the standard 12-lead ECG does not asses the right ventricle, which contributes to an "out of sight, out of mind" situation. However, increasing attention is being focused on RVI. The recognition of RVI is discussed in this chapter, while specific treatment of its complications is addressed in Chapter 4.

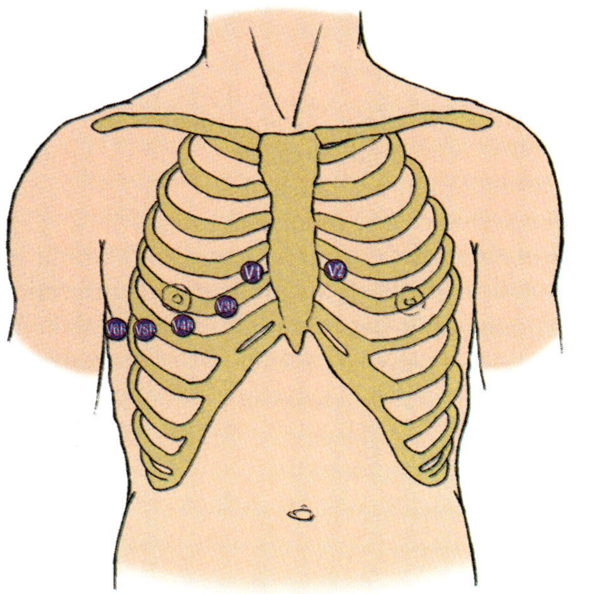

FIG. 3-15 Position of right-sided chest leads V3R through V6R.

Right ventricular infarctions complicate inferior wall infarctions more often than is generally realized—RVI has been noted with a frequency approaching 40% of all inferior wall infarctions. Right ventricular infarction is quite significant because it not only indicates a larger infarction, it also signifies that the infarction involves both ventricles. To be able to recognize RVI, one should be familiar with both its clinical and ECG manifestations.

The ECG evidence is simple enough to obtain. When the possibility of RVI exists, a set of chest leads can be applied to the right chest (Fig. 3-15). These leads then "look" directly at the right ventricle and can show the ST segment elevation created by the infarct. Fig. 3-16 shows ST segment elevation in leads II, III, AVF, V4R, V5R, and V6R. This tracing suggests that an occlusion of the right coronary artery has occurred (II, III, and AVF) and that this occlusion is proximal enough to involve the right ventricle (V4R, V5R, and V6R).

Researchers have investigated the usefulness of each right-sided chest lead in recognizing infarction. Their work has shown that V4R is the single most accurate (about 90% sensitive and 90% specific). Therefore, in the event that time does not permit for the acquisition of all six right-sided chest leads, or if any other circumstance exists in which only one right-sided chest lead can be obtained, then V4R is the single best choice. Since the evidence of RVI will never be found unless it is sought, it is very important to know when to obtain the extra lead(s). **Obtain lead V4R whenever ST segment elevation is noted in leads II, III and AVF**. In addition to ECG evidence, certain clinical signs also support the suspicion of RVI.

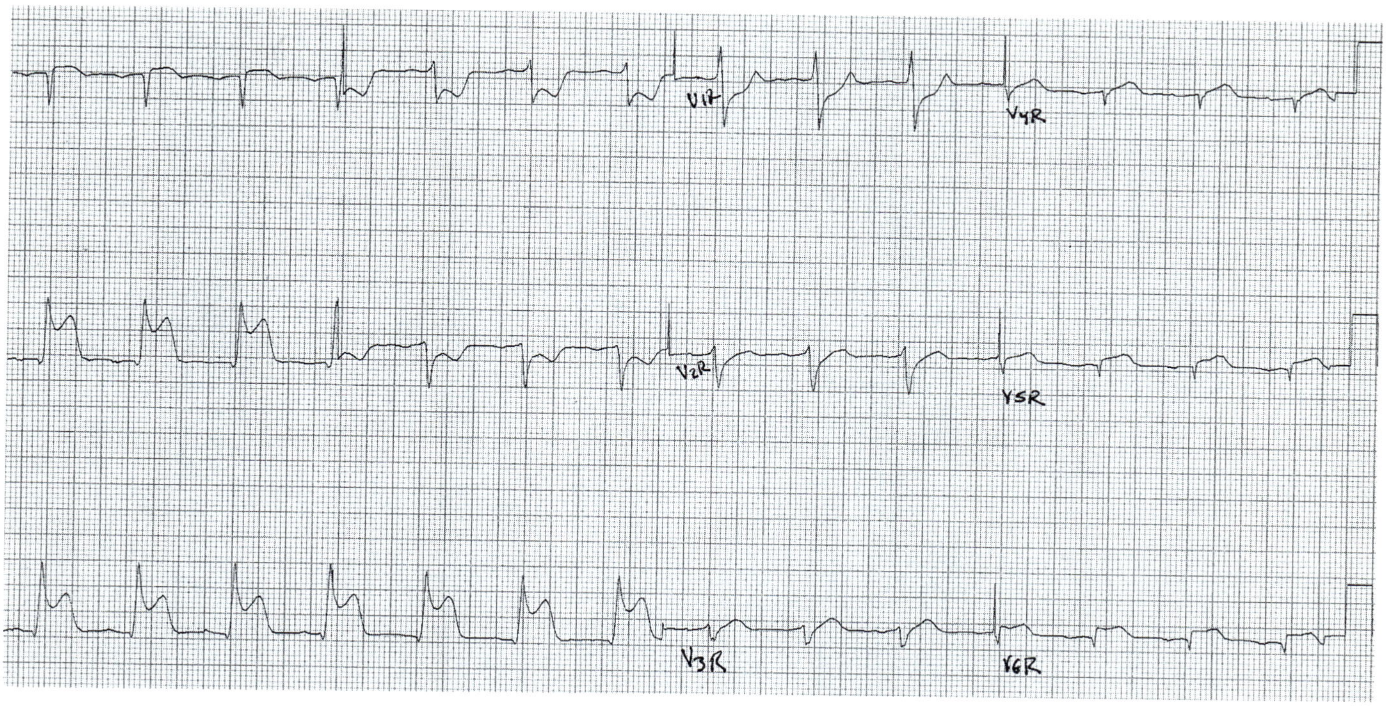

FIG. 3-16 A 12-lead obtained using the right-sided chest leads.

The clinical evidence of RVI involves three components: hypotension, jugular venous distention, and dry lung sounds. Each is examined and explained after a brief review of physiology.

As blood leaves the right atrium, it enters the right ventricle and is then pumped from the right ventricle into the lungs. While circulating through the pulmonary circuit, the blood is oxygenated and is delivered into the left atrium. From the left atrium, blood fills the left ventricle and is then forcefully sent into the systemic circulation. In the setting of RVI, the right ventricle may lose some of its ability to pump blood into the pulmonary circuit. When this happens blood "stalls" in the right ventricle and may begin to "back up." (Technically, the blood does not back up; the venous return exceeds ventricular output and blood begins to accumulate.). This stalling and backing up produce the hypotension, jugular venous distention, and absence of pulmonary edema (dry lung sounds) that are considered the clinical triad of RVI.

It is easy to understand why jugular venous distention is a part of the triad. As blood backs up from the right ventricle, the jugular veins become enlarged. Hypotension results from the decrease in blood volume moving into the lungs and left ventricle. The left ventricle can only pump as much blood as it receives, and if less blood reaches the left ventricle, less blood is pumped into the systemic circulation. The net effect of this reduction in left ventricular output is a decrease in blood pressure.

Often in the setting of myocardial infarction, hypotension is accompanied by pulmonary edema. However, this is not the case with RVI. In the setting of RVI, blood does not back up from the left ventricle into the lungs, so pulmonary edema is not expected. Shortness of breath may occur, but not as a result of pulmonary edema.

Just as infarctions of the left ventricle can occur without producing significant hemodynamic change, not every patient experiencing RVI will present with hypotension, jugular venous distention, and dry lung sounds. It has been estimated that about half of all RVIs will have significant hemodynamic compromise. When RVI is significant, care providers may opt to modify the standard treatment for chest pain, AV block, and hypotension. Those subjects are discussed in Chapter 4.

Practice ECGs

Review Figs. 3–17 through 3–22 and determine the following:

- Are indicative changes present?
- Where is the myocardial infarction?
- Where is the coronary artery occlusion?
- Are additional leads required?

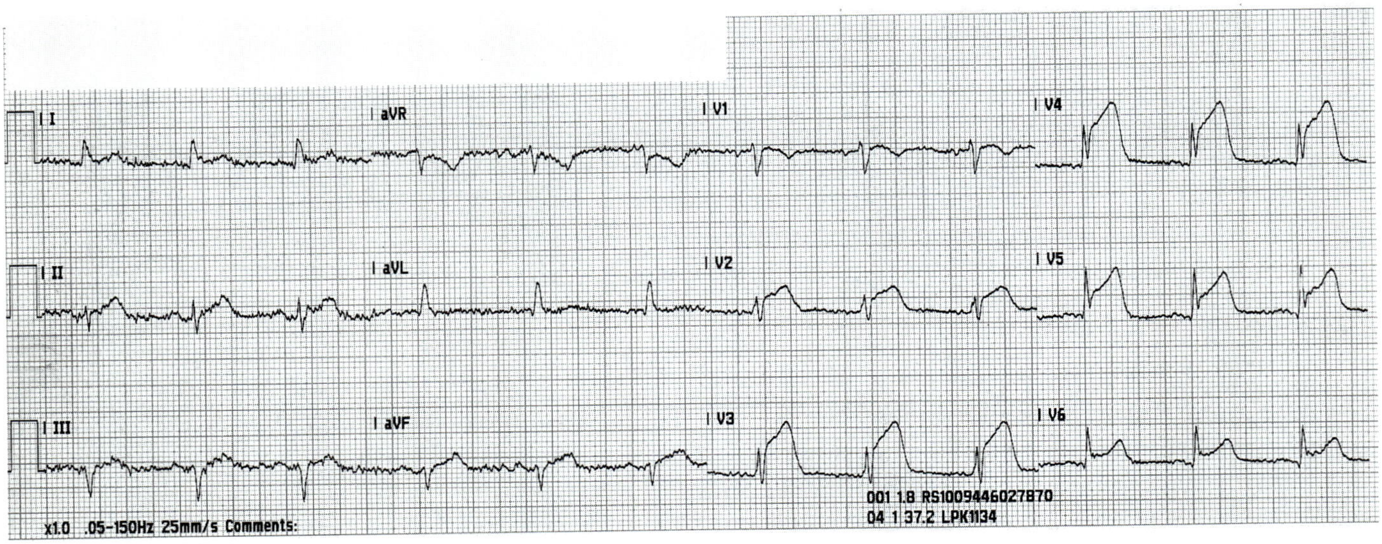

FIG. 3-17

Indicative changes noted in V2-V6, Q wave in AVL approaching 40 ms. Anterolateral infarct with septal extension. Left coronary artery occlusion. No further leads needed.

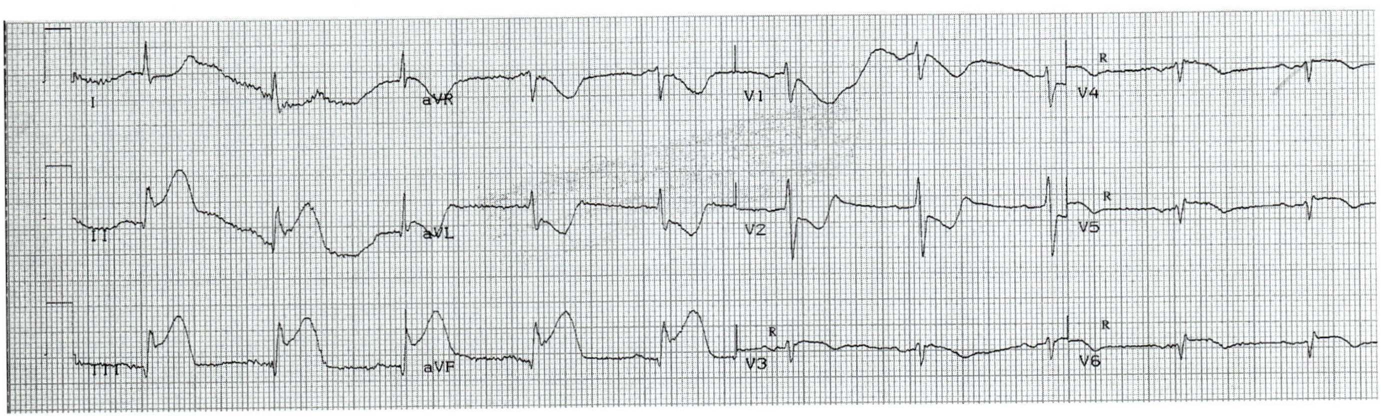

FIG. 3-18

Changes noted in II, III, and AVF. Inferior infarction. Right coronary artery occlusion. Changes in V4R-V6R suggest right ventricular infarction.

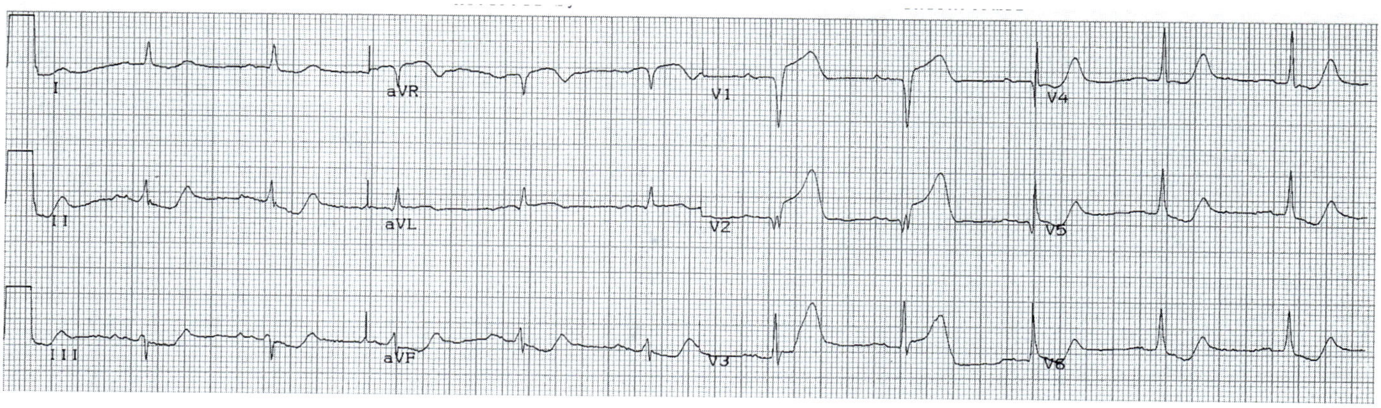

FIG. 3-19

Changes in V1 and V2 indicate septal infarct, changes in V3 suggest anterior extension. Left coronary occlusion. No additional leads required.

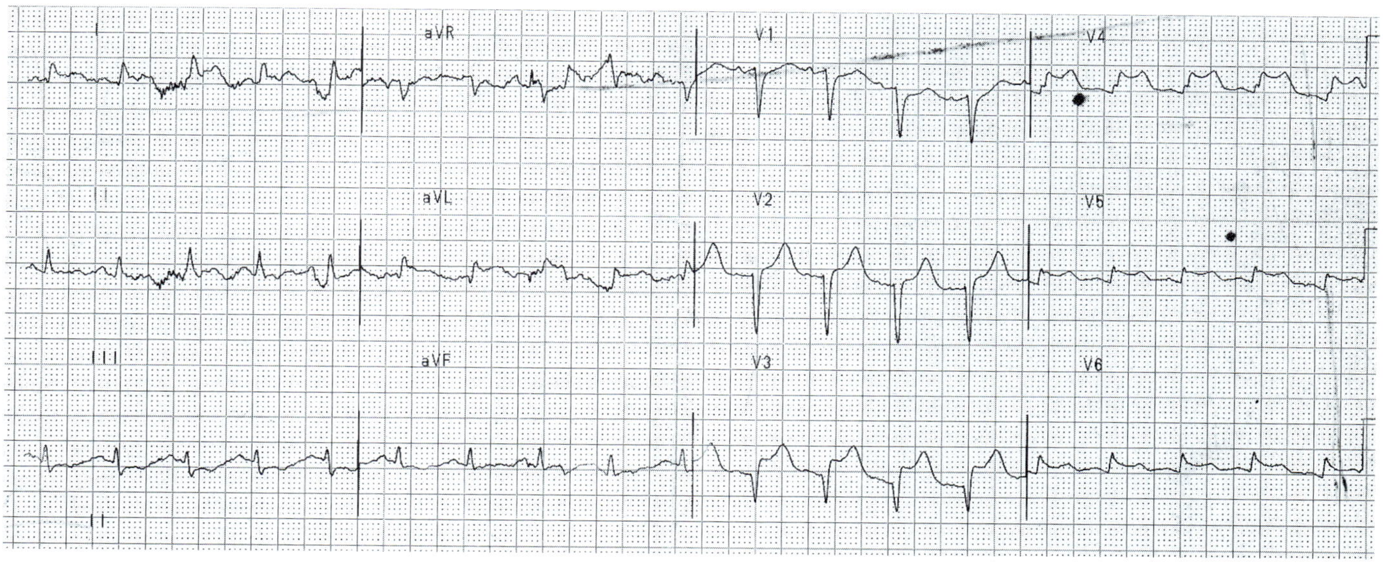

FIG. 3-20

Changes in I, AVL, and V2-V6 indicate extensive infarct involving septal, anterior extension. Left coronary occlusion. No additional leads required.

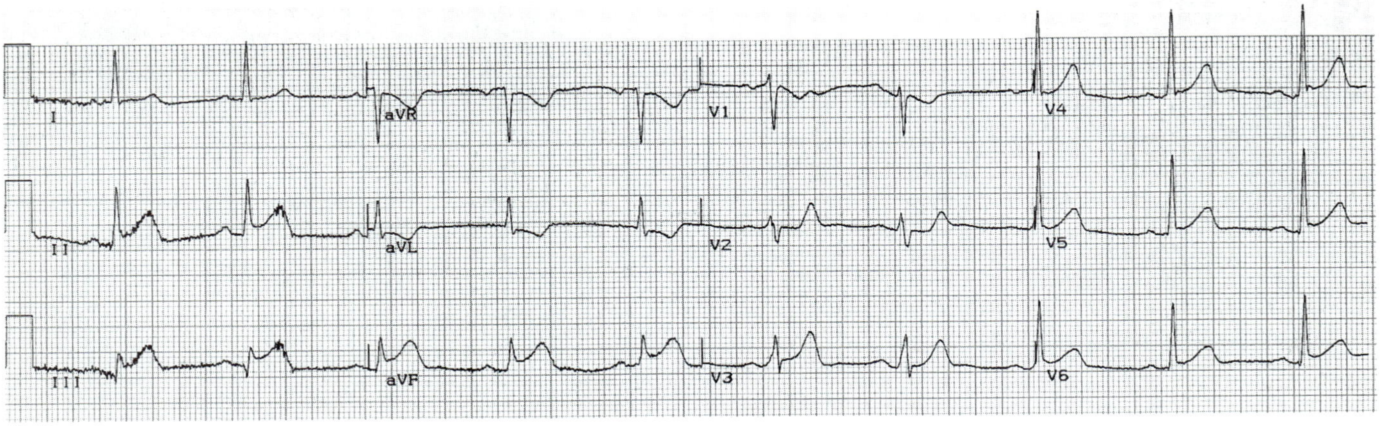

FIG. 3-21 Leads II, III, and AVF identify an inferior infarction. Right coronary artery occlusion. Right sided chest leads should be obtained. Subtle changes in V4-V6 suggest possible lateral extension.

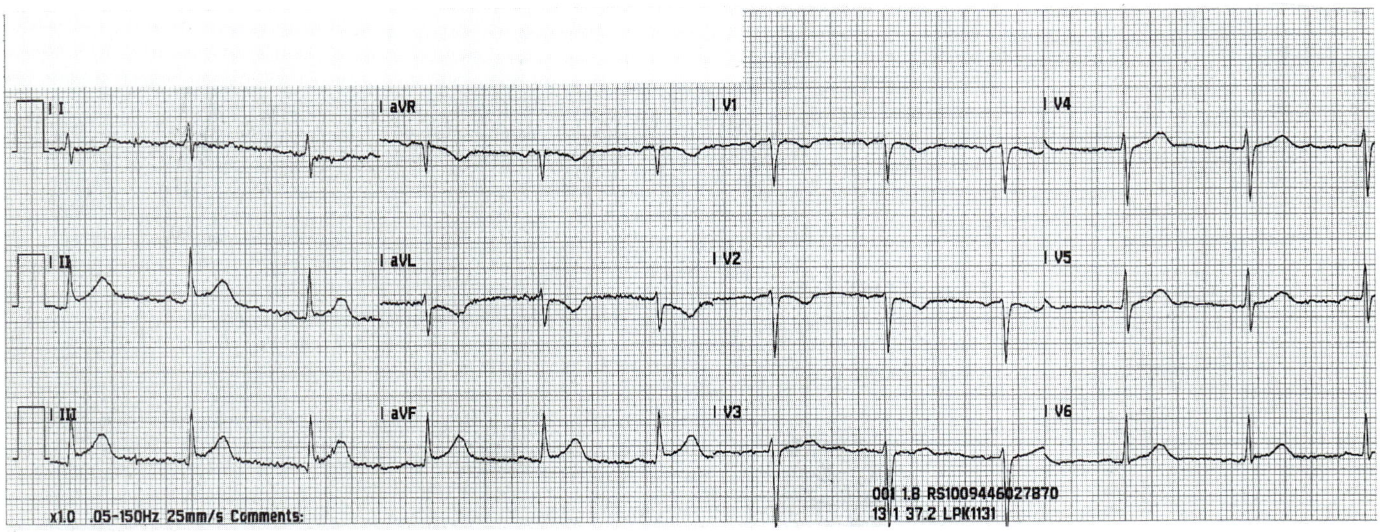

FIG. 3-22 Leads II, III, and AVF show indicative changes. Inferior infarction. Right sided chest leads should be obtained.

Posterior Wall Infarctions

Initially, the topic of posterior wall infarctions can be confusing, but this need not be the case. Most of the confusion generally stems from the fact that there are no leads in the standard 12-lead ECG which "look" at the posterior wall. While additional leads can be attached to the patient's back to improve the view, this is not always clinically feasible or practical. Fortunately, there are ways to suspect a posterior wall infarction using evidence provided by the standard 12-lead ECG. However, the evidence used to recognize posterior wall infarctions is not derived from the indicative changes previously studied. Rather, a whole new set of clues are

A

B

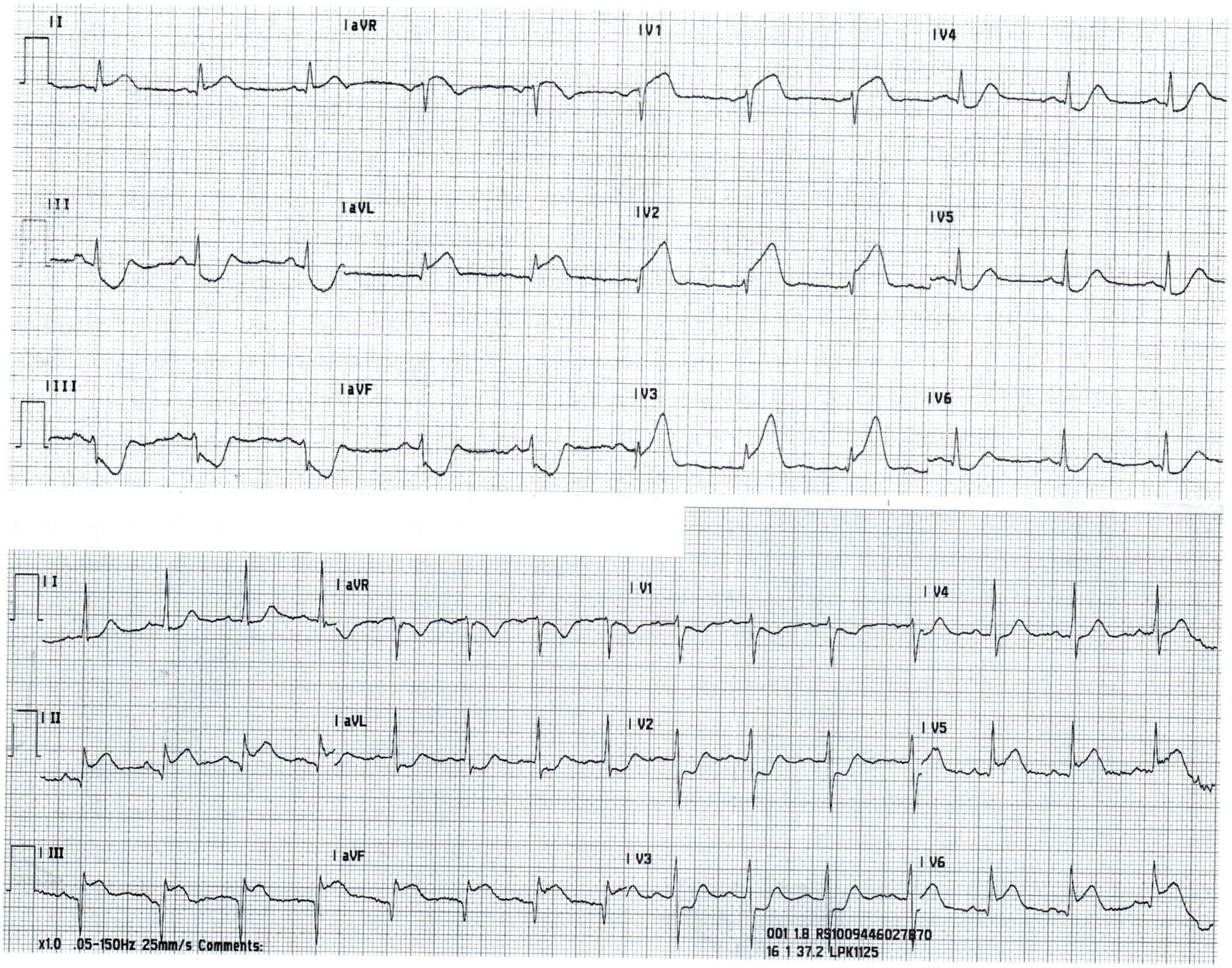

FIG. 3-23 A, Leads II, III and AVF look at the infarct indirectly and see ST segment elevation. The chest leads look at the infarct backwards and show ST segment depression. **B,** The chest leads display ST segment elvation because they see the infarct directly. Obvious ST segment depression is noted in leads II, III and AVF because these leads see the infarct backwards.

sought out when inspecting for a posterior wall infarction.

When leads "look" directly at the infarct site, ST segment elevation and Q waves may be seen. When leads look at the infarct site and see ST segment elevation, it is called an **indicative change**. However, often a different pattern is seen in those leads looking at the infarct site from the opposite perspective. When leads look at the infarct site backwards, instead of seeing ST segment elevation they often see ST segment depression. Likewise, when looking at the infarction backwards, instead of a Q wave (a negative deflection) being recorded, the R wave becomes taller (a positive deflection). These backward changes, which are only seen when looking at the infarct site from reverse, are called **reciprocal changes** (Figs. 3-23A and B.) Understanding the concept of reciprocal changes is the key to recognizing posterior infarctions because posterior wall infarctions are most commonly recognized by the presence of ST segment depression and tall R waves.

Since no electrodes are routinely placed on the patient's back, there are no leads which look directly at the posterior wall. Subsequently, in-

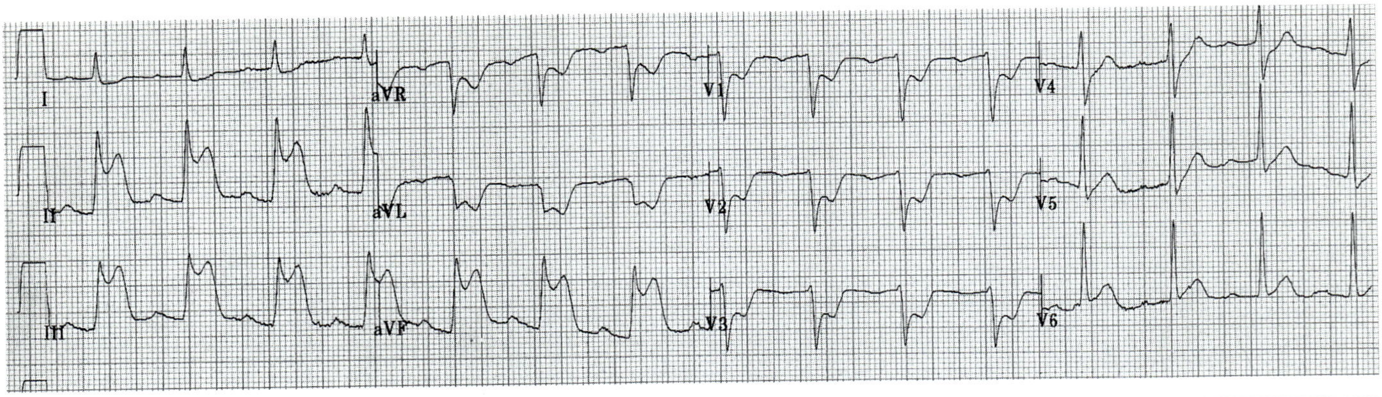

FIG. 3-24 An inferior wall infarction associated with a posterior wall infarction.

dicative changes on the standard 12-lead ECG are not expected as a result of posterior wall infarction. If indicative changes are not possible, then the next method to evaluate for the presence of a posterior wall infarction is to look for reciprocal changes (Fig. 3-24). As expected, when reciprocal changes are produced by a posterior wall infarction, they are noted in leads V1, V2, and V3, which look at the posterior wall backwards.

Causes of ST Segment Depression

Several of the previous examples of acute myocardial infarction not only demonstrated ST segment elevation, but displayed ST segment depression as well. There are many potential explanations for such ST segment depression and this section explores several of them.

In addition to the reciprocal changes noted above, the drug digitalis is very capable of producing ST segment depression. The digitalis effect is actually quite common. Another common cause of ST segment depression is ischemia.

During a stress test, the development of ST segment depression can be evidence of ischemic heart disease. In this case, the patient's exertion was the obvious cause of the ischemia. However, some causes are less obvious.

In the setting of acute myocardial infarction, ischemia may develop in one of two ways. First, there is often a zone of ischemia surrounding the injured and infarcting tissues (Fig. 3-25). While there may have been no physical exertion, ST segment depression may appear on the tracing. A second possibility is referred to "ischemia at a distance."

Considering that acute myocardial infarction generally occurs in an already diseased heart, it is not difficult to imagine that areas away from the infarct site might be experiencing an increased workload because they are forced to pick up the slack for the infarcting portion. As a result, these areas must work harder, but they do not have an adequate blood supply to provide the oxygen needed for this extra work, which produces ischemia and ST segment depression.

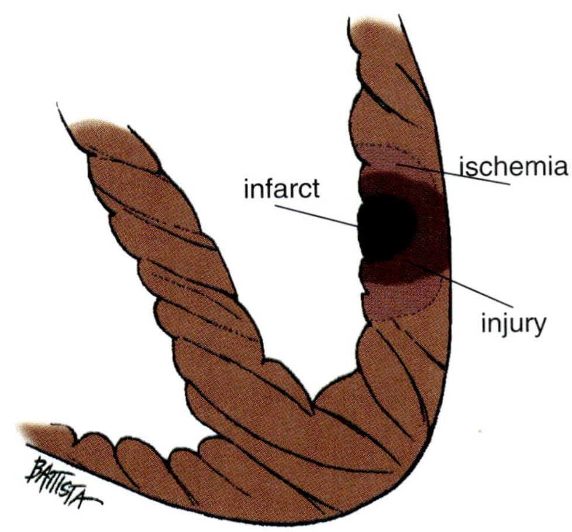

FIG. 3-25 A zone of ischemia surrounding the injured and infarcting tissue.

Exceptions

The indicative changes described in this chapter are by no means absolute and not every infarction follows this pattern. However, once these indicative changes are understood, they can be applied to each individual patient setting and used as a reference point. There are several notable exceptions to the "classic" pattern of indicative changes.

Indicative changes may occur in a different order or different time frame than described. Some infarctions do not develop a Q wave, while others may lose their Q wave sometime after the infarct. Some patients' ECGs continue to show persistent ST segment elevation indefinitely after the infarction.

A very significant deviation from the classic pattern occurs when an infarction does not produce recognizable changes in the ECG. This deviation underscores an important fact: **A normal ECG does not rule out the possibility of myocardial infarction!**

Other exceptions relate to the localization of the infarct. While ECG localization of the infarct site is possible, it is not perfect. For example, what appears to be a lateral wall infarct on the ECG may, in actuality, be an anterior wall infarct. This can occur with any location of infarct and is due, once again, to the fact that the ECG is nothing but a measurement of current flow on the patient's skin; factors including anatomic variations, patient position, and other underlying conditions may affect the perceived locations versus the actual location.

The patient's unique pattern of coronary artery distribution can also affect the location of infarct and so can the presence of collateral circulation. For these reasons, emergency cardiac care providers occasionally encounter infarcts which are difficult to localize into the previously mentioned regions. Two common variations are apical infarctions and inferolateral infarctions.

The apex of the heart is the ventricular area most distal to the atria, or the bottom "tip" of the heart. This region consists of anterior wall tissue (supplied by the left coronary artery) and inferior wall tissue (supplied by the right coronary artery). Therefore, depending upon the individual's coronary artery distribution, a right coronary artery occlusion may not only produce an

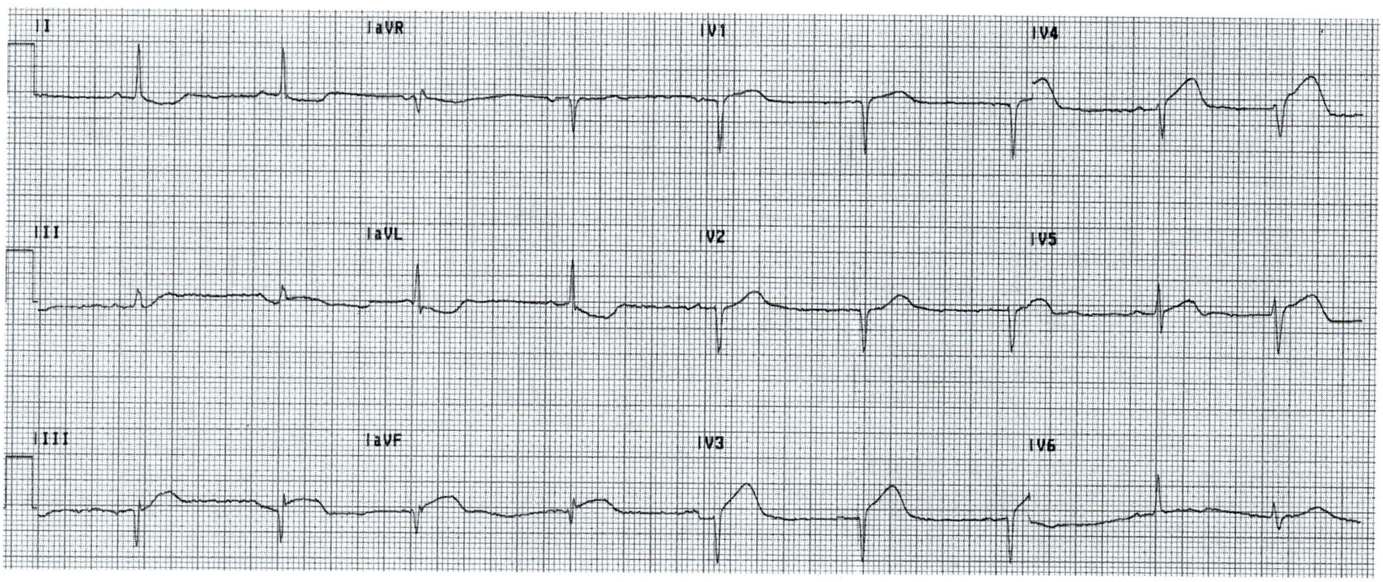

FIG. 3-26 "Combined" locations of infarct, apical infarction.

inferior infarction, but it may also affect a portion of the anterior wall. Likewise, a left coronary artery occlusion in some individuals will not only affect the anterior wall, but also extend into the inferior wall. These situations produce what is known as an apical infarction (Fig. 3-26).

Another common variation in coronary anatomy distribution may produce an inferolateral infarction. In the 10% of the population in which the left coronary artery supplies the inferior wall, an occlusion of that artery may produce an infarct which not only involves the inferior

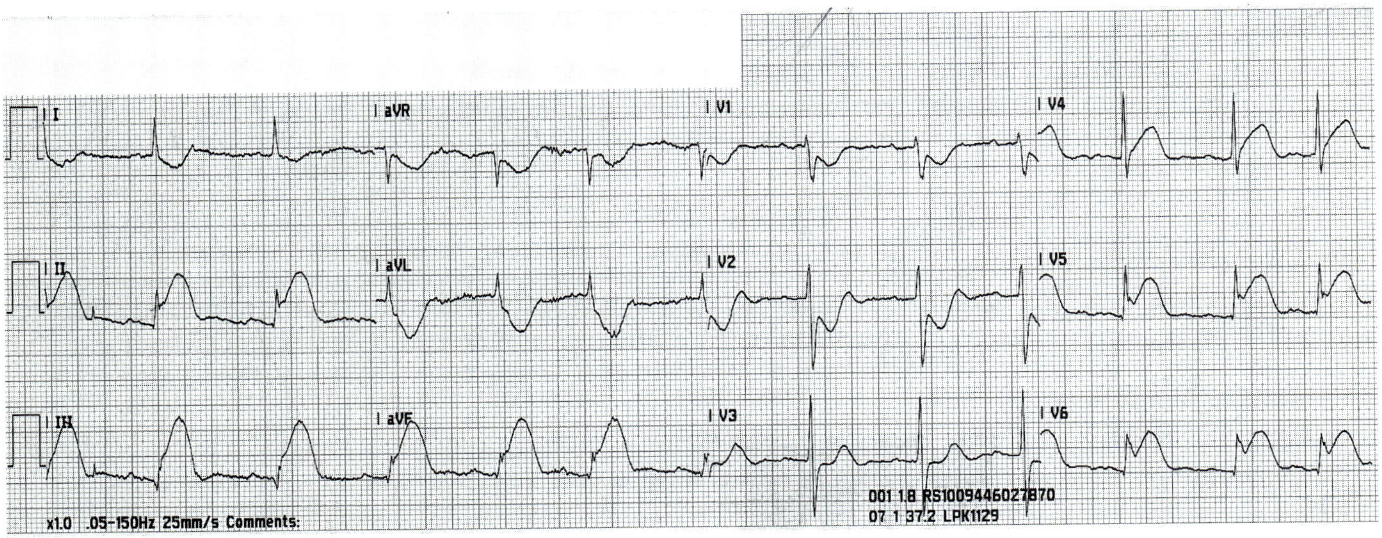

FIG. 3-27 "Combined" locations of infarct, inferolateral infarction.

wall, but the lateral wall as well. This is one explanation for the inferolateral infarction seen in Fig. 3-27.

Another possible explanation for both apical and inferolateral infarctions is the presence of extensive collateral circulation. In this situation, each coronary artery, to some extent, provides blood to tissues generally supplied by the other coronary artery. Therefore, an occlusion in either artery can produce injury in unexpected areas, and may produce indicative changes in leads typically supplied by the other coronary artery.

SUMMARY

- **Each lead in the 12-lead ECG provides a slightly different view of the myocardium.**
- **Infarct may produce certain recognizable changes (indicative changes) in the QRS complex and the ST segment.**
- **Infarction is suspected when indicative changes are seen in at least two anatomically contiguous leads.**
- **There is significant variance in coronary artery distribution among individuals, but it is possible to predict whether an occlusion is in the right or the left coronary artery.**
- **The more proximal an occlusion, the greater the infarct size.**
- **When the ECG shows indicative changes in many leads it suggests a larger infarction.**
- **The standard 12-lead ECG provides an excellent view of the portions of the left ventricle supplied by the left coronary artery.**
- **The standard 12-lead ECG provides only limited information about tissues supplied by the right coronary artery.**
- **In the setting of a suspected right coronary artery occlusion (inferior wall infarction), additional right-sided chest leads should be obtained.**
- **V4R is the single best lead to use when screening for a right ventricular infarction (RVI).**
- **Clinical signs of RVI include hypotension, jugular venous distention, and clear lung sounds.**
- **Possible causes of ST segment depression include digitalis, ischemia, and reciprocal changes seen in myocardial infarction.**
- **Posterior infarctions are suspected when an inferior infarction is accompanied by ST reciprocal changes in leads V1-V3.**
- **A normal 12-lead ECG does not rule out the possibility of an acute myocardial infarction.**

4

OBJECTIVES

Myocardial Infarction: Complications and Treatment

- Learn which coronary arteries supply the AV node and the bundle branches.
- Understand how determining the site of coronary artery occlusion can allow complications to be predicted in advance.
- Know when to use caution in administering nitroglycerin for chest pain.
- Differentiate nodal AV blocks from infranodal AV blocks.
- Predict which AV blocks are more likely to deteriorate and which are less likely to respond to atropine.
- Identify the need for standby pacing in the setting of myocardial infarction.
- Recognize the indications for vigorous fluid therapy in the treatment of hypotension due to right ventricular infarction.

CHAPTER 4

Complications of Myocardial Infarction

Any number of complications can present in the course of a myocardial infarction. Some of these complications are more likely to occur at particular times during the infarct process—lethal arrhythmias are most common in the first hour of infarct—while others are more specific to the site of infarction. Anyone who has managed such complications will agree that it is preferable to be warned in advanced of these complications so as to be ready to treat them should they present.

This chapter provides an increased understanding of the cardiac anatomy which, when combined with a knowledge of the coronary occlusion site, allows for certain complications to be anticipated. This same information can then be used to develop a more effective treatment plan for those complications should they develop. Chest pain, AV block, and hypotension are specifically examined.

Chest Pain

In the setting of acute myocardial infarction, pain may be lessened by two primary methods. First, analgesics mask the pain and decrease the catecholamine response, which otherwise could increase the heart's rate, force, and oxygen demand. Second, vasoactive drugs alter the hemodynamics of preload and afterload to reduce the workload of the heart and lower its oxygen requirement. For these reasons, a high priority is placed on the relief of cardiac chest pain.

The most common approach to the management of chest pain uses nitroglycerin as the initial agent, followed by morphine if chest pain persists. This complement is extremely effective and indicated in most chest pain patients. However, there is a subset of infarct patients who may require an altered approach to the management of chest pain.

Right ventricular infarction (RVI) presents an exception to the standard regimen for chest pain management. In the setting of RVI, the infarction can reduce the output of the right ventricle, with a subsequent reduction in left ventricular filling. Should such a decrease in preload occur, it could potentially decrease left ventricular output as well. This, of course, would result in a decrease in blood pressure.

Morphine and nitroglycerin are vasodilators and thus reduce preload. This reduction of preload, while usually beneficial, can be undesirable in the setting of RVI, and may cause profound hypotension. Therefore, one must be cautious when administering nitroglycerin and morphine to patients experiencing RVI. Should hypotension occur, it brings with it the serious consequence of a decrease in coronary artery perfusion.

Since the coronary arteries are supplied from the aorta, a decrease in blood pressure will reduce blood flow through the coronary arteries. When this occurs in an already infarcting heart, it can reduce collateral circulation to the infarcting areas and/or create ischemia in previously unaffected areas of the heart. Therefore, hypotension is more than just an inconvenience; it can reduce coronary artery perfusion and worsen the area of injury.

The hazards of nitroglycerin administration in the setting of RVI have long been known. In its 1987 *Textbook of Advanced Cardiac Life Support*, the American Heart Association (AHA) recommends that "vasodilator drugs should be avoided" when treating RVI. Similar recommendations are present in the scientific literature, as well as in AHA's 1994 *Textbook of Advanced Cardiac Life Support*. Therefore, hypotension secondary to pain management is a complication that may be anticipated when treating RVI. Please note that the concern over vasodilators exists only when there is evidence of RVI. The presence of an inferior wall infarction without any ECG or clinical evidence of RVI does not merit any additional caution with nitroglycerin or morphine.

AV Block Reclassification

While the degree system of AV block is still the most common method of classifying AV block, there are other criteria that may be used. Dr. Henry J.L. Marriott has contributed much to the understanding of AV block and to the development of alternate means of classification. Before discussing AV block, it is important to highlight a few elements of AV block reclassification.

Dr. Marriott points out that the term "degree," when applied to AV blocks, does not imply severity. What does that mean to the care giver? It means that unlike murder, which is worst in the first degree, and unlike burns, which are worst in the third degree, a second degree block is not necessarily any "worse" than a first degree block. Likewise, a third degree block is not necessarily "worse" than a second degree block. When determining the severity of an AV block, factors other than degree must be considered. These factors include the pathogenesis of the block, the underlying atrial rate, the location of the AV block, and the behavior of an AV block at that location. While this chapter does not attempt to convey all of the concepts of AV block reclassification, it does emphasize the significance of an AV block's location, as well as discuss other issues which affect the management of AV block.

AV Block Location

When the term AV block is used, the letters "AV" do not stand for atrioventricular node. Rather, AV block indicates that the electrical impulse originating in the atrium has somehow been blocked from depolarizing the ventricles. AV block can occur at the level of the AV node, at the level of the bundle branches, or at some site in between, such as the bundle of His. The two most common sites of AV block are the AV node (**nodal block**) and the bundle branches (**infranodal block**). Since these are the two most common sites of AV block, let us look at how each of them is supplied by the coronary arteries.

CORONARY ARTERY SUPPLY

The AV node's location in the heart is shown is Fig. 4-1. The vertical line in the illustration represents the division between the right and the left side of the heart, while the horizontal line represents the division between the atria and the ventricles. The point at which these two lines cross is called the **crux** of the heart—crux means cross in Latin—and it is below the crux that the AV node lies. When the coronary anatomy is superimposed over the crux, one can see that the right coronary artery is located nearest to the crux. It

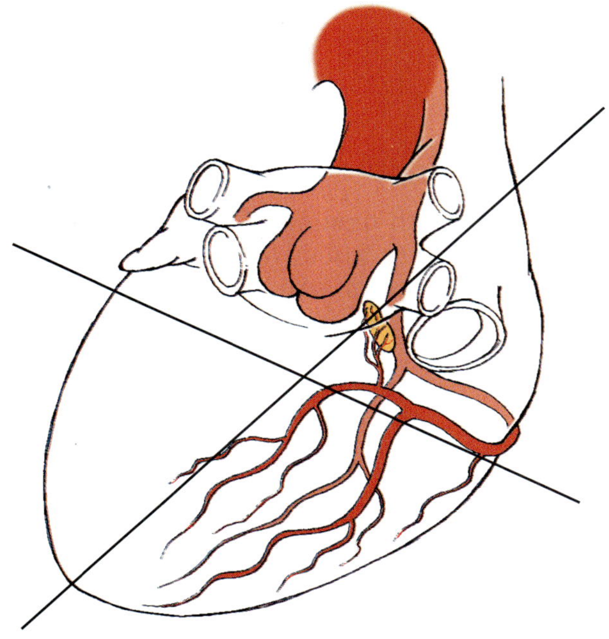

FIG. 4-1 The right coronary artery is the primary blood supply to the AV node in approximately 90% of the population.

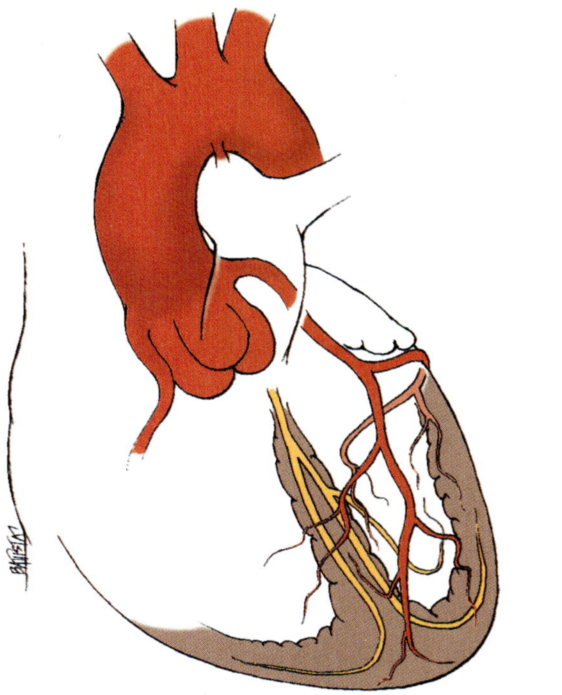

FIG. 4-2 It is the left coronary artery which supplies most of the bundle branch tissue.

is not surprising, therefore, to learn the right coronary artery supplies the AV node in 90% of the population. Thus, right coronary artery occlusions are associated with AV block occurring in the AV node.

The bundle branches are, for the most part, located near the ventricular septum (Fig. 4-2). While some portions of the bundle branches are supplied by the right coronary artery, it is the left coronary artery which supplies most of the bundle branch tissue. Therefore, when AV block occurs in the setting of a left coronary artery occlusion, the location of that AV block is generally in the bundle branches.

MECHANISM OF AV BLOCK

Another important aspect of AV block is the underlying cause. In this text, the only cause of AV block discussed is myocardial infarction. However, not all AV block is caused by infarction. Several conditions can produce an AV block including fibrotic disease and calcification of the conduction system. Certain medications, such as digitalis, can also produce an AV block. When infarction is the cause of AV block, the actual mechanism is due to either an increase in parasympathetic tone or a serious tissue injury.

The effect of the parasympathetic nervous system is to slow the conduction of electrical impulses through the AV node, while the effect of the sympathetic nervous system is to speed conduction of electrical impulses through the AV node. A balance normally exists between the two nervous systems which creates a needed delay in conduction through the AV node, long enough for the ventricles to fill before systole.

The rich supply of parasympathetic nerve endings in the AV node is demonstrated in Fig. 4-3. As previously mentioned, the right coronary artery supplies the AV node in approximately 90% of the population. In the instance of a right coronary artery occlusion, ischemia may develop in the AV node. As a result of this ischemia, there can be a disturbance in the balance between the parasympathetic and sympathetic nervous systems, resulting in an increase in parasympathetic tone. Once parasympathetic tone increases, conduction through the AV node is slowed. This

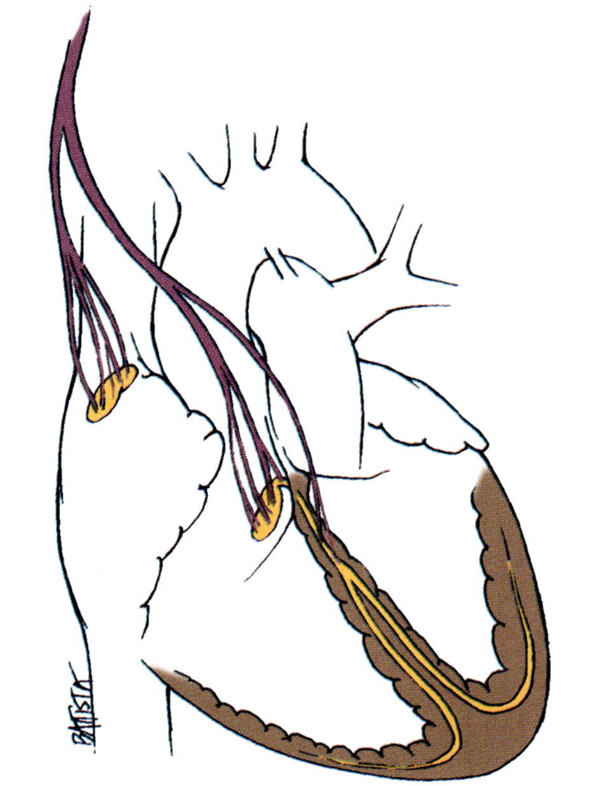

FIG. 4-3 Note the presence of parasympathetic nerve endings in SA and AV nodes. However, there are few, if any, parasympathetic nerve endings in the bundle branches.

slowing may manifest itself as a prolonged PR interval (first degree block) or beats may be dropped as a result (second degree or third degree block). Increase in parasympathetic tone is the cause of most AV blocks complicating right coronary artery occlusions (inferior wall infarctions and RVI). Of course, the occlusion can also lead to serious tissue injury or death of the AV node, but this happens much less frequently.

There is very little, if any, innervation of the parasympathetic nervous system in the bundle branches. With little or no parasympathetic nerve endings there, ischemia in the bundle branches usually does not result in AV block. Rather, when AV block occurs in the setting of a left coronary artery occlusion (septal and anterior infarctions), the block is usually located in bundle branches and most likely due to serious tissue injury or tissue death.

Overall, infarct produces AV block most frequently because of an increase in parasympathetic tone. Local ischemia around the AV node is all that is required to produce AV block. This type of block requires a less severe insult than an AV block caused by serious tissue injury or death. Blocks that are the result of serious tissue injury are usually the result of a more extensive infarction.

SUBSIDIARY PACEMAKERS

Both nodal and infranodal AV blocks may become serious enough to require the use of a natural subsidiary pacemaker. Should such an escape pacemaker become a necessity, nodal AV blocks have a tremendous advantage. If required, there is usually a reliable junctional pacemaker available that can fire at 40–60 beats a minute. However, when the location of an AV block is below the junction, the only available pacemaker may be a slow ventricular one, firing at 20–30 beats per minute. Not only are those ventricular pacemakers slow, they are prone to long pauses, making them less than reliable. Therefore, nodal AV blocks usually have a more effective and reliable escape pacemaker than do infranodal AV blocks.

QRS COMPLEX WIDTH

AV blocks that occur in the AV node usually produce a narrow QRS complex (just as a junctional rhythm does) and an AV block in the bundle branches usually produces a wide QRS complex (just as a ventricular rhythm does). While this rule is not absolute, it is another useful clue in determining the site of an AV block.

RESPONSE TO ATROPINE

Atropine is a parasympatholytic agent; it diminishes the parasympathetic effect. If an AV block

Table 4.1 Nodal and Infranodal Block

	NODAL BLOCK	INFRANODAL BLOCK
Coronary Supply	Right coronary artery	Left coronary artery
QRS Width	Narrow	Wide
Stability	Generally stable	Often unstable
Atropine Response	Usually improves	Often does not respond

is due to an increase in parasympathetic tone, as most AV blocks are, then atropine is ideally suited to correct the block. However, if the AV block is due to a serious tissue lesion, atropine will have little beneficial effect. In fact, the AHA notes that some experts consider atropine to be contraindicated in that setting. The concern lies in the possibility that the atropine will not improve the block but will increase the rate of discharge of the atria. This may trigger a situation in which even fewer impulses are conducted into the ventricle and the ventricular rate is further slowed. While this concern was noted by the AHA, the final guidelines did not include that contraindication. The AHA does recommend that a standby pacemaker be used in the setting of infranodal AV blocks, as is further discussed later in this chapter. Refer to Table 4-1 for further information on nodal and infranodal block.

Hypotension

A common approach to the treatment of hypotension secondary to myocardial infarction (not due to an inappropriate heart rate) has been to administer a small fluid bolus followed by an inotropic drug such as dopamine. The 1994 edition of the AHA *Textbook of Advanced Cardiac Life Support* includes an Acute Pulmonary Edema/Hypotension/Shock algorithm, with emphasis upon determining whether the underlying problem is a rate problem, a pump problem, or a volume problem. This approach forces the emergency cardiac care provider to conceptualize and evaluate the underlying problem. Right ventricular infarction is one such underlying factor that should be considered when treating a patient experiencing hypotension in the presence of an inferior wall MI.

When hypotension complicates inferior wall infarction, one must question whether the hypotension is secondary to a simultaneous RVI. As detailed in Chapter 2, whenever an inferior wall MI is suspected (indicative changes in leads II, III, and AVF) right-sided chest leads should be obtained to screen for an RVI. At a minimum, V4R should be obtained and the care provider should look for the clinical evidence of RVI: jugular venous distention, clear lung sounds, and hypotension. These signs signify the presence of a preload-dependent patient, one who may benefit from fluid therapy. Remember, the problem in this setting is that blood is "stalling" in the right ventricle resulting in the left ventricle being underfilled. Also included in the 1994 edition of the AHA *Textbook of Advanced Cardiac Life Support* is the following statement about hypotension in RVI: "Treatment requires judicious though often vigorous fluid therapy to raise the left ventricular filling pressure. . . ."

It is important to remember that while the RVI may respond to fluids, there also is a simultaneous infarction occurring in the inferior wall of the left ventricle. This coexistent infarction may reduce the left ventricle's pump function. When increased fluids are administered in the setting of decreased left ventricular pump function, the possibility of provoking pulmonary edema is a very real concern. Practical methods for treating hypotension in RVI are presented in the next section, along with treatment methods for chest pain and AV block.

Treatment

This section reviews the treatment strategies for the management of cardiac chest pain, hypotension, and AV block. The information has been obtained from a variety of texts, research papers, and journal articles, and is provided only as an overview. The treatments described here are not guidelines or recommendations. Each emergency cardiac care provider must follow the established treatment protocols in his or her own setting.

CHEST PAIN

Nitroglycerin and morphine are well-suited for the management of cardiac chest pain and are by far the most commonly used agents. However, in the setting of RVI, the vasodilatation produced by these agents may precipitate hypotension. The emergency cardiac care provider is thus faced with a dilemma. When does the risk of hypotension outweigh the benefit of pain management? In most cases, it is desirable to have physician input.

If the decision is made to administer vasodilators there are a few methods of administration which may lessen the hypotensive response. One option calls for the administration of a fluid bolus either before or along with nitroglycerin or morphine administration. This option attempts to increase preload and offset the upcoming decrease in preload. A similar approach is to administer an inotrope along with the vasodilators. The intent of this strategy is obvious: offset the decrease in preload with an increase in contractility. Finally, the physician may opt for the routine administration of nitroglycerin and morphine, or may choose not to administer any vasodilators at all.

It is important to recognize that not every patient experiencing RVI will fall into deep hypotension after nitrate administration. Just as there are verifying degrees of severity in left ventricular infarctions, RVI is not always so extensive as to manifest great hemodynamic significance. It is estimated that about 50% of all patients with RVI will develop hemodynamic compromise.

AV BLOCK

Locating the probable site of an AV block plays a critical part in developing an effective treatment plan for AV block. Remember, when AV block is associated with inferior wall infarction and produces a narrow QRS complex, it is probably located in the AV node. However, when anterior wall infarction produces AV block it usually occurs in the bundle branches (infranodal) and displays a wide QRS complex.

Nodal AV blocks resulting from inferior infarctions tend to be the result of increased parasympathetic tone, and are generally stable. Because the nodal AV blocks are stable, treatment is often not required and the blocks tend to be self-limiting. If the block does become more severe and an escape pacemaker is required, frequently a lower site in the AV junction will produce a ventricular rate of 40–60. In the event that a nodal AV block does require treatment and the ventricular rate must be increased, either atropine or pacing are appropriate.

If an IV has already been established, atropine may be the first choice. In that case, atropine administration could be accomplished more

Table 4.2 AV Block Summary

	INFARCT SITE	CORONARY ARTERY	CAUSE	SUBSIDIARY PACEMAKER	QRS WIDTH	ATROPINE RESPONSE
Nodal AV Block	Usually inferior or right ventricular	Usually right	Usually parasympathetic tone	Junctional, usually reliable	Often narrow	Likely
Infranodal AV Block	Usually septal or anterior	Usually left	Usually serious tissue injury	Ventricular, often unreliable	Often wide	Unlikely

quickly than transcutaneous pacing, and would probably be tolerated better by the patient. Since nodal AV block complicating an inferior wall infarction is probably due to increased parasympathetic tone, a parasympathetic agent such as atropine is often very effective. However, there are still some situations in which transcutaneous pacing may be preferable.

According to the AHA, in the 1994 *Textbook of Advanced Life Support*, "Transcutaneous pacing is indicated for the treatment of hemodynamically significant bradycardias that have not responded to atropine therapy or when atropine therapy is not immediately available." Thus, when treating a hemodynamically compromised patient, transcutaneous pacing may be provided more readily than atropine if an IV has not yet been established. Of course, if the patient is unresponsive to atropine, transcutaneous pacing should be attempted immediately. While nodal AV blocks are sometimes unresponsive to atropine, infranodal AV blocks are often unresponsive to atropine. Therefore, transcutaneous pacing plays a larger role in the treatment of infranodal AV block.

Infranodal AV block, which occurs far less frequently than nodal AV block, is generally the result of serious tissue injury secondary to anterior wall infarction. Atropine is often ineffective at increasing the ventricular rate of infranodal AV block and, theoretically, may produce a paradoxical slowing of the ventricular rate. Furthermore, the onset of an infranodal AV block complicating anterior infarction is a poor prognostic sign.

Not only does the onset of an infranodal AV block indicate a more serious infarction but infranodal AV blocks may quickly progress to a near-asystole state (see pages 62 and 63). Therefore, standby pacing is indicated when infranodal AV block complicates anterior wall MI. The rationale behind this strategy is obvious. If an AV block is known to be unstable and unlikely to respond to atropine, then applying the pacemaker on standby—even when the AV block is presently stable—is the best defense.

Should atropine be used in the treatment of infranodal AV block? The issue is still a matter of debate but the AHA recommends, in the *Textbook of Advanced Cardiac Life Support*, that "Atropine can be used in these situations, but watch closely for paradoxical slowing." Likewise, if the infranodal AV block does not respond quickly to atropine, then pacing should be immediately attempted. See Table 4-2 for further explanation of nodal and infranodal AV block.

HYPOTENSION

A conventional approach to treating hypotension secondary to MI calls for the administration of a 200–500 cc fluid bolus, followed by an inotrope if needed. The fluid bolus begins to correct any relative hypovolemia and may increase cardiac output by increasing the fill of the ventricles. As the ventricles are filled to a greater degree, each myocardial cell is stretched, resulting in a more forceful contraction (Frank Starling mechanism). However, the benefit of this approach is limited because as the amount of fluid infused increases, so does the risk of pulmonary edema. Therefore, if the hypotension is not completely corrected by a limited fluid challenge, an inotrope must be used.

The conventional approach just described and the AHA algorithm previously mentioned are both general approaches to hypotension.

Table 4.3 Significant Features of Right and Left Coronary Artery Occlusions

	LEFT CORONARY ARTERY OCCLUSIONS	RIGHT CORONARY ARTERY OCCLUSIONS
Leads Showing Indicative Changes	V1 - V6, I, AVL	II, III, AVF V4R-V6R (RVI)
Localization	Septal Anterior Lateral Posterior	Inferior Posterior Right ventricular
Pain Control	Nitroglycerin and morphine appropriate	Nitroglycerin and morphine used with caution **if** RVI present
AV Block	Infrequent Usually wide QRS Often unstable Atropine may be ineffective Use standby pacing	Frequent Usually narrow QRS Generally stable Atropine often effective May not require treatment
Hypotension	200cc-500cc fluid bolus Inotrope	Vigorous fluid therapy **if** RVI present Inotrope

While these approaches apply to a broad category of patients, right ventricular infarction presents a possible exception to these approaches. Previous treatment discussions focused on the differences between right and left coronary occlusions. However, the following discussion of hypotension applies only to right ventricular infarctions and does not apply to distal occlusions of the right coronary artery (inferior wall infarction without RVI) not affecting the right ventricle. In other words, hypotension is treated identically for both right and left coronary occlusions unless an RVI is present. Refer to Table 4-3 for further information concerning significant features of right and left coronary artery occlusions.

Hypotension secondary to RVI may be particularly responsive to fluid therapy. The AHA states that, "A careful fluid challenge with normal saline may be lifesaving for these [RVI] patients." A liter or more of fluids may be required to sufficiently increase ventricular filling. Since pulmonary edema is still a significant concern, the fluid may be administered in small increments, reassessing the lung sounds after every 200–300 cc of fluid administration. Fluid therapy should be discontinued if pulmonary edema develops.

Inotropes are still effective in RVI. Since they increase contractility through a different mechanism than does fluid therapy, the two approaches may be used simultaneously. Interestingly, several sources state that dobutamine may be more effective than dopamine in treating hypotension in the setting of RVI.

It is important to remember that the use of a vigorous fluid challenge is only appropriate in the setting of RVI. Inferior wall infarction without clinical or electrocardiographic evidence of an RVI *does not* warrant the use of fluids in large quantities.

Infranodal AV Block

In the setting of infarction, infranodal AV block is usually associated with left coronary artery occlusions. As mentioned, the degree of AV block does not necessarily equate to the severity of AV block. In fact, the location of the block may better indicate the severity. Exclusive reliance on the degree system may cause some emergency cardiac care providers to assume that first degree AV blocks are not serious and consider it an incidental finding until the block progress to the second degree. In this section, it is demonstrated how a first degree infranodal AV block can quickly progress to either asystole or a third degree AV block with a slow ventricular rate.

The left coronary artery, which supplies the septal and anterior walls of the left ventricle, is also the blood supply for the bundle branches. When an AV block occurs as a result of this type of infarct it is usually located in the bundle branches, an infranodal location. The cause of infranodal AV block is probably not attributed to increased parasympathetic tone because there are few, if any, parasympathetic nerve endings at that location. Therefore, the probable cause of an infranodal block is a serious tissue lesion.

In the ventricular conduction system, there are three pathways by which the electrical impulses are distributed to the myocardium. Ventricular depolarization can occur as long as one of these pathways is functioning. Therefore, as shown in Fig. 4-4, even when the infarct has produced tissue injury which prohibits conduction through two of the pathways, no AV block results.

If the infarct then produces an incomplete tissue lesion in the remaining pathway, conduction is still possible, but the impulse may encounter a delay. This delay is represented as a prolonged PR interval on the ECG, and is classified as a first degree AV block (Fig. 4-5).

If this condition does not progress, then the degree of AV block is not expected to change. However, if the lesion in the last remaining fascicle becomes complete, then conduction into the ventricles will be stopped. At this point the patient is completely reliant on a ventricular escape rhythm to sustain cardiac output (Fig. 4-6). These escape rhythms may only fire at 20–30 times per minute and may be irregular, with long pauses between beats. If no ventricular rhythm intervenes, then ventricular asystole is the result.

In treating this patient, the use of atropine may prove to be ineffective. The block itself

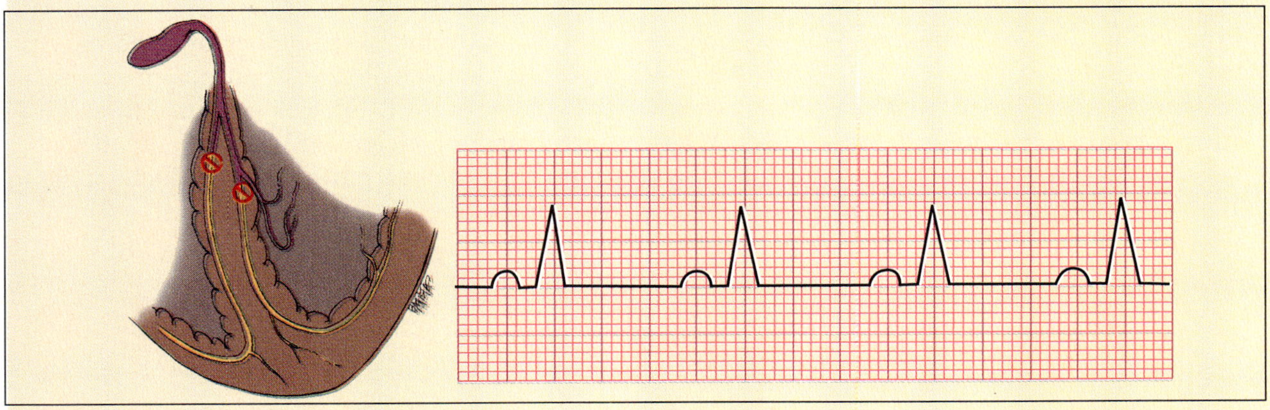

FIG. 4-4 Normal sinus rhythm.

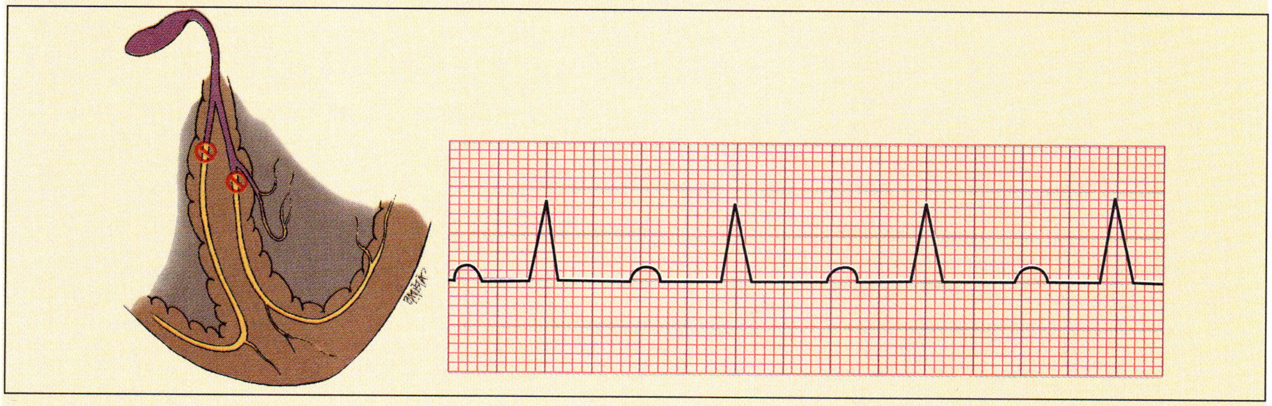

FIG. 4-5 First degree AV block.

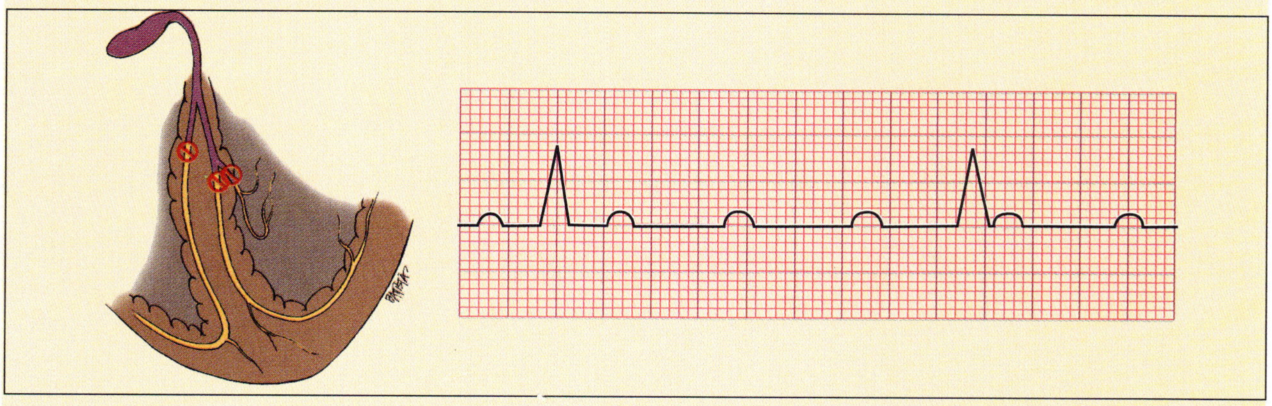

FIG. 4-6 Third degree AV block, ventricular escape rhythm.

is not due to parasympathetic tone and, therefore, atropine is unlikely to improve conduction throughout the tissue lesions. Furthermore, atropine has a limited ability to increase the rate of the ventricular escape rhythm. According to the AHA, it is not wrong to try atropine in this setting, but it is best to realize in advance that it may not be effective so that pacing can be quickly employed. In fact, once this situation is recognized, it is appropriate to apply the external pacemaker on standby, even before the patient becomes unstable.

SUMMARY

- Once the site of the coronary artery occlusion has been predicted, a knowledge of the tissues supplied by that artery make it possible to anticipate certain complications.
- The treatment of chest pain, AV block, and hypotension can be made more effective when tailored to the site of coronary occlusion.
- Nitroglycerin and morphine should be used with caution in the setting of RVI.
- Nodal AV block is frequently seen in right coronary artery occlusions, especially if RVI is present, and is generally stable.
- Nodal AV block is usually due to increased parasympathetic tone and atropine is often effective.
- Infranodal AV block is seen less frequently, usually in association with anterior infarction.
- Infranodal AV block is usually due to serious tissue injury and atropine is often ineffective.
- Infranodal AV block due to infarction is unstable and standby pacing is indicated, even when vital signs are normal.
- A narrow QRS favors nodal AV block while a wide QRS favors infranodal AV block.
- A judicious, but vigorous, fluid therapy may be very effective in treating hypotension secondary to RVI.

5

CHAPTER

Thrombolysis

OBJECTIVES

- Review the pathophysiology of myocardial infarction.
- Discuss the mechanisms of action, indications, contraindications, and complications of thrombolytic agents.
- Examine strategies for reduction of "door-to-drug" time in the emergency department.
- Review the scientific research relating to the prehospital 12-lead ECG and prehospital thrombolysis.

This chapter examines the pathophysiology of myocardial infarction, its various clinical presentations, and the current role of thrombolytic agents. Answers are provided to frequently asked questions regarding prehospital 12-lead electrocardiography and its impact on thrombolysis. Strategies that can reduce the time required for emergency department administration of thrombolytic agents are also included.

The Pathophysiology of Myocardial Infarction

Coronary thrombosis, a blood clot in a coronary artery, is the most frequent cause of myocardial infarction. Frequently, the underlying circumstances involve diseased coronary arteries that have accumulated atherosclerotic plaque. This plaque not only makes the arteries harder and more fragile, it also reduces the inner diameter of the coronary artery and thereby limits the volume of blood supplied by that artery. This reduction in flow may lead to the development of ischemia whenever additional oxygen demands are made by the heart. The increased demand for oxygen in the face of a fixed supply of blood produces chest pain. The pain generally prompts the patient to rest, thus reducing the oxygen demand and relieving the pain. This scenario of simple angina does not, in itself, produce a loss of muscle tissue.

A blood clot in an already narrowed coronary artery can lead to a total occlusion of that coronary artery. Cardiac tissue, like all other tissues of the body, can temporarily survive without blood flow, but cannot do so indefinitely. If a spontaneous lysis of the clot occurs, and blood flow is quickly restored, then tissue death may be avoided. However, if the clot does not dissolve, or is not other-

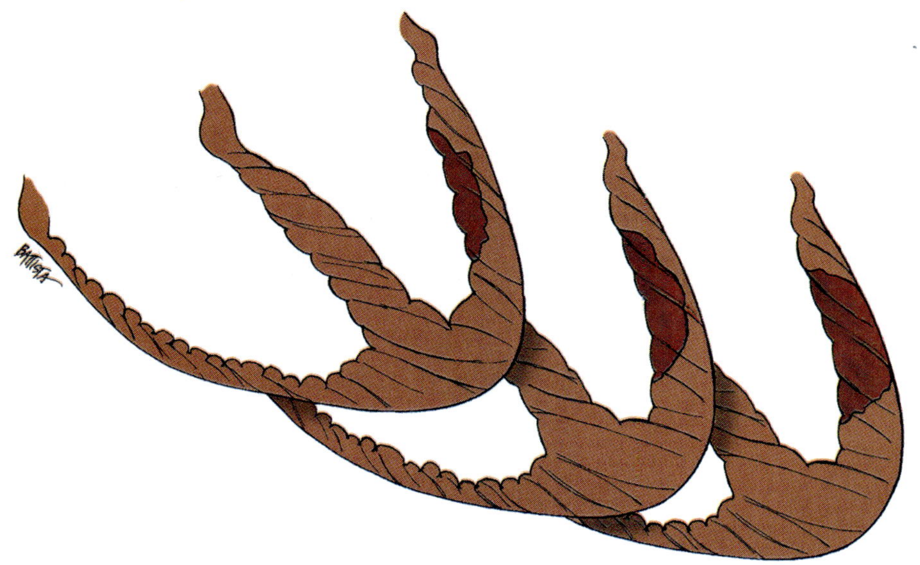

FIG. 5-1 Wave front expansion of myocardial infarction progresses from endocardium to epicardium.

wise eliminated, the myocardium will start to experience necrosis.

Once the process of tissue death begins it continues quickly. The progress of tissue death has been described as a "wave" that begins in the endocardium and spreads to the epicardium. As the wave extends, the infarction becomes larger (Fig. 5-1). The only way that the infarction can be halted is if the source of the coronary artery occlusion can be eliminated. Since the most frequent cause of coronary occlusion is a blood clot, definitive treatment must somehow eliminate the clot.

Thrombolytic Agents

Until very recently, there was no widely available treatment that could halt the progress of an acute myocardial infarction and restore circulation to the infarcting heart. While percutaneous transluminal coronary angioplasty (PTCA) has been on the scene for over a decade and is quite effective, not every hospital can afford the equipment and staffing necessary to perform PTCA. In fact, in many communities there is not even an accessible facility to which the AMI patient can be referred for timely angioplasty. Therefore, the problem with PTCA is not one of efficacy but of availability.

With the advent of pharmacologic agents capable of lysing the blood clot causing the infarction, every emergency department can now provide a treatment with the potential to stop the infarction in its tracks. The availability of these agents literally revolutionizes the treatment of myocardial infarction. This section discusses thrombolytic agents, their mechanism of action, indications, contraindications, and complications. Before beginning a discussion of these clot busters, an overview of the normal clotting process is beneficial.

When we have a small cut and blood is drawn, a clot quickly forms. The formation of the clot is not due to exposure of the blood to air. In fact, if blood were to be carefully drawn from a vessel so that it did not contact the damaged portion of the vessel, and then placed on a smooth plastic dish, it would not clot. What causes blood to clot?

Clotting involves two essential elements: damaged tissue and damaged platelets. The tissue damage generally occurs first and releases certain chemicals. The platelets in circulation may then run into the damaged tissue and become damaged themselves. Both the tissue and the platelet release chemicals which together initiate a chain reaction, leading to the formation of a clot. The complete process is actually quite complex and involves several steps in which one substance is produced, then acts as a catalyst in the production of another substance, which stimulates another reaction, and so on, until finally a substance called fibrin is formed. Fibrin forms a fibrous mesh which traps red cells, white cells, and platelets. This mesh contracts and squeezes the plasma out of it. This squeezing may pull the walls of the vessel closer together. A simplified representation of the clotting process is presented in Fig. 5-2.

In the case of AMI, the tissue damage results from a rupture of atherosclerotic plaque which has accumulated inside the coronary artery. When the plaque ruptures and platelets are exposed to it, both release chemicals that start the formation of a blood clot in the coronary artery.

MECHANISM OF ACTION

Though differences exist among the exact mechanisms that trigger the reduction of blood clots, all thrombolytic agents result in an increased

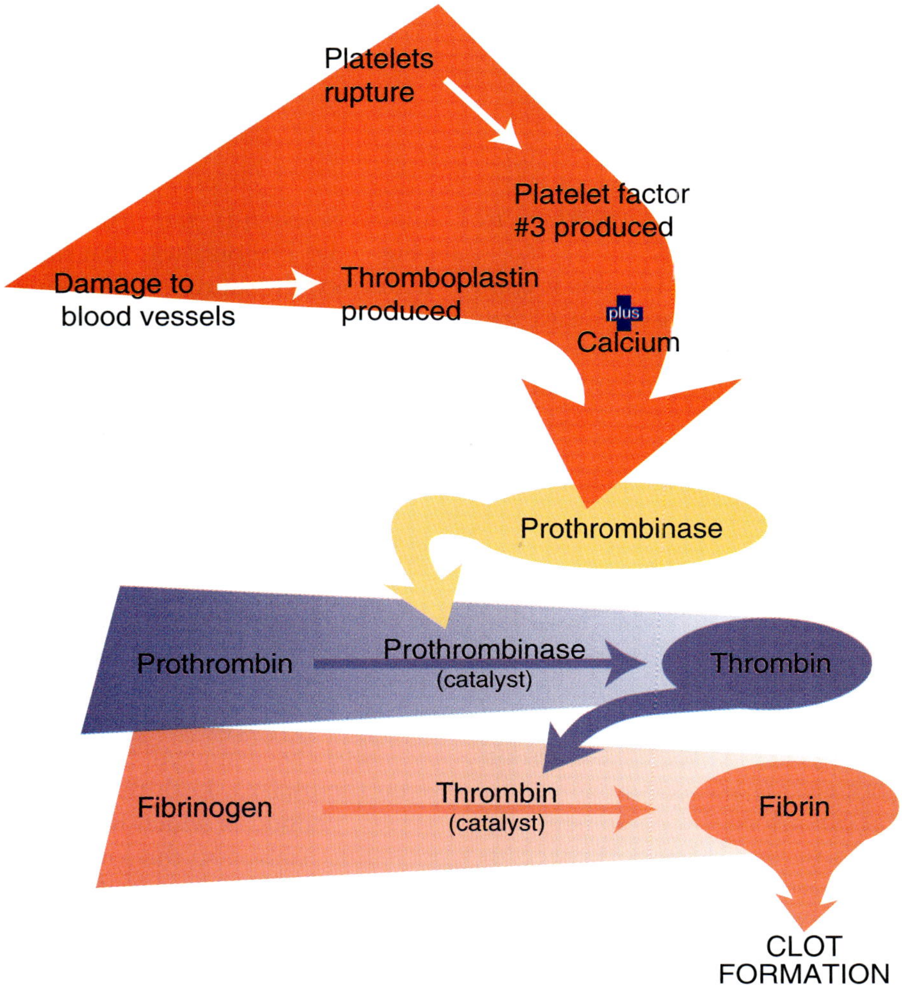

FIG. 5-2 The process of clot formation.

production of plasmin. When the concentration of plasmin increases around the clot, the plasmin begins to break down fibrin, which then causes the clot to dissolve.

INDICATIONS

Thrombolytic therapy is indicated when AMI is suspected by both clinical presentation and ECG evidence. Since thrombolytic therapy is intended to interrupt the process of myocardial infarction, it is counterproductive to wait for definitive evidence of tissue death, i.e., Q waves. Elevation of the ST segment is the most frequently used marker to indicate the presence of myocardial injury leading to infarction. A new onset bundle branch block in the setting of suspected AMI is considered by some to also be an indication for thrombolytic therapy.

CONTRAINDICATIONS

Many contraindications to thrombolytic therapy exist, most relating to bleeding complications. Both the AHA and the National Heart Attack Alert Program (NHAAP) have published contraindications to thrombolytic therapy, both absolute and relative. Their recommendations are included in Tables 5-1 and 5-2 for comparison. A comparison of the two recommendations shows that though some minor differences exist, in general they are very similar.

Age has been suggested as a potential contraindication. Several of the large thrombolytic

Table 5-1 Absolute Contraindications to Thrombolytic Therapy

AMERICAN HEART ASSOCIATION	NATIONAL HEART ATTACK ALERT PROGRAM
Active internal bleeding	Altered consciousness
Suspected aortic dissection	Active internal bleeding
Known traumatic CPR	Known spinal cord or cerebral arteriovenous malformation or tumor
Severe persistent hypertension despite pain relief and initial drugs (greater than 180 systolic or 110 diastolic)	Recent head trauma
Recent head trauma or known intracranial neoplasm	Known previous hemorrhagic CVA
History of CVA in the past 6 months	Intracranial or intraspinal surgery within 2 months
Pregnancy	Trauma or surgery within 2 weeks, which could result in bleeding into a closed space
	Persistent BP 200/120
	Known bleeding disorder
	Pregnancy
	Suspected aortic dissection
	Previous allergy to a streptokinase product (but not a contraindication to use of other thrombolytic agents)

trials excluded chest pain patients older than 75 years. This exclusion stemmed from the recognition that the elderly have a higher incidence of CVA and other serious complications as a direct result of the thrombolytic therapy. However, age is itself a very poor prognostic sign in AMI and the elderly experience a high mortality rate secondary to AMI. Therefore, the group that is most likely to experience a serious complication from treatment is also the group most likely to die from the infarct. At least two studies which did not use age as a contraindication noted that the benefit of reduced mortality from thrombolytic treatment outweighed the increased incidence of iatrogenic complications.

Ultimately, the decision whether to administer thrombolytic agents is made by weighing the potential benefits against the possible risks. Patients presenting with an absolute contraindication to thrombolytic therapy, or several relative contraindications, may be good candidates for PTCA or coronary artery bypass grafting (CABG).

COMPLICATIONS

Remember that blood clots are normally beneficial to the body and become a concern only when occurring in areas such as the heart, brain, and lungs. While some thrombolytic agents are

Table 5-2 Relative Contraindications to Thromobolytic Therapy

AMERICAN HEART ASSOCIATION	NATIONAL HEART ATTACK ALERT PROGRAM
Recent trauma or major surgery	Active peptic ulcer disease
Initial blood pressure greater than 180 systolic or 100 diastolic that is controlled by medical treatment	History of ischemic or embolic CVA
Active peptic ulcer or guaiac-positive stools	Current use of anticoagulants
History of CVA, tumor, injury, or brain surgery	Major trauma or surgery after 2 weeks and up to 2 months
Known beeding disorder or current use of warfrin	History of chronic, uncontrolled hypertension (diastolic greater than 100 mmHg), treated or untreated
Significant liver dysfunction	Subclavian or internal jugular venous cannulation
Exposure to streptokinase or ansitreplase during the preceding 12 months (these agents only)	
Known cancer or illness with possible thoracic, abdominal, or intracranial abnormalities	
Prolonged CPR	

more specific to clots within the coronary artery, all exert some influence on fibrin throughout the body. Therefore, the potential for bleeding is the chief concern when administering thrombolytic therapy. The incidence of serious bleeding complications is about 5% in all treated patients. The incidence of intracranial bleeding is about 1% in patients younger than 75 years. However, the rate of inhospital stroke complicating AMI was about 3% before the advent of thrombolytic therapy. While the rate of stroke is actually lower in the group receiving thrombolytic therapy, those patients more often experienced intracranial hemorrhage as the cause of stroke, while the untreated group usually experienced stroke due to embolism.

Another complication is that of allergic reaction, particularly when streptokinase or a streptokinase containing agent such as anistreplase (APSAC) is used. Allergic reactions are more common in patients who have had streptococcal infections and/or received a streptokinase product within 1 year. The allergic reaction can be managed with antihistamines and corticosteroids, but often the allergic reaction results in a destruction of streptokinase.

Hypotension and reperfusion dysrhythmias are frequently seen with thrombolytic therapy. Hypotension may be treated with fluids and/or elevation of the feet. When administering a streptokinase product, hypotension may be dose-related. When hypotension occurs, a reduction in the rate of administration may reduce the hypotension. Reperfusion dysrhythmias are commonly seen with thrombolytic therapy, generally occurring about 60–90 minutes after administration of the agent. These dysrhythmias may include accelerated idoventricular rhythms, bradycardias, and heart blocks. These dysrhythmias should be observed and treated if necessary.

DOSAGE

Each thrombolytic agent has its own recommended dosage and administration procedures.

ADJUNCTIVE THERAPY

Aspirin can rival thrombolytic therapy in its impact on mortality reduction. The fact that aspirin is effective, inexpensive, available, and produces few side effects explains why the AHA recommends that the care giver ". . . treat virtually all patients with suspected MI with a chewable 160 mg aspirin tablet." In the emergency setting, chewable aspirin allows for quicker absorption. Therefore, flavored children's chewable aspirin may be better accepted by the patient over standard aspirin tablets.

Allergy to aspirin is an absolute contraindication, and active ulcer disease or asthma are relative contraindications. Many asthma patients may report an "allergy" to aspirin but upon questioning have never experienced an allergic reaction. Because aspirin can induce bronchospasm in the asthmatic, many physicians advise asthma patients not to use aspirin. These patients may perceive this as an allergy when in fact bronchospasm is the true concern. During infarct, the physician may consider the potential bronchospasm a relative contraindication and order aspirin for the infarcting asthmatic.

Anticoagulants have at least two roles in the treatment of AMI. First, as an adjunct to thrombolytic therapy and, second, as aid in preventing embolic complications such as pulmonary embolism and cardiac thrombi. Thrombolytic agents dissolve clots but new ones may form and reocclude the coronary artery. Anticoagulants such as heparin help to prevent such reocclusions. The use of heparin is especially important when using alteplase (TPA) but should be avoided when using APSAC.

EFFICACY

The ability of a medication or treatment to achieve its intended result is considered its **efficacy**. Several factors contribute to the efficacy of thrombolytic therapy, but probably the most significant is the duration from symptom onset to treatment. It is conceded that the benefits of thrombolytic therapy are time-dependent. Remember, time is muscle.

In canine studies, it has been estimated that 50% of tissue loss occurs within 2 hours of coronary occlusion. Tissue death may be noted as early as the first 20 minutes of infarction, and studies estimate that approximately 90% of tissue loss occurs within the first 6 hours. Therefore, if myocardium is to be saved, the occlusion must be eliminated before irreversible tissue death occurs. Fig. 5-3 shows the relationship between the duration of coronary artery occlusion and myocardial salvage in the canine heart.

The results from thrombolytic trials suggest that a similar pattern occurs in humans. Fig. 5-3 also shows the reduction in mortality in patients receiving thrombolytic therapy as compared to the time from symptom onset to administration of the drug. Note how strikingly similar the myocardial salvage curve is to that of the mortality rate. This illustrates the importance of early treatment and demonstrates that very early treatment provides the greatest reduction in mortality.

Fig 5-3 demonstrates the rate of myocardial tissue loss and the time-related benefits of thrombolytic therapy. Notice that the rate of myocardial loss is greatest within the first 2 hours. After that, the rate of loss slows until it is essentially complete at the 12-hour point. The curve displaying mortality rates demonstrates that administering thrombolytic agents within the first 2 hours provides the most significant benefit.

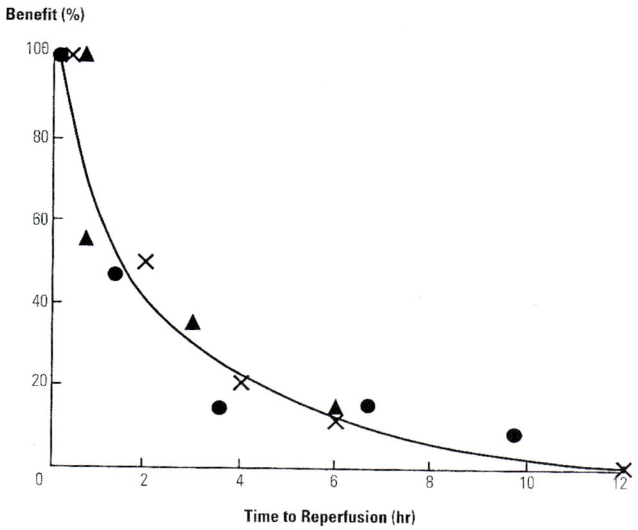

FIG. 5-3 The time-related benefits of thrombolytic therapy in the canine heart. *(From the National Heart Attack Alert Program Coordinating Committee, 60 Minutes to Treatment Working Group: Emergency department: Rapid identification and treatment of patients with acute myocardial infarction, Annals of Emergency Medicine, February 1994: 23:311-329.)*

The curves in Fig. 5-3 illustrate that the canine studies reveal that 12 hours after coronary occlusion, myocardial loss was complete. The curve from the thrombolytic data shows a reduction in mortality up to the 12-hour point. Several investigators have asked, "when is it too late to administer thrombolytic therapy?" It has been established that treatment up to 12 and even 24 hours after symptom onset can produce a reduction in mortality. This improved survival rate, even after the point of extensive myocardial loss, suggests that factors other than reduction of infarct size are responsible for the reduced mortality. It is theorized that late thrombolytic therapy may allow for a more stable electrophysiologic environment and may benefit the process of myocardial healing.

On average, all thrombolytic agents are about 85% effective at reestablishing coronary artery patency when measured at the 24-hour point. Prior to that point, differences in patency rates between thrombolytic agents exist. It is important to realize that thrombolytic therapy does not always reestablish normal coronary artery patency.

Door-to-Drug Time

Every emergency department has an enormous challenge on its hands. Despite the large numbers of patients continuously streaming into the emergency department, the NHAAP has challenged hospitals to rapidly identify acute infarct patients and administer thrombolytic therapy within 30 minutes of patient arrival. Given the ratio of patients to staff in most emergency departments, it is not surprising that few emergency departments are able to meet this objective on a regular basis. In one study, fewer than 5% of patients received thrombolytic therapy within 30 minutes of their arrival. The task can seem monumental. One may wonder where to even begin trying to reduce the door-to-drug time. Fortunately, some answers have emerged.

Several recurring steps are noted when assessing the flow of events from the time an infarct patient enters the hospital until the time thrombolytic therapy is administered. These recurring steps have been grouped by the NHAAP into the following four phases: Door, Data, Decision, Drug. Fig. 5-4 diagrams several of the components of each step and lists them in the most typical order of occurence. To further elaborate on each phase and demonstrate the potential time loss at each step along the way, let's follow an imaginary patient entering the hospital. Along the way, every potential point of delay will be indicated. As you read the following information, please remember that the intent of this exercise is to account for (not judge) the delays in time.

The **Door** phase begins as the patient walks into the emergency department. A few minutes may pass while the patient waits for an available registration clerk (first delay). Depending upon the clinical presentation, the registration clerk may or may not recognize the complaint as possibly cardiac in nature (second delay). Even with additional training, the registration clerk may not recognize an atypical infarct presentation. If the patient is not immediately recognized as potentially experiencing an infarct, the patient is asked to sit in the waiting room until the triage nurse calls for him or her (third delay). When called to the triage area, the nurse recognizes the potential infarct and the patient is transferred to the treatment area (fourth delay).

Once in the treatment area, the **Data** phase begins as the nurse assigned to the bed continues the assessment. Despite the nurse's suspicion that an infarct may be in progress, in some emergency departments only the physician has the authority to order an ECG (fifth delay). Once the physician orders the 12-lead, the ECG technician may need to be paged (sixth delay) so that when they have completed their present assignment (seventh delay) the 12-lead machine can be brought to the emergency department (eighth delay) and the tracing obtained (ninth delay). Once the ECG technician completes the tracing, it is added to the patient's chart and may sit there for a period of time before the physician is available to read it (tenth delay).

As the physician picks up the chart containing the 12-lead and other lab work, the **Decision** phase begins. In some instances, it is easy to recognize the evidence of infarct in progress, while in others it may be more difficult (eleventh delay). A cardiologist may need to be called for a consult

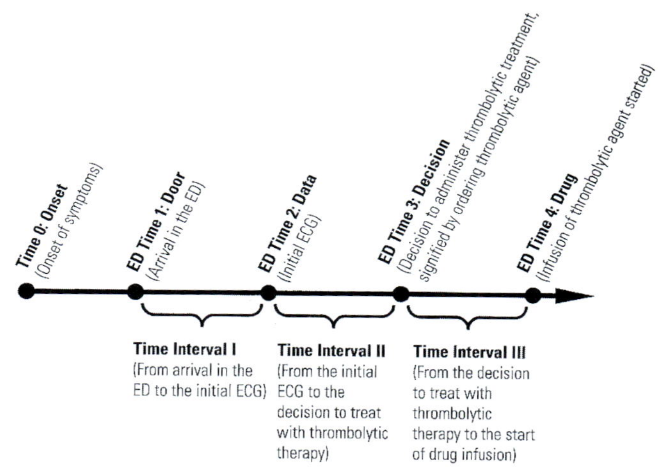

FIG. 5-4 The "Four Ds" represent common steps in the process of infarct recognition and treatment with thrombolytic agents. *(From the National Heart Attack Alert Program Coordinating Committee, 60 Minutes to Treatment Working Group: Emergency department: Rapid identification and treatment of patients with acute myocardial infarction, Annals of Emergency Medicine, February 1994: 23:311-329.)*

(twelfth delay) to make the decision of whether to administer thrombolytic therapy (thirteenth delay).

The **Drug** phase begins when the decision is made to administer thrombolytic therapy. The patient must be informed of the potential risks (fourteenth delay). In some institutions, either the drug must be requested from pharmacy (fifteenth delay) and/or the patient must be transferred to the CCU for thrombolytic administration (sixteenth delay).

We have just identified sixteen potential points of delay that can slow the administration of thrombolytic therapy. If we assume only a 3-minute delay at each step, this would translate into a total of 45 minutes in delays. Remember, that it is not a 45-minute door-to-drug time, rather it adds 45 minutes to the door-to-drug time. This is, of course, a worst case scenario, but it serves to illustrate the potential for delay at each step in the process and identifies areas of potential time savings.

Reducing the Delay

In each of the four phases, policy and procedures can be structured in a way that speeds up the process of infarct recognition and management. Following are suggestions for streamlining each phase.

DOOR

Generally, the first staff person that the patient encounters is the registration clerk. While typically not trained as a medical provider or technician, the registration clerk is placed in the position of recognizing the possibility of myocardial infarction. Registration clerks can be trained to identify chest pain patients for immediate evaluation and a list of other "atypical" signs and symptoms may be prepared for the registration clerk. If a patient presents with any of these signs or symptoms, then the triage nurse should be immediately notified.

DATA

When infarction is suspected, a 12-lead ECG should be considered a part of the patient's vital signs. In recognition of the fact that the acquisition of a 12-lead ECG can be a time drain, the NHAAP states that "ED nurses should be provided with a standing order to obtain a 12-lead ECG on any patient suspected of having an AMI."

However, the ability to order an ECG is of little consequence if the ECG machine and/or technician are unavailable. Therefore, keeping a 12-lead ECG machine in the emergency department makes the most sense. If the ECG machine is not immediately available, it should be available within 5 minutes of paging. Since a 12-lead ECG can go unnoticed for a significant period of time before a physician is able to read it, the NHAAP recommends that "emergency nurses should be trained to recognize ECG changes indicative of AMI, particularly if they are responsible for obtaining the tracing."

DECISION AND DRUG

Nurses will have less direct influence over the Decision and Drug phases than over the Door and Data phases. However, the nurse can influence time reductions in these last two phases. A checklist for specific thrombolytic indications/contraindications can be completed during the nursing history and may serve to identify potential thrombolytic candidates. This approach has proven to be very effective in the prehospital setting. Nurses can also participate in the development of hospital policies which directly affect the management of infarct patients.

PREHOSPITAL IDENTIFICATION OF AMI PATIENTS

If the emergency department and the emergency medical services are working cooperatively, the results can dramatically reduce the door-to-drug time. It has been established that a prehospital 12-lead ECG coupled with a checklist to determine the eligibility for thrombolytic therapy can reduce the door-to-drug time by as much as 60 minutes.

In terms of obtaining patient information, the advantage of the EMS agency over the emergency department is obvious—in the prehospital setting, the staff outnumbers the patients. The paramedic is in a unique position to quickly gather much of the data necessary to allow the physician to make a rapid decision regarding thrombolytic therapy. When the clinical and ECG evidence suggest that an infarction is present and the patient appears to be a good candidate for thrombolytic therapy, an "Infarct Alert" is issued to the receiving facility before the patient arrives. This approach allows for the mobilization of staff and equipment so that when the patient arrives, the infarct may be treated quickly and appropriately. One of the most effective ways an emergency department can improve its door-to-drug time is to participate with emergency medical services in an infarct alert program. This, along with questions relating to the prehospital identification of the infarct patient, are explored in the next section.

Prehospital Thrombolytic Studies

Given the fact that very early treatment of AMI with thrombolytic therapy provides the greatest reduction in mortality, it is logical to suspect that administering thrombolytic agents in the prehospital setting may provide the greatest reduction in mortality. This hypothesis has been investigated and the results are both interesting and surprising. In this section, four fundamental questions are asked and answered as an introduction to the body of research that investigates prehospital thrombolysis and prehospital 12-lead ECG.

QUESTION 1

Can thrombolytic agents safely be administered in the prehospital environment?

Yes, thrombolytic agents can be safely administered outside of the hospital. Initial research was aimed at assessing the fidelity of the prehospital 12-lead ECG and the ability of paramedics to use a checklist to identify patients eligible for thrombolytic therapy. All of the researchers agreed that prehospital caregivers could obtain an ECG of equal quality to one obtained in the hospital, transmit it without a loss of fidelity for physician interpretation, and use a checklist to evaluate inclusion/exclusion criteria for thrombolytic therapy.

A later study randomized eligible AMI patients to either receive thrombolytic therapy in the field or in the hospital. After the study was complete, the investigators concluded that no evidence existed suggesting that prehospital administration was associated with more complications. The results, therefore, indicated that thrombolytic agents can be administered safely outside of the hospital.

Many studies designed to answer the same research question have been completed in Europe. These studies also noted that thrombolytic agents could be safely administered outside the hospital. However, it is important to point out that physicians typically staffed the emergency medical service vehicles that were used in these studies.

QUESTION 2

Is there a benefit to prehospital administration of thrombolytic therapy?

While the research clearly showed that thrombolytic therapy could be safely administered in the field, it did not demonstrate a significant benefit to this strategy. In the Myocardial Infarction Triage and Intervention (MITI) trial, 360 chest pain patients met the criteria for thrombolytic therapy and had ECG evidence of AMI. Of the 360 patients, 175 were randomized for prehospital treatment and 185 were randomized for hospital treatment. The outcome of these two groups was very similar in terms of left ventricular ejection fraction, infarct size, and mortality. The result was that no significant difference in outcome was measured between these two groups. Given the notion that time is muscle, these results may be surprising. A possible explanation lies within another benefit of the prehospital 12-lead ECG — its ability to reduce the door-to-drug time at the emergency department.

In the MITI trial, as in numerous other studies, it was demonstrated that the ability to obtain a 12-lead ECG and to perform a simple checklist to determine how suitable the use of thrombolytic therapy is can greatly reduce the door-to-drug time at the hospital. In the case of the MITI trial, the patients randomized for hospital treatment received thrombolytic agents within an average of 20 minutes of arrival. However, during the time of the trial, the nonrandomized patient receiving thrombolytic therapy in the same hospital averaged a 60-minute wait for treatment. This represents a 40-minute decrease in the door-to-drug time for patients receiving a prehospital 12-lead ECG. Such a significant reduction in door-to-drug time may overshadow any potential benefits from field administration of thrombolytic therapy.

Therefore, the evidence from the only large American study of prehospital thrombolytics seems to indicate that, at least in the urban setting, prehospital administration of thrombolytic therapy does not provide any additional benefit over hospital administered therapy. No work has yet examined the efficacy of prehospital thrombolytic administration in rural settings, with long transport times. Future studies may shed more light on the usefulness of prehospital thrombolysis.

QUESTION 3

If there is no benefit to field administration of thrombolytic therapy, is there any reason to obtain a prehospital 12-lead ECG?

Yes. As mentioned in the previous question, the prehospital 12-lead ECG can be instrumental in reducing the door-to-drug time for thrombolytic administration within the hospital. This benefit has been very well–documented by a number of investigators.

The average door-to-drug time reported by many investigators ranges between 60-90 minutes. These times reflect the task that most emergency departments face in attempting to identify the AMI patients from among the scores of patient complaining of chest pain. The majority of patients that complain of chest pain are not experiencing AMI. The challenge facing most emergency departments is to process all of these patients, along with every other patient, gather information so that a decision can be made as to whether infarction is present, and determine if treatment with thrombolytic therapy is appropriate. Considering the ratio of patients to staff, it is understandable that the process is time-consuming. However, despite the difficulty, and in light of the need for rapid treatment of AMI, the AHA recommends that eligible patients receive thrombolytic therapy within 30–60 minutes of their arrival. The NHAAP suggests the more ambitious goal of a 30-minute door-to-drug time.

The evidence is clear that a prehospital 12-lead ECG can reduce the door-to-drug time by up to 1 hour. The reduction in time can be partially explained by the fact that outside the hospital, emergency cardiac care providers outnumber the patients. This allows attention to be focused on one individual complaining of chest pain. A team approach can be applied to gathering necessary information and relaying it to the receiving facility, so that before the patient arrives, the likely candidate for thrombolytic therapy can be identified. This preselection makes the goal of a 30-minute door-to-drug time much more feasible.

QUESTION 4

How much time does a prehospital 12-lead ECG add to the treatment time?

The amount of additional patient contact time required to obtain a 12-lead ECG has been measured in many studies. The increase in time ranges from essentially no increase in patient contact time, to approximately a 5-minute increase. This is significant because the prehospital treatment of the cardiac patient can be a source of delay, and every effort must be made to quickly treat and transport the infarcting patient.

When assessing whether the time investment required to obtain the prehospital 12-lead ECG is worthwhile, one need only recall the reduction in door-to-drug time. Reductions of the order of 20–60 minutes in door-to-drug time have been attributed to the prehospital 12-lead ECG and a protocol approach to identifying the AMI patient. Even when assuming a 5-minute increase in patient contact time, the longest documented increase in the studies, a potential reduction of up to 60 minutes clearly justifies expending the additional time. In fact, those few minutes provide an excellent return on investment.

It is noteworthy that several EMS systems participating in a prehospital 12-lead study were able to obtain and transmit the tracing with only an additional 2–3 minutes of patient contact time. Paramedics in one study accomplished this task with only the addition of 20 seconds to their average patient contact time. These times underscore the fact that a few additional moments on the scene are justified when offset by a significant reduction in door-to-drug time.

The Bottom Line

Significant reductions in door-to-drug time are possible. When an emergency department couples a prehospital infarct identification program with efforts aimed at reducing delays to treatment, the result can be dramatic. Some of the emergency departments that have made great efforts to eliminate delays and participate in a prehospital infarct identification program, relay incidents of 7–15-minute door-to-drug times when ST segment changes were recognized in the field.

Fig. 5-5 was obtained from a prehospital chest pain patient. The prehospital 12-lead obviously

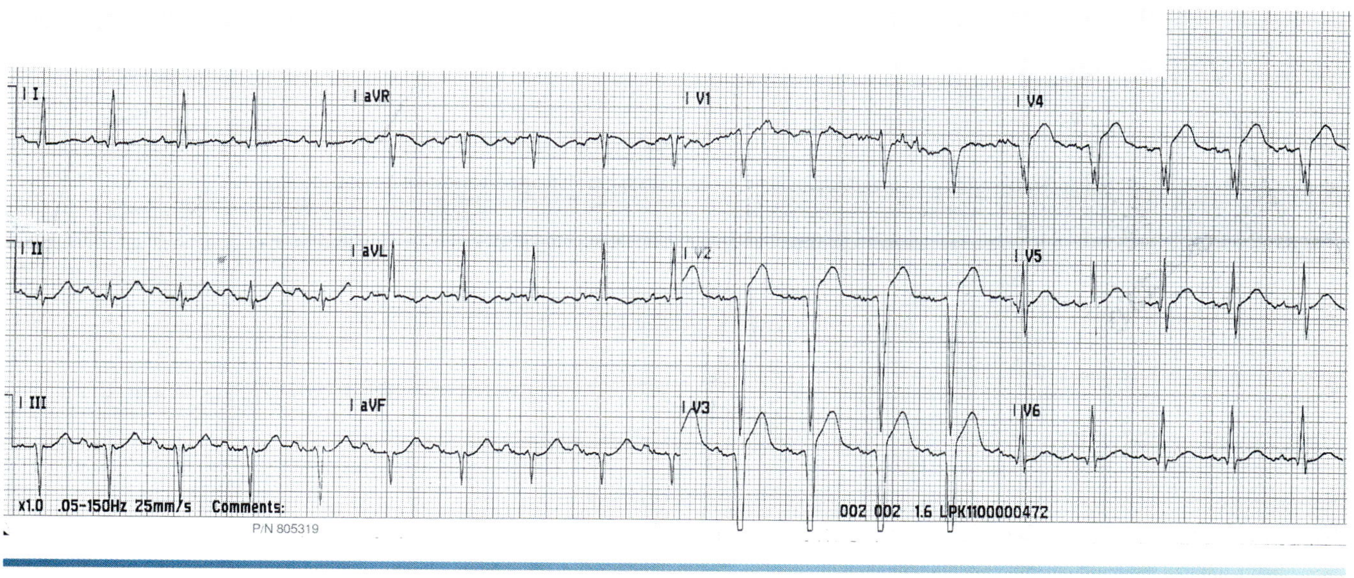

FIG. 5-5 Prehospital identification of AMI resulted in a 7 minute door-to-drug time.

suggested the presence of acute myocardial infarction and the results of the thrombolytic checklist suggested that the patient was a good candidate for treatment. The emergency department was notified of the infarct before the patient arrived at the hospital and the thrombolytic team was notified. When the patient arrived at the emergency department, the thrombolytic team had been assembled and was waiting. In this scenario, because the thrombolytic team was alerted in advance, the patient received thrombolytic therapy within **7 minutes** of arrival.

While this is only anecdotal evidence and this performance cannot be repeated with every patient, it does serve to illustrate how a team approach can significantly reduce time to treatment.

SUMMARY

- **Thrombolytic therapy and PTCA offer a means of stopping the infarct and restoring blood flow to the dying myocardium.**
- **The benefits of thrombolytic therapy and PTCA are time-dependent, with most of the myocardial salvage occurring when treatment is begun within the first 2 hours of the infarct process. However, some benefits has been demonstrated even when thrombolytic agents were administered 12–24 hours after the onset of infarction.**
- **The phrase "Door-to-Drug" time refers to the elapsed time between the point at which the patient enters the hospital and when thrombolytic therapy is initiated.**
- **Because of the time-dependent nature of thrombolytic therapy, emergency departments must strive for a short door-to-drug time. The American Heart Association recommends a 30–60 minute door-to-drug time, while the National Heart Attack Alert Program recommends a 30-minute door-to-drug time.**
- **When the process of infarct recognition and thrombolytic administration is analyzed, four distinct phases can be identified: Door, Decision, Data, and Drug.**
- **The cumulative effect of even minor delays at each step in the patient treatment process can add up to a considerable increase in door-to-drug time. Many of these delays can be eliminated or shortened, thus reducing the time to treatment.**
- **The prehospital 12-lead ECG has been shown to reduce the emergency department's door-to-drug time by as much as 1 hour.**
- **Emergency departments and emergency medical systems should work cooperatively in the development of a prehospital "infarct alert" program which utilizes a prehospital 12-lead ECG and a thrombolytic checklist to identify infarct patient who are good candidates for thrombolytic therapy.**

Chapter 6: Bundle Branch Block

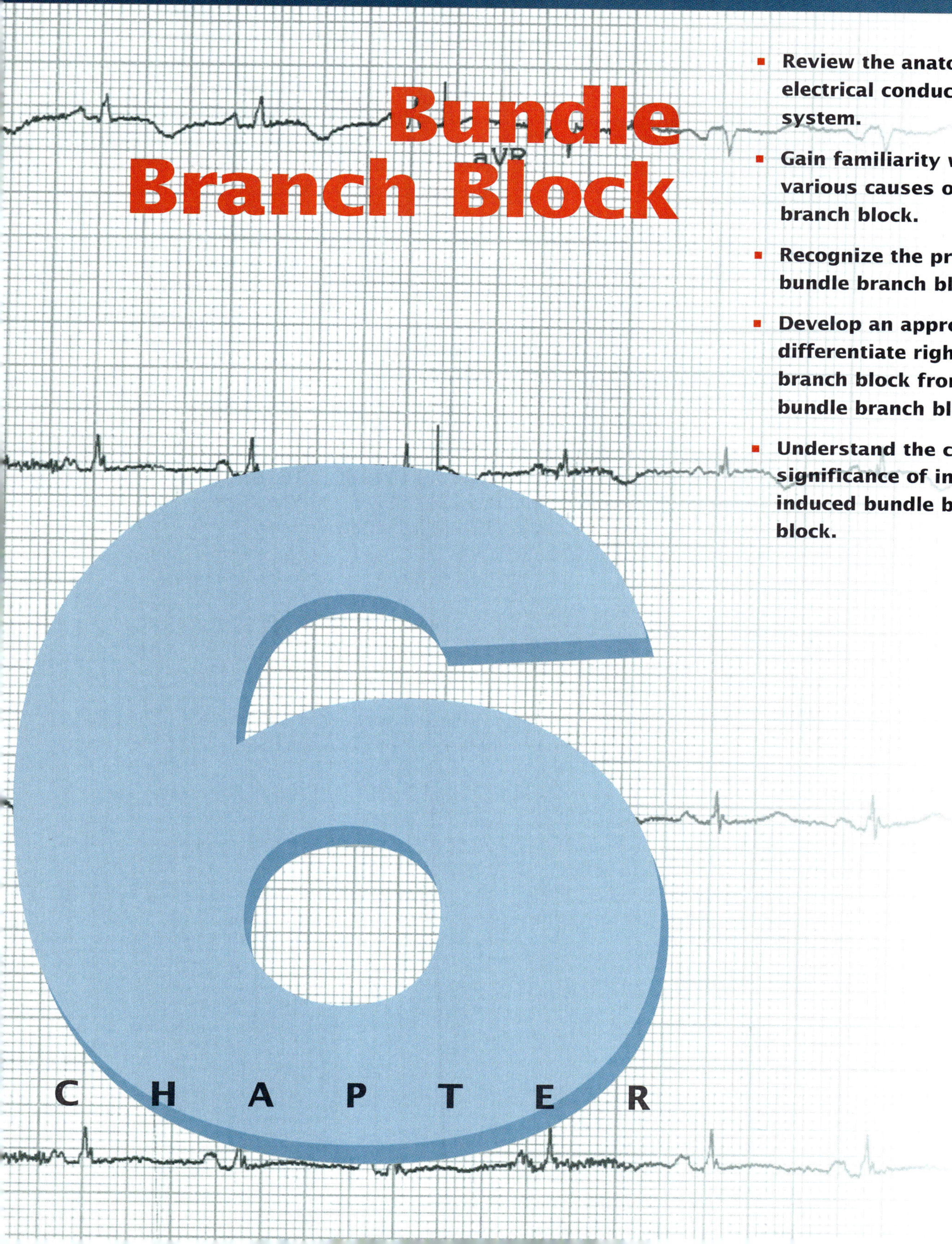

OBJECTIVES

- Review the anatomy of the electrical conduction system.
- Gain familiarity with the various causes of bundle branch block.
- Recognize the presence of bundle branch block.
- Develop an approach to differentiate right bundle branch block from left bundle branch block.
- Understand the clinical significance of infarct induced bundle branch block.

Significance of Bundle Branch Block

In the setting of myocardial infarction, a new onset of bundle branch block (BBB) is a very significant finding. Infarct-induced BBB carries with it an increased mortality rate of between 40% and 60%. The rate of cardiogenic shock increases as well, up to 70%. It is not the BBB itself that causes these outcomes. Rather, the new onset BBB indicates extensive infarct, and it is the tissue lost to the infarct that produces the increase in mortality and cardiogenic shock.

Since the left anterior descending artery supplies much of the bundle branches, patients experiencing septal and anteroseptal infarctions are most likely to develop BBB. Of course, an infarcting patient presenting with BBB may have had it as a preexisting condition. Unless a previous ECG is available for comparison, or the BBB develops during the infarction, it can be difficult to determine which came first, the infarct or the BBB.

Bundle branch block in the setting of infarction also identifies patients with a higher likelihood of developing complete heart block. These patients are actually developing a form of infranodal heart block. This is the reason that infranodal AV block often has a wide QRS complex. Standby pacing is indicated when BBB complicates infarction. Like the infranodal AV block discussed in Chapter 4, when BBB is caused by infarct, it can quickly progress to a more complete block with a slow ventricular rate.

Another significant aspect of BBB is its ability to mimic the infarct pattern on the ECG. In particular, LBBB can produce ST segment elevation and wide Q waves that look remarkably similar to infarction. Chapter 7 is devoted to conditions that can elevate the ST segment and simulate myocardial infarction.

Anatomy of the Conduction System

A simplified graphic representation of the electrical conduction system is shown in Fig. 6-1. In a normally functioning heart, impulses from the atria enter the ventricular conduction system via the atrioventricular (AV) node. Those impulses, which were conducted at about 1000 mm/sec in the intraatrial pathways, now slow to approximately 200 mm/sec. This delay is intentional and allows the atria to contract fully, thus maximizing the ventricular filling.

As the impulse leaves the AV node, it enters the Bundle of His. It is here that the fibers that will form both bundle branches begin to organize (Fig. 6-1). Those fibers that first became discrete in the Bundle of His begin to bifurcate as they proceed distally. At the first bifurcation, the right and left bundle become separate. Shortly thereafter, the left bundle divides again into two halves called fascicles. Both fascicles together constitute the left bundle branch. The right bundle branch, with its single division, is said to be rope-like or cord-like. The left bundle's form is said to be ribbon-like.

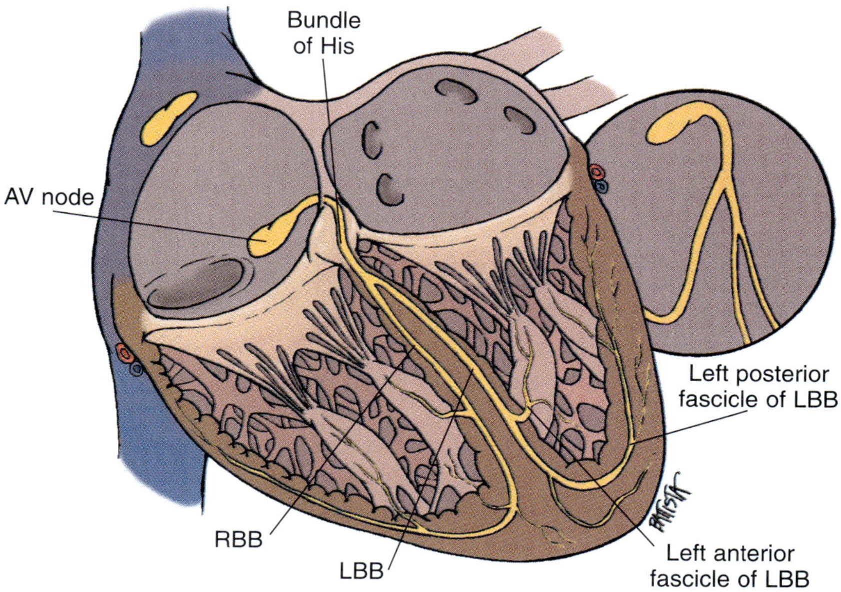

FIG. 6-1 The electrical conduction system.

Causes of Bundle Branch Block

Not unexpectedly, if an occlusion occurs in a coronary artery that supplies one of the bundle branches, a bundle branch block may result. Infarction, therefore, is one cause of bundle branch block. However, not every bundle branch block is the product of infarction or even the result of ischemic heart disease. In fact, many nonischemic diseases, such as Lev's disease and Lenègre's disease, are capable of producing a bundle branch block.

Lev's disease produces bundle branch block through a calcification of the heart's fibrous skeleton. The fibrous skeleton is the infrastructure to which the muscles and valves are attached. Portions of the conductive system are located near the fibrous skeleton or may pass through it. If the fibrous skeleton begins to calcify, then part of the electrical conduction system may become "pinched," resulting in a block.

Lenègre's disease is a more diffuse sclerodegenerative disease that tends to affect the distal portions of the conduction system, but may affect the more proximal portions as well. This process occurs with age, is not related to ischemic heart disease, and is sometimes referred to as the "graying" of the electrical conduction system.

While many other conditions do produce bundle branch block, the three most common are ischemic heart disease, Lev's disease, and Lenègre's disease. Whatever the cause, bundle branch block is relatively easy to identify on the ECG.

Recognizing Bundle Branch Block

The first rule of BBB recognition is to forget about the notch! While BBB can put a notch on the QRS complex it does not always do so, and, when present, the notch is certainly not seen in every lead. Conversely, a notch seen on the QRS complex does not necessitate the presence of a BBB. There is a pervasive association between notching and bundle branch block. People do not easily give up the association, despite its unreliability. Fortunately, there is a simple and reliable method for detecting BBB, the first criteria of which is a widened QRS complex.

When one of the bundles becomes blocked, the impulse that is normally conducted by that bundle branch is interrupted and does not depolarize the intended ventricle. Meanwhile, the other bundle branch is conducting its impulse and depolarizing its respective ventricle. How does the other ventricle depolarize? Very slowly.

In order for the second ventricle to depolarize, the electrical impulses must trudge through myocardial cells, which are not specialized for electrical conduction. Thus, the impulses from one ventricle must be transmitted, cell by cell, to the other ventricle. Since the impulses are wading through the muck and mire, and not traveling down the superhighway, ventricular depolarization takes longer to occur. This delay is evidenced in the form of a wide QRS complex. A QRS complex that is 120 ms wide (three small boxes), is a sign of abnormal ventricular conduction. However, BBB is not the only cause of abnormal ventricular conduction; ventricular rhythms are another common cause of wide QRS complexes. Consequently, an additional criterion must also be met to suspect BBB as the cause, as opposed to a ventricular rhythm.

Criteria for Bundle Branch Block Recognition

1. A QRS duration of 120 ms or more.
2. QRS complexes produced by supraventricular activity.

Since BBB implies that a supraventricular impulse was aberrantly conducted, and ventricular rhythms are not the result of supraventricular activity, evidence of atrial activity producing the QRS complex rules out the possibility of a ventricular rhythm. Therefore, the second criterion for BBB recognition is evidence of atrial activity producing the QRS complex.

There are two important points to remember when examining any ECGs. The first is not to trust your eyes. Complexes that are biphasic or triphasic can look more narrow than they truly are. Some complexes appear narrow in some leads, but, when measured, are just as wide as the other leads. **Measure QRS complex duration. Do not trust only your eyes.**

The second point is that the QRS complex may indeed be wider in one lead than it is in another. Variation in QRS duration from lead to lead is often seen and may produce confusion about whether the complex is or is not wide. As a rule, use the widest QRS complex to determine width. Be careful to accurately pinpoint the exact beginning and end of the QRS complex. This can be difficult to do and is sometimes impossible. Therefore, **when measuring for bundle branch block, select the widest QRS complex with a discernible beginning and end.**

The criteria for BBB recognition may be found in any lead of the ECG. However, when differentiating RBBB from LBBB, pay particular attention to the QRS morphology in specific leads. Lead V1 is probably the single best lead to use when differentiating between the two forms of bundle branch block. Before describing the characteristic pattern of each bundle branch block, a review of some basic monitoring principles is required.

Principles of Monitoring

The form of the QRS complex in any given lead is determined by the direction of electrical current in relation to that lead's positive electrode. If an electrical current moves toward the positive electrode, a positive defection is recorded. When current moves away from the positive electrode, a negative deflection is recorded. If the electrical current travels perpendicular to the positive electrode, an equiphasic complex is seen. In an equiphasic complex, the net upward deflection equals the net downward deflection. An equiphasic complex may produce a QRS in which the total upward deflection equals the downward deflection, or it may take the form of an isoelectric line (Fig. 6-2).

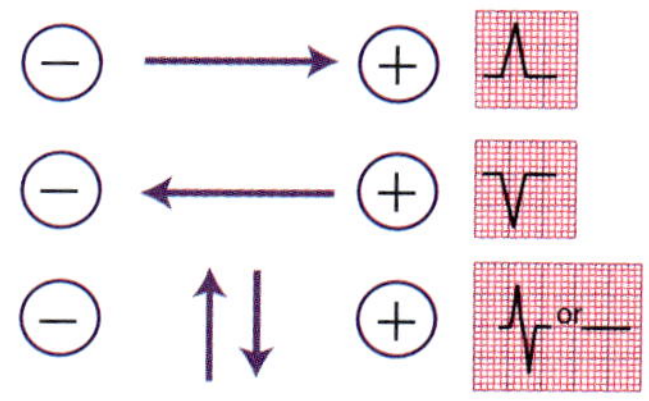

FIG. 6-2 Basic principles of monitoring.

Differentiating RBBB from LBBB

Once the presence of BBB is suspected, an examination of V1 can reveal whether the block affects the right or the left bundle branch. Following are descriptions of how each type of block affects the direction of electrical current and produces its own, distinct QRS morphology.

RIGHT BUNDLE BRANCH BLOCK

In RBBB, the electrical impulse travels through the AV node into the left bundle branch, but not into the right one. Electrical impulses from the left bundle branch depolarize the septum in a left-to-right direction (event 1 in Fig. 6-3). Thus, septal depolarization moves in a left-to-right direction, which is toward V1, and produces the initial small R wave. As the left bundle continues to conduct impulses, the entire left ventricle is depolarized (event 2). This produces a movement away from V1 and results in a negative deflection. Now, the impulses that depolarized the left ventricle conduct through the myocardial cells and depolarize the right ventricle (event 3). This depolarization creates a movement of electrical activity in the direction of V1, and so a second positive deflection is recorded.

The RSR' pattern seen here is characteristic of right bundle branch block. **Whenever the two criteria for BBB have been met, and V1 displays an RSR' pattern, RBBB is suspected.**

LEFT BUNDLE BRANCH BLOCK

In LBBB, the septum is depolarized by the right bundle branch as is the right ventricle. The septum is part of the left ventricle and, thus, the wave of myocardial depolarization has begun with the net movement of current going away from V1 (event 1 in Fig. 6-4). This movement of current continues to move away from V1 as the rest of the left ventricle is depolarized (event 2), and the QRS complex continues in its negative direction.

Thus, LBBB produces a QS pattern in V1. **When BBB is known to exist and a QS pattern is seen in V1, LBBB is suspected.**

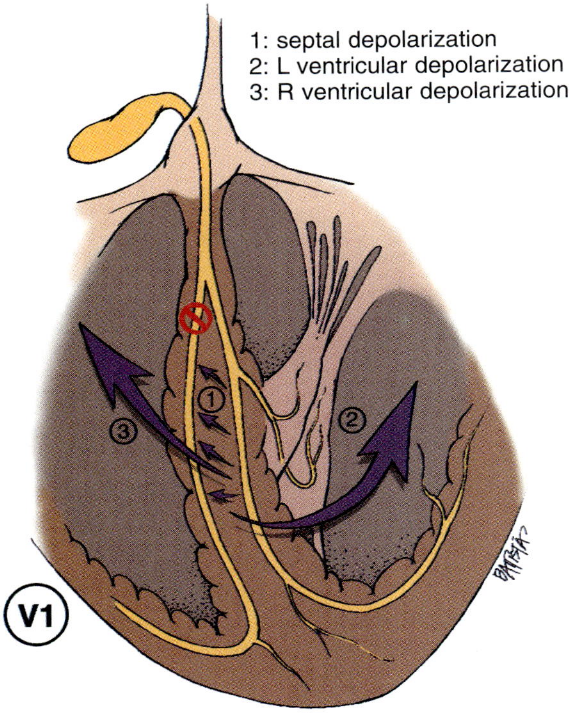

FIG. 6-3 The RSR' pattern, characteristic of right bundle branch block.

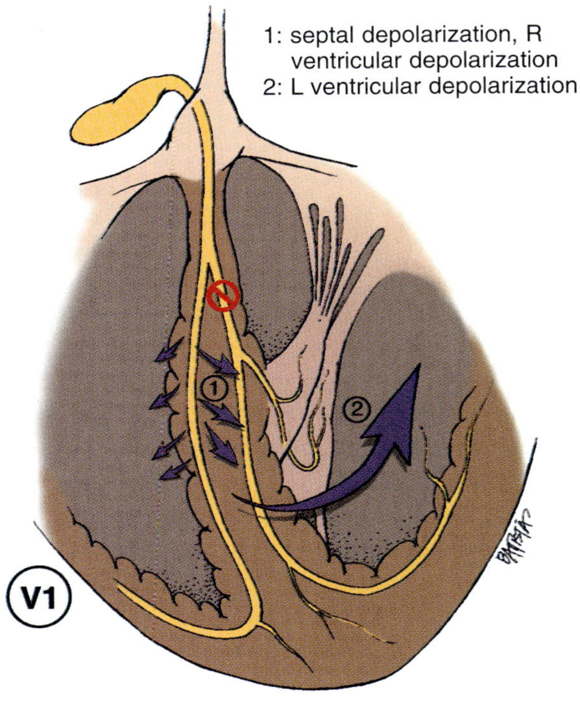

FIG. 6-4 A QS pattern in V1, characteristic of left bundle branch block.

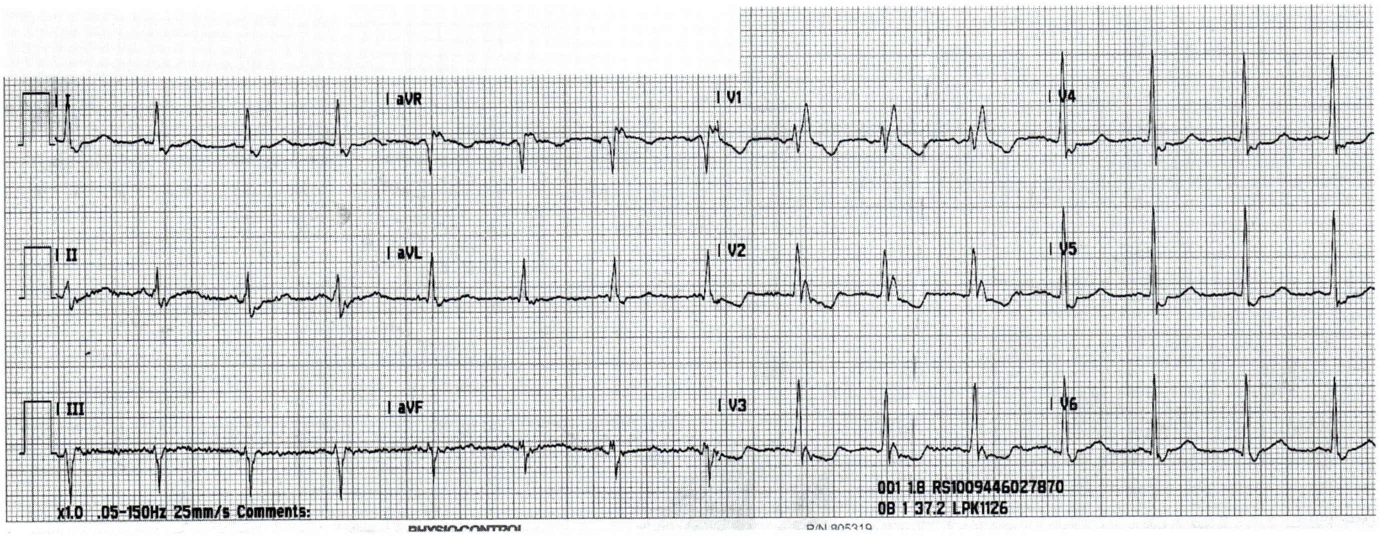

FIG. 6-5 An example of RBBB.

EXAMPLE ECGs

Notice the ST segment elevation found in the examples of left bundle branch block (Figs. 6-5 to 6-8). While the ST segments are very definitely elevated, there is no myocardial infarction in progress. This ST segment elevation is due only to the presence of the LBBB. In Chapter 7, management strategies for this situation and others like it are discussed.

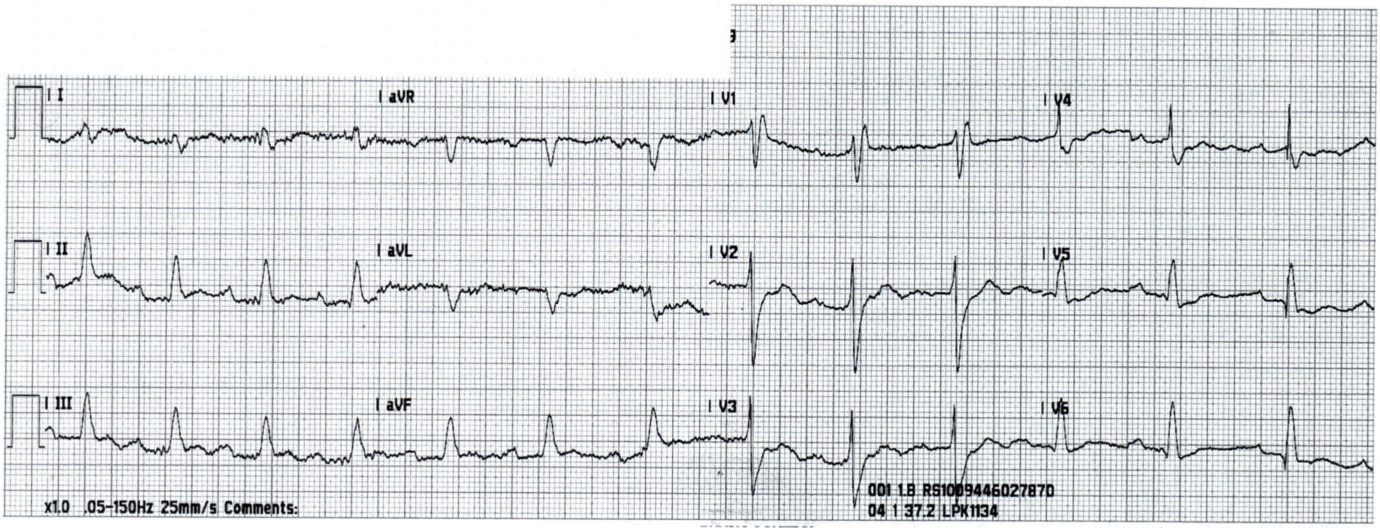

FIG. 6-6 An example of RBBB.

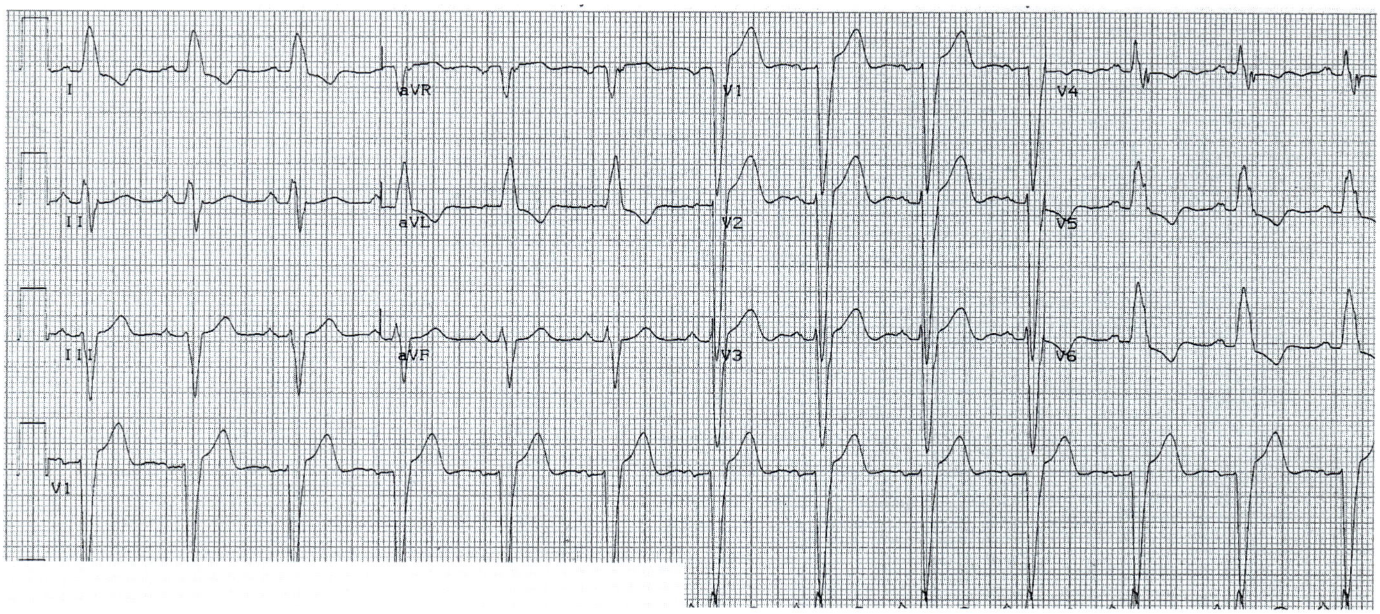

FIG. 6-7 An example of LBBB.

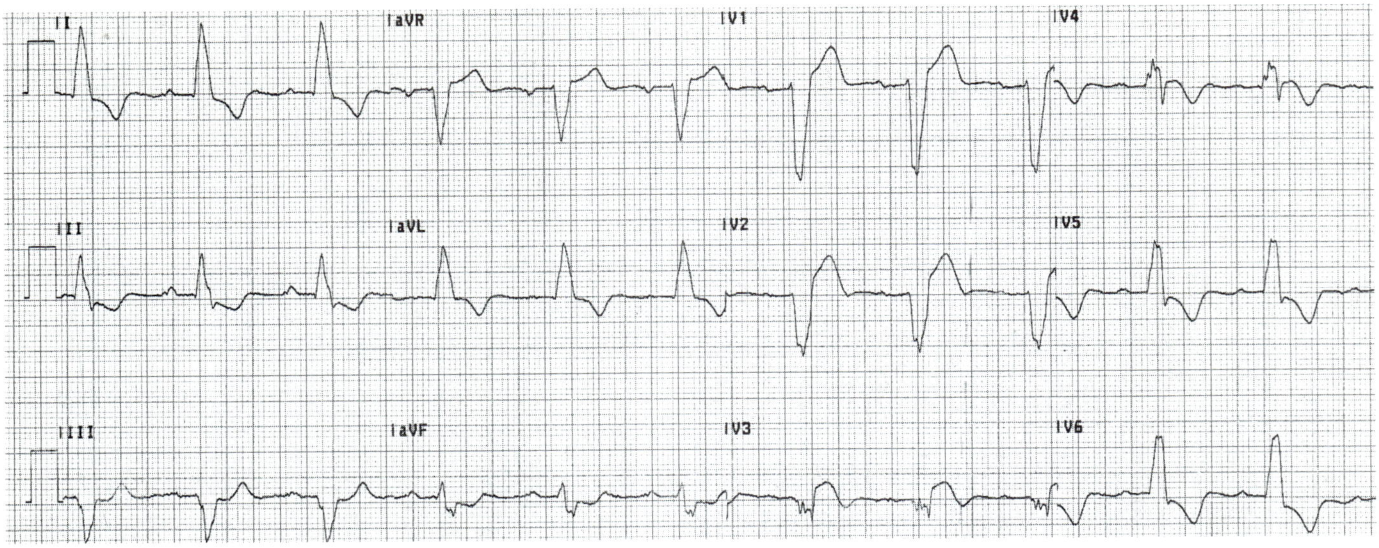

FIG. 6-8 An example of LBBB.

An Easier Way

Unfortunately, not every bundle branch block presents with a clear RSR' or QS pattern in V1. Often, the pattern more closely resembles a qR pattern or an rS pattern (Fig. 6-9), making the differentiation less clear. When this occurs, it is time to focus on the terminal force of the QRS complex.

Remember that in the setting of bundle branch block, the ventricles are not depolarized in their normal simultaneous manner. Instead, they are depolarized sequentially. The last ventricle to be depolarized is, of course, the ventricle with the blocked bundle branch. Therefore, if it is possible to determine the ventricle that was depolarized last, it becomes possible to determine the bundle branch that was blocked. For example, if the right ventricle was depolarized last, it is because the impulse traveled down the left bundle branch, depolarized the left ventricle first, then marched through and depolarized the right ventricle.

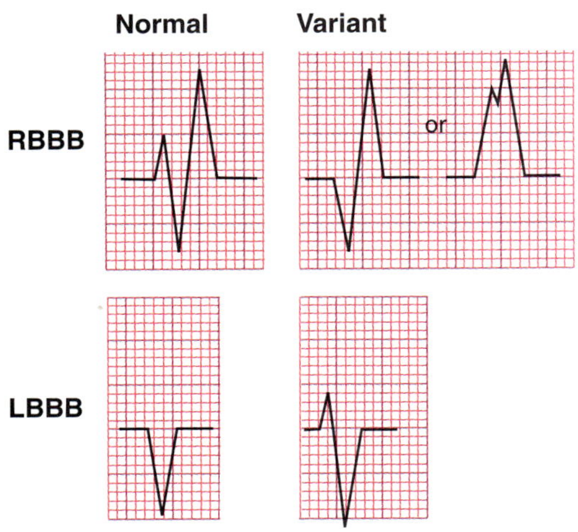

FIG. 6-9 Variant patterns of BBB as seen in lead VI.

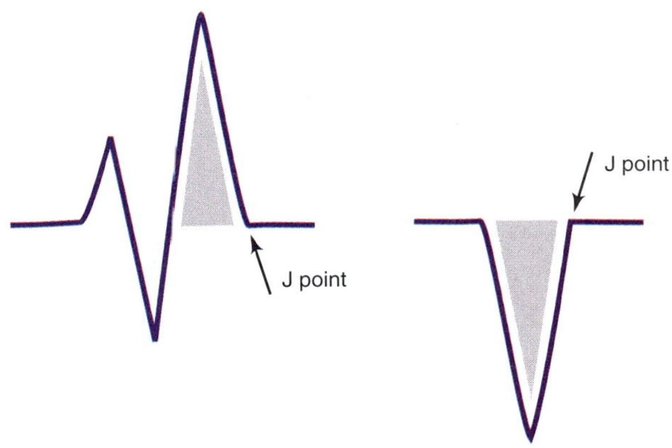

FIG. 6-10 Determining the direction of the terminal force. Move from the J point back into the QRS complex and note whether final electrical activity produced an upward or a downward deflection.

It stands to reason that if one ventricle is depolarized late, its depolarization makes up the later portion of the QRS complex. Examination of the terminal force of the QRS complex reveals the ventricle that was depolarized last, and, therefore, the bundle that was blocked.

The final portion of the QRS complex is referred to as the **terminal force**. To identify the terminal force, first locate the J point. From the J point, move backward into the QRS and determine if the last electrical activity produced an upward or downward deflection. An example of the terminal force in both RBBB and LBBB is illustrated in Fig. 6-10.

If the right bundle branch is blocked, then the right ventricle will be depolarized last and the current will be moving from the left ventricle to the right. This will create a positive deflection in the terminal force of the QRS complex in V1.

If the left bundle branch is blocked, the left ventricle will be depolarized last, and the current will flow from right to left. This will produce a negative deflection in the terminal force of the QRS complex seen in V1.

Therefore, to differentiate RBBB from LBBB, look at V1 and determine if the terminal force of the QRS complex is directed upward or downward. If it is directed upward, an RBBB is present (the current is moving toward the right ventricle and toward V1). An LBBB is present when the terminal force of the QRS complex is directed downward (the current is moving away from V1 and toward the left ventricle). This rule is especially helpful when RSR' and QS variants are present (Fig. 6-9).

A simple way to remember this rule has been suggested by Mike Taigman and Syd Canan, and is demonstrated in Fig. 6-11. They recognized the similarity between this rule and the turn indicator on a car. When a right turn is made, the turn indicator is lifted up. Likewise, when an RBBB is present, the terminal force of the QRS complex points up. Conversely, left turns and LBBB are directed downward.

Use the "turn signal" method to determine if the following examples of bundle branch block (Figs 6-12 to 6-15) represent LBBB or RBBB.

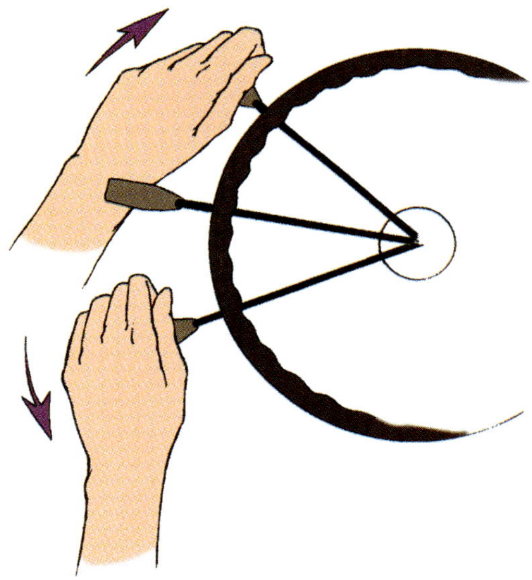

FIG. 6-11 Differentiating between RBBB and LBBB. Remember that right is up and left is down.

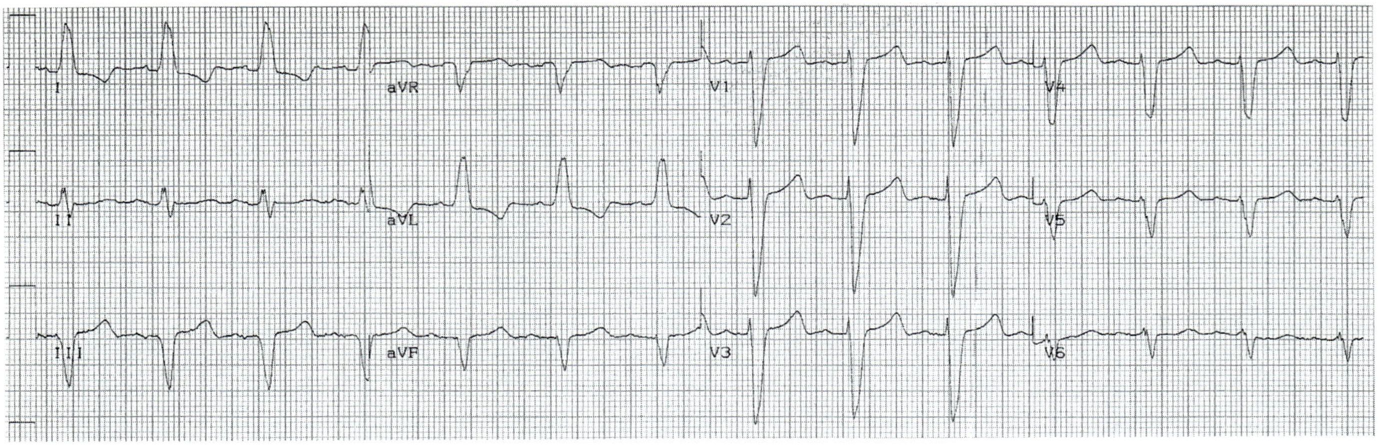

FIG. 6-12 LBBB.

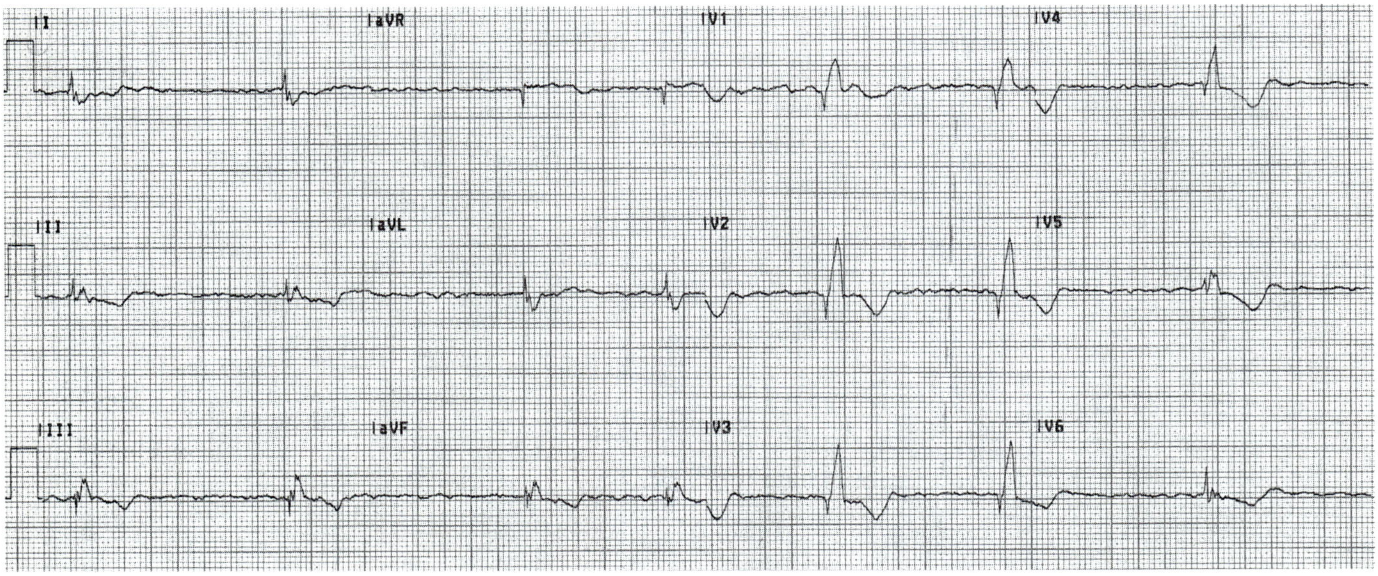

FIG. 6-13 RBBB.

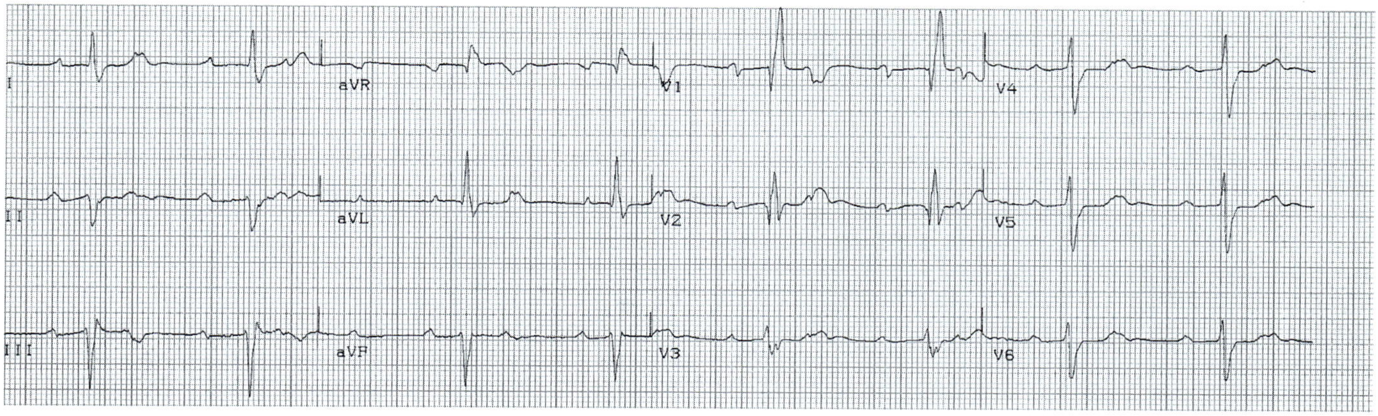

FIG. 6-14 RBBB.

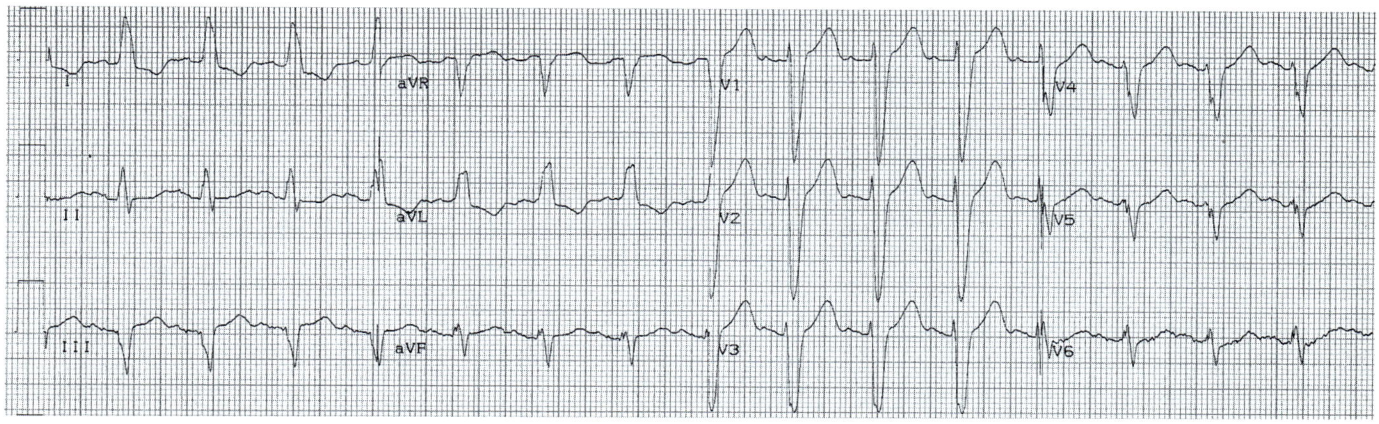

FIG. 6-15 LBBB.

Exceptions

Two notable exceptions must be mentioned to complete the discussion of BBB. The first involves the criteria used to recognize BBB, while the second relates to differentiating LBBB from RBBB.

The criteria used to recognize BBB are valid, but lack some sensitivity and specificity. The sensitivity can be limited by junctional rhythms because there may be no discernible P waves when the AV junction is the pacemaker site. While the AV junction is a supraventricular pacemaker, this presents as an exception to the two-part rule of BBB recognition. Specificity is limited by Wolff-Parkinson-White syndrome (WPW) and other conditions that produce wide QRS complexes resulting from atrial activity. If the characteristic delta wave and shortened PR interval are recognized, then WPW can be suspected. This exception should not present too great a concern because the incidence of WPW is in the range of 0.1%. Similarly, hyperkalemia and other conditions that can widen the QRS are relatively infrequent.

As for differentiating LBBB from RBBB, a third category exists—nonspecific Intraventricular Conduction Delay (NSIVCD). These blocks do not display the typical V1 morphologies generally produced by BBB. Their origin may not be due to a complete BBB, but are often the result of several factors, of which incomplete BBB may be one. Atypical patterns of BBB can be attributed to NSIVCD.

SUMMARY

- **Bundle branch block may be caused by a variety of conditions, including myocardial infarction.**
- **Bundle branch block produces a wide QRS complex because there is a delay in the ventricular activation.**
- **If a wide QRS complex is produced by atrial activity, bundle branch block is suspected.**
- **Right bundle branch block produces an RSR' pattern in V1.**
- **Left bundle branch block produces a QS pattern in V1.**
- **The terminal force of the QRS complex is produced by the ventricle with the blocked bundle branch.**
- **Like a turn indicator, the terminal force of the QRS complex points up in right bundle branch block and down in left bundle branch block.**
- **When infarction is the cause of bundle branch block, the mortality rate is 40%–60% and cardiogenic shock occurs with a frequency of 60%–70%.**
- **Left bundle branch block can mimic infarction.**

CHAPTER 7

Infarct Imposters

OBJECTIVES

- Realize that many conditions other than infarction may produce ST segment elevation.
- Identify the ECG criteria for left bundle branch block, ventricular rhythms, left ventricular hypertrophy, pericarditis, and early repolarization.
- Recognize the manner in which the ST segment is altered by left bundle branch block, ventricular rhythms, and left ventricular hypertrophy.
- Describe the clinical presentation of pericarditis.

ST Segment Elevation

Thus far in the text, virtually every example of ST segment elevation has been due to myocardial infarction. This isolation was a strategy to allow the reader to gain familiarity with the pattern(s) of myocardial infarction. However, if every instance of ST segment elevation was interpreted as myocardial infarction, a gross overdiagnosis would result.

ST segment elevation is not caused by myocardial infarction per se. While the theories are complex, suffice it to say that ST segment elevation is caused by changes which affect ventricular repolarization and/or ventricular depolarization. Myocardial infarction produces ST segment elevation because the infarction affects ventricular repolarization and/or depolarization. Likewise, any condition that affects ventricular repolarization and/or depolarization can also produce ST segment elevation.

There are a number of conditions that can cause ST segment elevation. Hypothermia, increased intracranial pressure, electrolyte inbalance, and medications are just a few of the conditions that can produce ST segment elevation. This chapter emphasizes five conditions which can mimic myocardial infarction by producing ST segment elevation: left bundle branch block (LBBB), ventricular rhythms, left ventricular hypertrophy (LVH), pericarditis, and early repolarization. These five conditions were selected for either the frequency with which they occur or the degree to which their mimicry is convincing.

A Common Feature of LBBB, LVH, and Ventricular Beats

Awareness of the particular feature shared by LBBB, LVH, and ventricular beats is helpful before progressing to the specific criteria for each. The common feature relates to an ECG pattern in which the QRS complex and the T wave are oppositely directed. In other words, when the QRS complex points down, the T wave points up, and vice versa.

This phenomenon would hardly be noteworthy in a discussion of infarction except for one important fact: The T wave often "drags" the ST segment along with it. Thus, when the QRS complex is primarily negative, the T wave will be positively deflected, and it can drag the ST segment up with it. This is how LBBB, LVH, and ventricular rhythms can masquerade as an infarction. Fig. 7-1 demonstrates this pattern.

Note how the T wave "drags" the ST segment along with it. This phenomenon produces ST segment elevation in leads with a negatively deflected QRS complex. Additionally, the negative deflection may produce a Q wave or QS complex equal to or more than 40 ms in duration. This further clouds the interpretation by giving the appearance of pathologic Q waves.

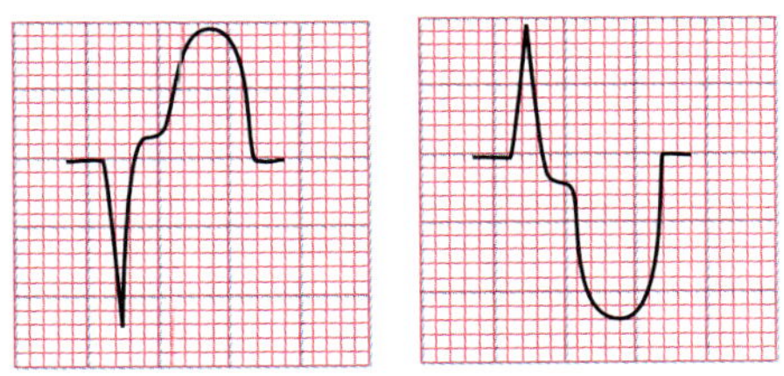

FIG. 7-1 When LBBB, ventricular rhythms, and LVH are present, the T wave is opposite in direction from the QRS complex. Note how the ST segment is shifted in the direction of the T wave.

Left Bundle Branch Block

ECG RECOGNITION

Essentially two conditions must exist to suspect bundle branch block. First, the QRS complex must have an abnormal duration (120 ms or more in width), and second, the QRS complex must arise as the result of supraventricular activity (this excludes ventricular beats). If these two conditions are met, a delayed ventricular conduction is assumed to be present, and bundle branch block is the most common cause of this abnormal conduction.

Once a bundle branch block has been detected, lead V1 may be used to differentiate right from left bundle branch block. In lead V1, determine the direction of the terminal (last) force of the QRS complex. If the terminal force points up, suspect a right bundle branch block. If the terminal force points down, suspect a left bundle branch block. The recognition criteria for bundle branch block is more completely discussed in Chapter 6.

When bundle branch block is present, ST segment elevation is often seen in leads with negatively deflected QRS complexes. This situation occurs most frequently in the presence of left bundle branch block and is generally seen in leads V1, V2, and V3, but sometimes extends to V4 and beyond. Fig. 7-2 demonstrates this pattern.

Right bundle branch block rarely produces ST segment elevation because most of the leads remain positively deflected. Occasionally, when the inferior leads (II, III, and AVF) happen to be negatively deflected, a right bundle branch block may produce ST segment elevation in those leads, and may occasionally mimic an inferior

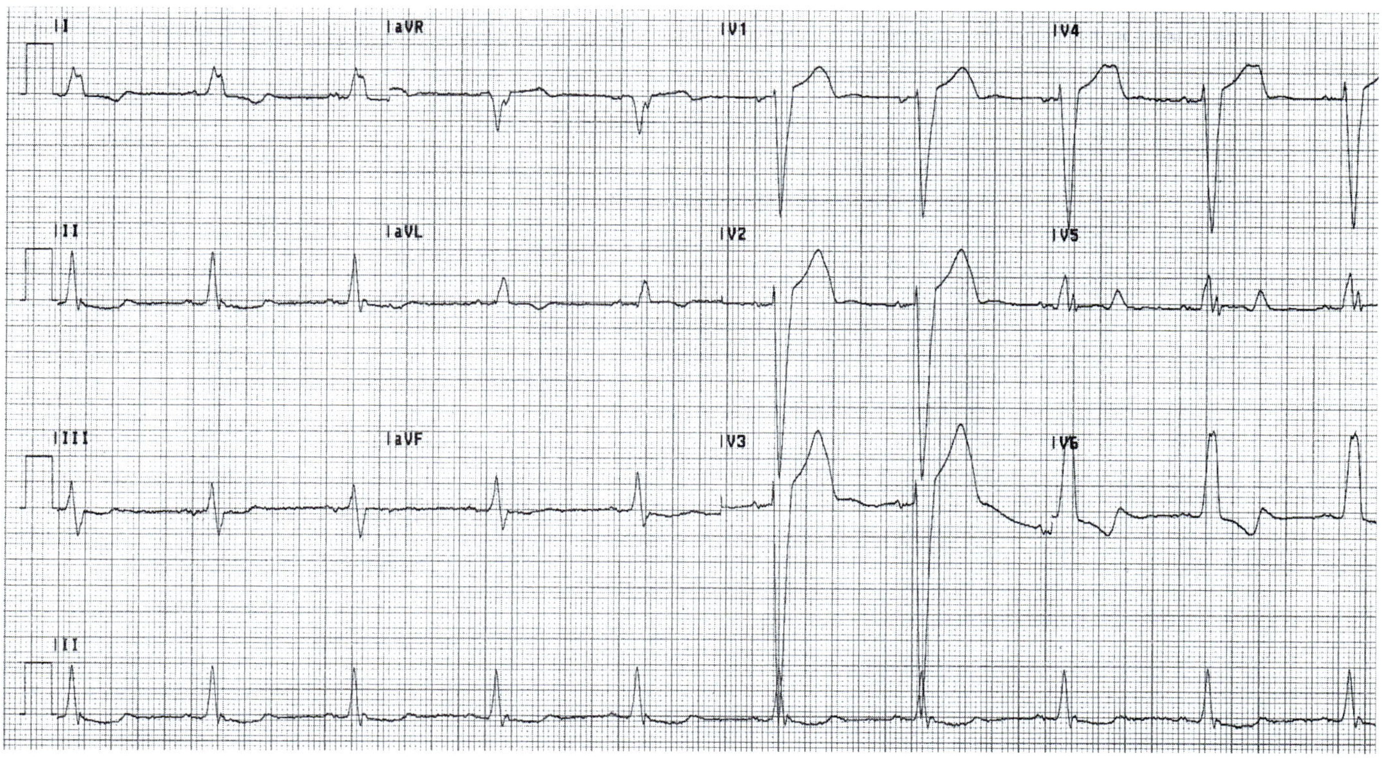

FIG. 7-2 LBBB is present. Note the ST segment elevation in the leads with negatively deflected QRS complexes.

wall infarction. While this combination is possible, left bundle branch block is by far the more common cause of ST segment elevation.

CLINICAL PRESENTATION

The clinical presentation is of little value in recognizing bundle branch block because a ventricular conduction delay itself does not produce any clinical signs or symptoms. The underlying cause of the presence of a bundle branch block may present with specific symptoms, but it does not help to identify the presence of a bundle branch block. Therefore, rely on the ECG criteria to recognize the presence of bundle branch block.

Ventricular Rhythms

Impulses originating in the ventricles may be the result of either natural pacemaker sites or of implanted pacemakers. Just as with bundle branch block, ventricular rhythms may exhibit ST segment elevation that is not due to any infarct-related causes. This spurious ST segment elevation is seen when the QRS complex is negatively deflected.

VENTRICULAR PACED RHYTHM

In many ways, a ventricular paced beat is a man-made left bundle branch block. Consider that when left bundle branch block occurs, the electrical impulse travels down the right bundle branch, depolarizes the right ventricle, and the impulse spreads through the myocardium to depolarize the left ventricle. Pacemakers are most often introduced into the right ventricle attached to the right ventricular wall. When a pacemaker fires, it sends its impulse into the right ventricle, which depolarizes, and the impulse is spread through the myocardium to depolarize the left ventricle. The similarity between the two is shown in Fig. 7-3.

Similarly, spontaneous impulses originating in the ventricles can produce ST segment elevation, which is often seen accompanying a negatively deflected PVC. If a ventricular rhythm is present, the ECG may show ST segment elevation in the leads that are negatively deflected (Fig. 7-4).

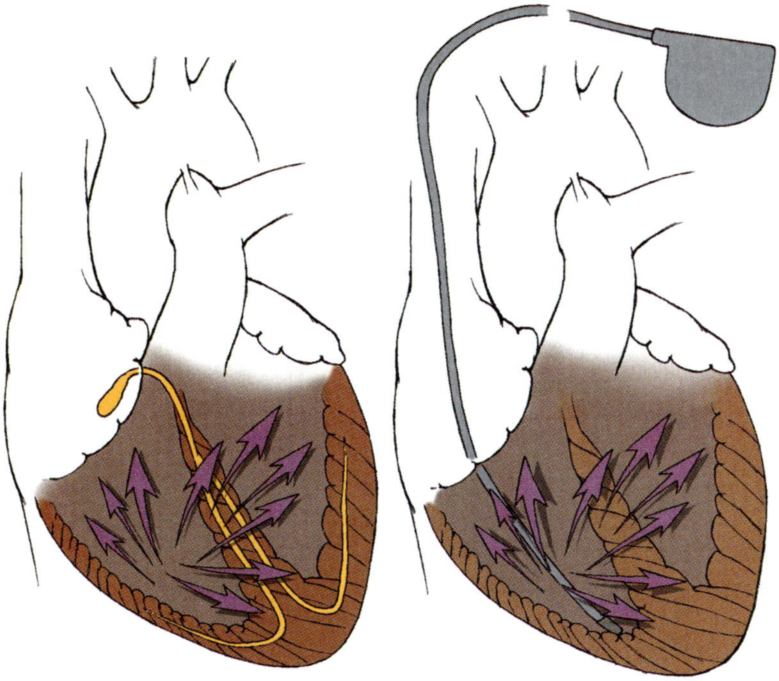

FIG. 7-3 The patterns of LBBB and a ventricular pacemaker are similar because in both cases the ventricular impulse begins in the right ventricle and conducts throughout the myocardium to depolarize the left ventricle.

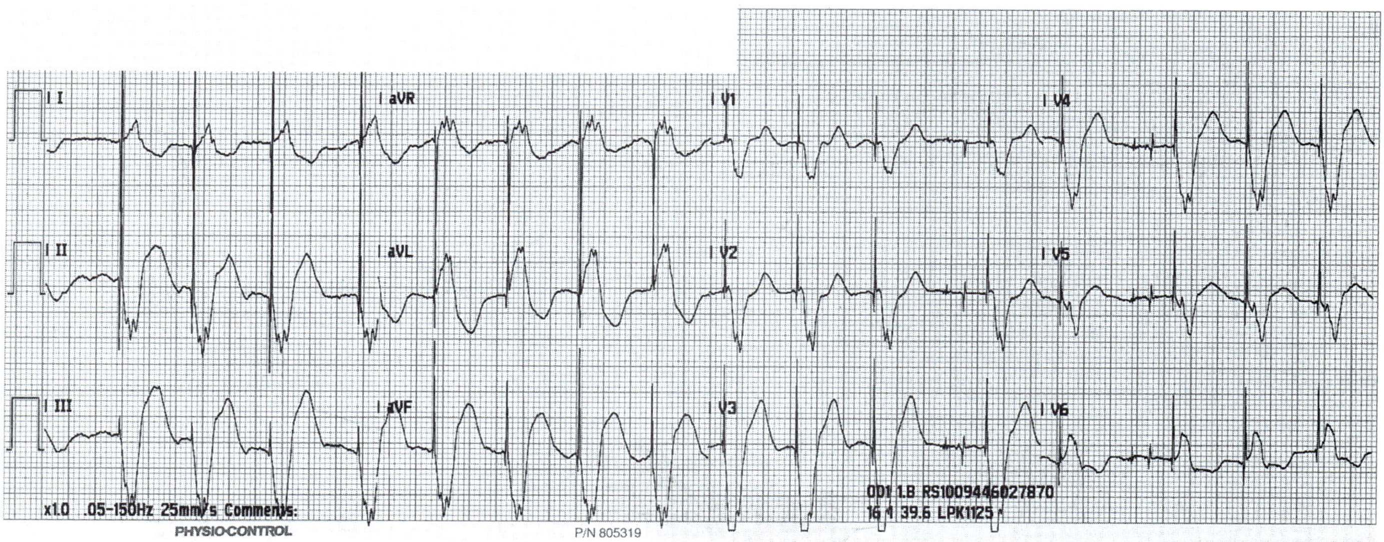

FIG. 7-4 An example of a ventricular rhythm producing ST segment elevation.

Left Ventricular Hypertrophy

As its name implies, left ventricular hypertrophy is an enlargement of the left ventricle. The enlargement results from a prolonged state of overfilling in the left ventricle, or from its pumping against increased resistance. The ECG does not detect every case of LVH, but there are clues which, when present, strongly favor its presence.

ECG CRITERIA

Several formulas exist for the ECG recognition of LVH. The formula presented here was selected because it is easy to remember and may be used to quickly check for the presence of LVH.

While bundle branch block increases the width of the QRS complex, LVH increases the amplitude because of the increase in electrical activity. To detect evidence of LVH on the ECG use the following method. Remember that LVH does not produce a wide QRS complex.

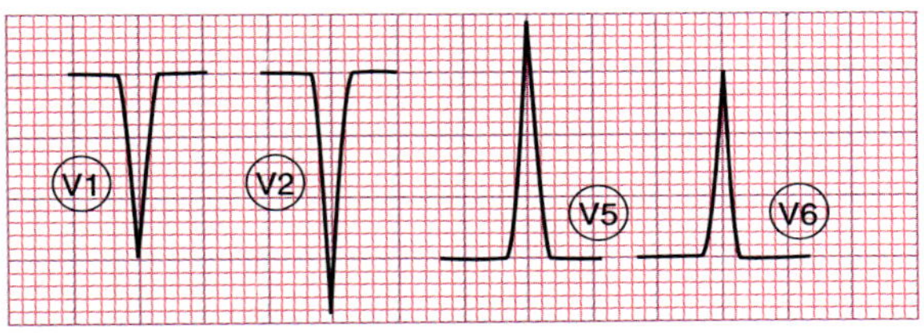

FIG. 7-5 Step 1, In comparing V1 and V2, the S wave is greater in V2 and equals about 19 mm in depth. **Step 2,** The R wave in V5 is taller than in V6. The height of the R wave equals 19 mm. **Step 3,** The sum of the depth of the S wave plus the height of the R wave is 19 + 19 = 38. The voltage criteria for the LVH has been met.

Step 1

- Compare V1 and V2 and determine which lead has the deepest S wave.
- Determine the depth of the deeper S wave in millimeters (count the small boxes—one box equals 1 mm).

Step 2

- Compare V5 and V6 and determine which lead has the tallest R wave.
- Determine the height of the taller R wave in millimeters (count the small boxes).

Step 3

- Add the height of the taller R wave and the deeper S wave.
- If the number is equal to or greater than 35, suspect LVH. Use the example in Fig. 7-5 to practice this method.

The ECG shown in Fig. 7-6 meets the voltage criteria for LVH. Note that the ST segment is elevated in leads V1, V2, and V3. Also note the ST segment depression shown in leads V5 and V6. This conforms to the pattern described earlier in which negatively deflected QRS complexes display ST segment elevation while positively directed QRS complexes show ST segment depression.

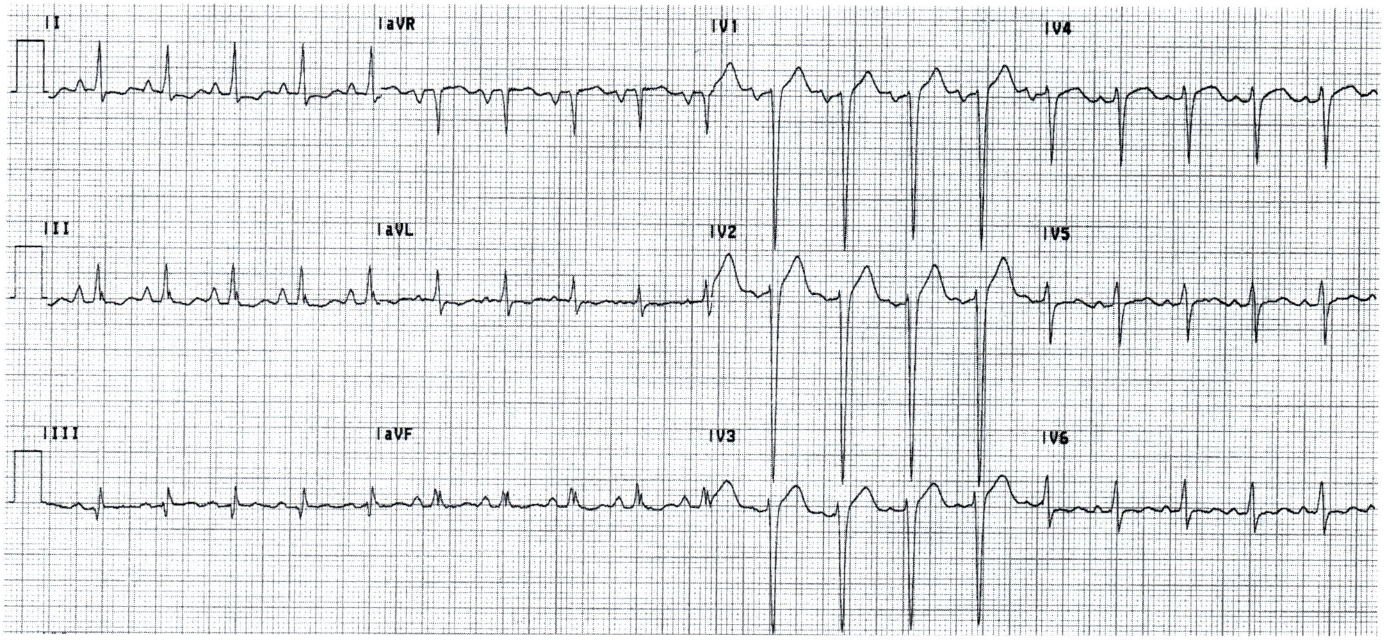

FIG. 7-6 ST segment elevation noted in the presence of left ventricular hypertrophy.

Pericarditis

Another cause of counterfeit ST segment elevation is the condition known as pericarditis. In this case, portions of the pericardium become inflamed, as does the adjoining epicardial surface of the heart. When ST segment elevation occurs as the result of that inflammation, it is not due to coronary artery disease. Anyone can develop pericarditis, but post-MI and postcardiac surgery patients are especially prone.

ECG CRITERIA

Pericarditis is capable of producing a number of changes in the ECG. ST segment elevations occurs frequently and may be noted in any lead. Since the ST segment elevation is related to diffuse patches of inflammation around the pericardium, and not due to an occluded coronary artery, ST segment elevation is usually diffuse and not strictly grouped into leads which are anatomically contiguous.

In addition to the ST segment, pericarditis can also produce PR segment depression. When the ST segment is compared to a depressed PR segment, it can give the appearance of ST segment elevation. Using both the TP segment and the PR segment to establish the isoelectric line will minimize this illusion.

Another change that pericarditis may bring to the ECG is a notching of the J point. While not exclusive to pericarditis, J point notching signifies the possibility of a noninfarct cause of ST segment elevation. In the following example (Fig. 7-7), the ECG strip demonstrates how some leads show examples of true ST segment elevation, other leads appear elevated due to PR segment depression, and a few display J point notching.

CLINICAL PRESENTATION

Chest pain is commonly the chief complaint in pericarditis. The pain is often described as "sharp" (the term "sharp" is intended to convey a knife-like pain, not to convey intensity) unlike the more typical "pressure" or "heaviness" often

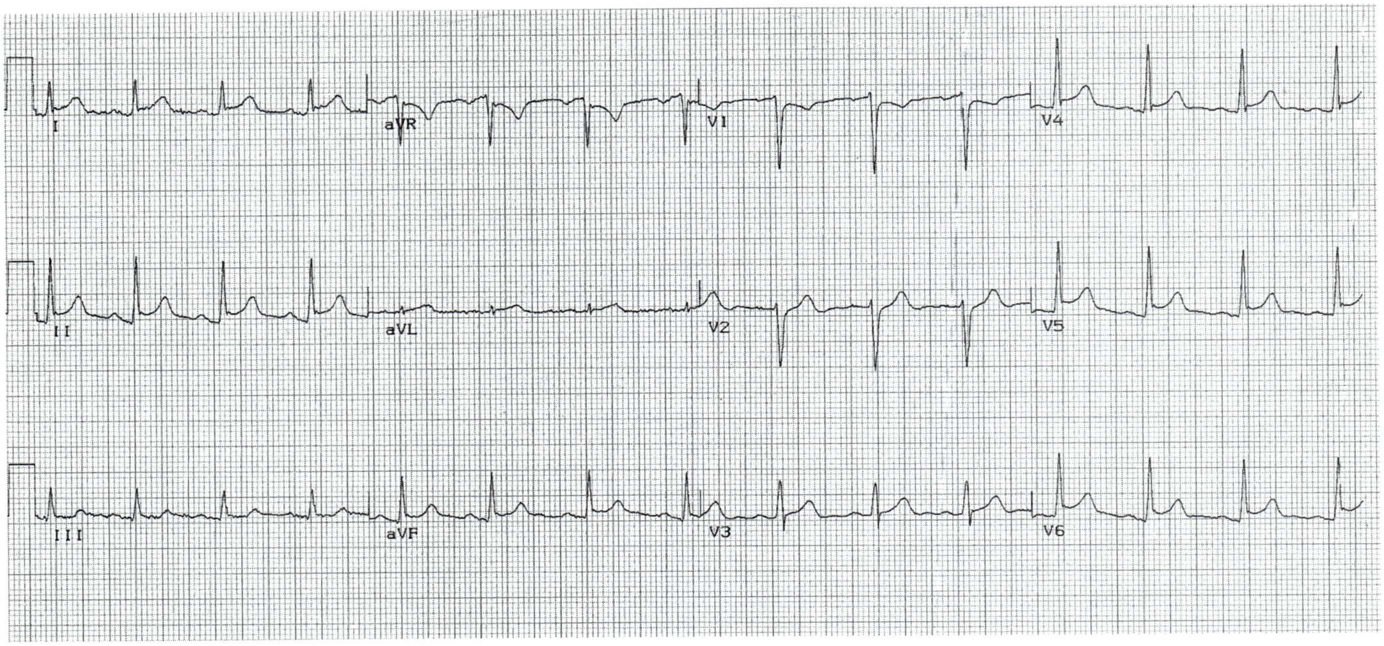

FIG. 7-7 The pattern of pericarditis. Note the diffuse pattern of ST segment elevation, PR segment depression in lead II, and J point notching in leads II, V5, and V6.

Table 7-1 The Clinical Presentation of AMI and Pericarditis

	MYOCARDIAL INFARCTION	PERICARDITIS
Chest Pain (nature)	Pressure	Stabbing
Chest Pain (radiation)	Left arm, shoulder, jaw	Base of neck, trapezious area
Chest Pain (aggravation)	Unaffected by movement and respiration	Affected by movement, respiration, swallowing, etc. May improve when leaning forward
ST Segment Elevation	Appears in anatomically contiguous leads	Diffuse across ECG
PR Segment Depressions	Uncommon	Common, may give appearance of ST segment elevation

accompanying infarction. The pain tends to be affected by movement, respiration, and position. The patient may state that the pain is minimized by leaning forward and intensified by lying supine. Drinking fluids may also provoke an increase in pain. If radiation occurs, the patient may report that it is felt about the base of the neck or the area between the shoulder blades.

The recognizable ECG features of pericarditis are subtle and can easily be overlooked or misinterpreted. Therefore, it is often the clinical presentation of pericarditis which is first recognized. Once pericarditis is suspected, the ECG can be closely examined (or reexamined) for substantiating evidence. Table 7-1 compares the ECG and clinical features of myocardial infarction and pericarditis.

Early Repolarization

Early repolarization produces an infarct-like pattern on the ECGs of healthy, asymptomatic patients. Early repolarization is considered to be a normal variant and does not indicate any underlying pathology.

ECG CRITERIA

Like all of the other conditions included in this chapter, early repolarization produces ST segment elevation which, in this case, is most often seen in the chest leads. Additionally, early repolarization produces tall T waves resembling those seen in the hyperacute phase of myocardial infarction. This combination creates a pattern on the ECG which closely resembles that of anterior or anterolateral infarction.

Like pericarditis, early repolarization can produce a notch at the J point. Just as with pericarditis, a notch at the J point causes one to consider noninfarct conditions as possible explanations for the ST segment elevation.

CLINICAL CRITERIA

Early repolarization is a completely normal and benign finding. The prevalence of early repolarization varies with age and ethnic background, with the highest prevalence occurring in young black males. Some researchers reported a frequency of less than 3% in whites males and as high as 27% in 20–40-year-old black males. The incidence of early repolarization is also higher among athletes. The pattern of early repolarization is shown in Fig. 7-8. Table 7-2 presents an overview of five conditions and how they mimic infarct.

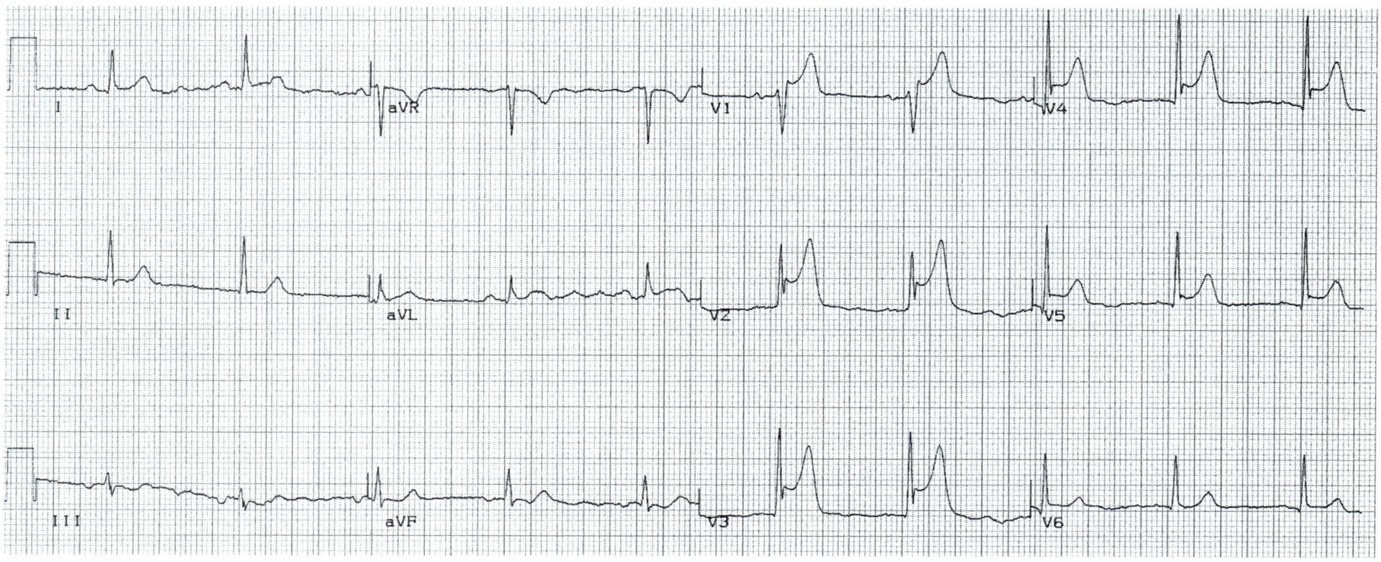

FIG. 7-8 An example of ST segment elevation due to early repolarization.

Table 7-2 Overview of the Infarct Imposters

CONDITION	INFARCTION RESEMBLANCE	RECOGNITION
LBBB	• ST segment elevation in the negatively deflected leads, usually V1-V3 • QS complexes in the negatively deflected leads, usually V1-V3	• QRS Complex ≥ 120 ms. • QRS complex produced by supraventricular activity. • QS complex, or negative terminal force in V1
Ventricular rhythms	• ST segment elevation in the negatively deflected leads • QS complexes in the negatively deflected leads	• Wide QRS complex following pacer spikes (if noticeable) • Negative terminal force in V1 (right ventricle paced)
LVH	• ST segment elevation in the negatively deflected leads, usually V1-V3	• Choose deepest S wave from V1 and V2 • Choose tallest R wave from V5 and V6 • Add deflections of tallest R wave and deepest S wave • Suspect LVH if total ≥ 35
Pericarditis	• Elevates ST segments in multiple leads	• ST segment elevation not in anatomical grouping • PR segment depression • Notching of the J point
Early repolarization	• ST segment elevation, particularly in anterior or anterolateral leads • Tall T waves	• Notching of the J point • Patient may be asymptomatic • Most common in young adult black males.

What Should You Do Now?

At times it is very difficult to differentiate between infarct and noninfarct causes of ST segment elevation. Some cases can only be decided after hours of observation, serial ECGs, and extensive testing. Therefore, it is not reasonable to expect that a single ECG will always provide enough information to determine the cause of ST segment elevation.

Chapter 1 stressed that the ECG is simply a recording of electrical current on the patient's skin. For that reason the ECG is not always sensitive enough to detect subtle changes, and is not always specific enough to differentiate between certain conditions. While the clinical presentation can be very helpful in differentiating between the causes of ST segment elevation in some cases, it does not always settle the matter.

How then can the ECG best be used when treating cardiac patients in the early hours of chest pain? **A realistic initial goal for the emergency cardiac care provider is to recognize situations when ST segment elevation could be due to either a myocardial infarction or some other condition.** For example, left bundle branch block can very closely simulate the ECG pattern of an anterior wall infarction. However, emergency cardiac care providers need not attempt to determine if the cause of the ST segment elevation is due to infarction or one of its imposters. In these instances, simply note the presence of ST segment elevation, recognize that it could be attributed to infarct or one of its imposters, and bring it to the attention of the physician for review. When the patient's clinical presentation is suspicious enough to motivate the emergency cardiac care provider to obtain a 12-lead, the presence of ST segment elevation and an infarct imposter should prompt an immediate review by the physician.

In the emergency department setting, the physician can determine whether or not the patient should be worked up as a cardiac patient. Outside of the hospital, the preference is for paramedics to transmit the ECG for physician interpretation. In the event that transmission is not possible, the objective findings can be relayed via radio or phone to the physician. For example, one may state that there is 4–5 mm of ST segment elevation in V1 through V3, and a LBBB pattern is present. Given that minimal information, the physician will immediately realize the interpretive predicament. The physician can determine whether the paramedic should proceed with the thrombolytic screening, aspirin, and multiple IVs.

In some ways this approach may seem inappropriate, but it is not. In fact, sometimes the phrase, "I don't know" is the most intelligent and sophisticated response that an emergency care provider can give. In situations in which there is simply not enough information to make a reasonable interpretation, it is far better to defer to the physician than to assign an interpretation without sufficient evidence. Often the physician will not have an immediate answer either. It may be only after comparative and serial ECGs are available, cardiac enzymes are analyzed, and the patient is observed over time, that the physician will feel comfortable applying a definitive interpretation. Therefore, emergency cardiac care providers should not be disheartened by this predicament.

SUMMARY

- ST segment elevation is not always due to myocardial infarction.
- LBBB, LVH, ventricular rhythms, pericarditis, and early repolarization are five noninfarct conditions which can elevate the ST segment.
- LBBB, LVH, and ventricular beats share a common pattern which typically produces ST segment elevation in leads V1-V3 and ST segment depression in leads V4-V6.
- The clinical presentation is often the crucial element which causes the emergency cardiac care provider to suspect pericarditis. The ECG is then reviewed for the characteristic changes of pericarditis.
- Early repolarization is a normal variant which produces a pattern very similar to the hyperacute phase of an anterior or anterolateral infarction.
- When confronted with an ECG containing ST segment elevation and evidence for one of the infarct imposters, present the tracing to the physician for review and determination of the patient's triage priority.

8

CHAPTER

Systematic Analysis

OBJECTIVES

- Develop a systematic approach for infarct recognition on the ECG.
- Gain experience using the Five Step Approach to:
  - —recognize myocardial infarction
  - —localize the infarct site
  - —predict the occluded coronary artery
  - —determine the need for additional leads
  - —apply the patient's clinical presentation to the findings of the ECG
  - —identify the presence of non-infarct conditions which may produce ST segment elevation
- Consider which complications are associated with occlusions of each coronary artery.
- Describe how the treatment strategies for the management of chest pain, AV block, and hypotension differ with various locations of coronary artery occlusion.

A consistent approach is essential when using the 12-lead ECG in the setting of the chest pain patient. A good approach is one that forces the interpreter to seek additional information when needed, to screen for the presence of non-infarct conditions that can cause ST segment elevation, and to incorporate the patient's clinical presentation into the ECG interpretation. One such approach is described in this chapter and is shown in Fig. 8-1. Several case studies are included to allow familiarization and application of this approach.

FIVE STEP ANALYSIS

for Infarct Recognition

1 Rate and Rhythm
- Treat life-threatening arrhythmias

2 Infarction
- Presence of indicative changes?
- Localize
- Coronary artery involved

3 Miscellaneous Conditions
- LBBB
- Ventricular rhythms
- LVH
- Pericarditis
- Early repolarization

4 Clinical Presentation
- Maintain a high index of suspicion, especially with diabetics and the elderly
- Remember, females infarct too

5 Acute Infarction?
- Early notification
- Anticipate complications
- Develop treatment plan

LEAD	LOCATION	CORONARY ARTERY
I, AVL, V5 and V6	Lateral wall	L
II, III, AVF	Inferior wall	R
V1, V2	Septal wall	L
V3, V4	Anterior wall	L
V4R, V5R, V6R	Right ventricle	R

FIG. 8-1 The five step analysis for infarct recognition.

The Five Steps

STEP 1 Rate and Rhythm

The topic of dysrhythmia recognition has not been covered in this text under the assumption that ACLS providers (the target audience of this text), are already familiar with the subject. However, this lack of attention is not a reflection of significance. **Determining rate and rhythm is the first priority when interpreting the ECG.** The treatment of life-threatening dysrhythmias initially takes precedence over the acquisition and interpretation of the 12-lead ECG. Yet, this does not mean that the 12-lead ECG is of no value when determining rate and rhythm.

The most simple benefit from the use of multiple leads when assessing rhythm is this: important interpretive criteria may be virtually undetectable in one lead, yet clearly present in another. For example, a lead II rhythm strip may contain no evidence of P waves, but after a quick glance at lead V1 their presence becomes obvious. A premature ventricular complex (PVC) may be obvious in one lead. However, in another lead, PVC may appear deceptively small or look remarkably like the complexes of the underlying rhythm. This benefit of multilead usage occurs simply as a function of additional "eyes" looking at the problem.

Another advantage of the 12-lead ECG in rhythm identification is in differentiating wide complex tachycardias. When using only a single lead it can be difficult or impossible to differentiate ventricular tachycardia from a supraventricular tachycardia with aberrant conduction. The clinical presentation is of little help in differentiating the two because the patient's hemodynamic stability is often due more to the ventricular rate than to the origin of the impulse. Therefore, a patient experiencing a fast SVT with aberrant conduction may look "sick" while a patient with a slower ventricular tachycardia may look remarkably well.

These are only a few examples of how multiple leads can clarify the process of rhythm identification. Regardless of how many leads are used, the initial determination of rate and rhythm takes precedence over infarct recognition.

STEP 2 Infarction

Once the underlying rate and rhythm are determined, examination for evidence of myocardial infarction is the next logical step when interpreting the ECG of a chest pain patient. Wide Q waves occurring in anatomically contiguous leads are the most specific evidence of myocardial infarction, but they do not occur in the earliest hours of infarction. Elevation of the ST segment is the most reliable marker during the first hours of infarction, and may be recognizable before significant tissue loss has occurred. Therefore, each lead, with the exception of AVR, should be examined for the presence of indicative changes with special emphasis on ST segment elevation and pathologic Q waves. Evidence must be found in at least two anatomically contiguous leads.

If acute myocardial infarction is suspected, one should mentally picture the cardiac anatomy to localize the infarction and predict which coronary artery is occluded. The relative extent of the infarction can be gauged by the number of leads showing ST segment elevation. In right coronary artery occlusions, right-sided chest leads should be obtained to help gauge the extent of the infarct and identify possible right ventricular infarction.

Remember that many infarctions do not produce identifiable changes on the ECG. In addition, certain conditions other than infarction can produce ST segment elevation. It is crucial that **the ECG is NEVER used to rule out an infarction,** especially within the first few hours of symptom onset. Conversely, conditions other than infarction may be the cause of ST segment elevation. Therefore, it is important to look for specific evidence of their presence before developing a working diagnosis of infarction.

STEP 3 Infarct Imposters

When changes indicative of myocardial infarction are noted on the ECG, it is important to ascertain if other conditions are present that might also account for the changes. To accomplish this task, a working list of these conditions is needed. While such a list would be quite extensive, several of the more common imitators of infarction are specifically listed in Step 3. In cases where these conditions are present, the emergency cardiac care provider should never rule out infarct, but rather should recognize that these noted changes may be due either to infarction or one of the infarct impostors. Remember, infarction can still occur in the presence of each of these conditions. Therefore, when the emergency cardiac care provider is screening potential infarct patients, recognition of indicative changes in the presence of one of the infarct impostors warrants an immediate physician overread.

One of the most distracting and frequent imitators is left bundle branch block (LBBB). The ECG changes of LBBB look much like those of infarction and are often pronounced enough to quickly gain the attention of the emergency care provider. Left ventricular hypertrophy (LVH) occurs more often than does LBBB, but usually provides a less striking resemblance of infarction. Ventricular rhythms, whether occurring spontaneously or as the result of a ventricular pacemaker, are not uncommon and often produce both Q waves and ST segment elevation.

Two less common conditions are pericarditis and early repolarization. The ECG changes produced by pericarditis are very subtle and recognition can be quite difficult. Often it is the clinical picture which causes the clinician to suspect pericarditis. Once suspected, the specific ECG evidence becomes more apparent. Early repolarization produces no clinical symptoms; it does produce an ECG resembling that of infarction, particularly anterior or anterolateral infarction. Early repolarization accounts for many of the tracings that indicate infarct obtained from young, healthy patients.

STEP 4 Clinical Presentation

Discovering the patient's clinical presentation is a priority for the clinician. The inclusion of the clinical presentation at this point does not imply that it is the first time that the care provider should obtain patient information. Rather, it is assumed that the clinician will already have obtained the relevant subjective and objective information from the patient. The specific inclusion of the clinical presentation is included here to emphasize the importance of integrating the clinical presentation into the ECG interpretation.

When incorporating the clinical picture into the ECG interpretation, remember that not all infarct patients present with substernal chest pain. Diabetics and the elderly are two groups that may not describe chest pain as their primary complaint when infarcting. During infarction, these patients may complain only of epigastric distress, arm/neck/jaw pain, shortness of breath, general weakness, or similar, vague complaints. While most of these complaints are frequently encountered and generally are not caused by infarction, it is important to include infarction in the differential diagnosis. Many "silent MIs" are not so much silent as they are atypical. Therefore, a high index of suspicion is always warranted, especially when treating either diabetics or the elderly.

Female patients are another exception to the classic presentation of acute myocardial infarction. It is commonly recognized that men experience myocardial infarction much more often than women do. However, this information can be misleading. Granted, estrogen does seem to provide a protective effect to the myocardium, resulting in a lower incidence of infarction in women. However, after menopause, that benefit is lost unless supplemental estrogen is taken. The incidence of heart attack in postmenopausal women may approach that of men. Interestingly, during myocardial infarction, women often rate their chest pain at a lower intensity than do men. The combination of a perceived lower incidence of infarction and a lower estimation of chest pain intensity may prompt emergency cardiac care providers to incorrectly assume that a noninfarct condition is the cause of chest pain. Do not lower your index of suspicion simply because of the patient's gender.

Complicating the effort to recognize infarction is the fact that only a minority of nontraumatic chest pain is due to infarction. Pericarditis is one cause of non-infarct chest pain that has previously been mentioned. Other causes of non-infarct chest pain include aneurysm, musculoskeletal pain, a variety of pulmonary conditions, and gastrointestinal disorders, as well as various emotional and psychologic states. Clearly, the task of early infarct recognition can be challenging. A well-trained emergency cardiac care provider should recognize infarction when it is easily identifiable. The emergency cardiac care provider should also determine which patient requires immediate physician attention to ascertain if infarction is present. It is the physician's task to ultimately differentiate infarction from other conditions.

STEP 5 Interpretation

While only the physician can make the final diagnosis of infarction, the emergency cardiac care provider is charged with the responsibility of recognizing infarction and taking steps to speed the process of data collection, physician evaluation, and, when appropriate, thrombolysis. The reality of this expectation is that nurses, paramedics, and all other cardiac care providers must be able to develop a "working diagnosis" of infarction. This working diagnosis must be confirmed by a physician before definitive treatment may begin, but it has been clearly demonstrated that the early recognition of infarction by the nonphysician can greatly reduce the time-to-treatment. The reduction in time-to-treatment is the emergency cardiac care provider's most compelling reason to become familiar with the 12-lead ECG.

Once a working diagnosis of infarction has been made, strategies for reducing time-to-treatment vary with setting. In the emergency department, nurses should have immediate access to a 12-lead ECG monitor. When the 12-lead shows evidence of infarction, or causes the nurse to suspect infarction, the tracing should be immediately brought to the attention of a physician. A team approach similar to the one used for trauma patients should be in place. Much of the routine lab work should be made a standing order so that the nursing staff can begin to collect data for physician review. This process allows the nurse to identify patients with a high likelihood of infarction and then to quickly gather the data necessary for physician review. Should infarction be confirmed and thrombolysis ordered, the team can rapidly carry out the order.

Paramedics should alert the receiving facility as soon as possible and communicate that a probable infarct patient is en route. A simple checklist (developed in conjunction with the receiving facility) is used to determine the appropriateness of thrombolytic therapy. When a patient meets all of the inclusion criteria and no contraindications are present, additional steps may be performed. The preferences of the receiving facility and system protocols determine which preparatory steps are appropriate but, in general, aspirin is administered, additional IV lines are established (possibly with multilumen catheters), and blood is drawn for necessary lab work.

Because nurses and paramedics are actively involved in the management of chest pain, AV block, and hypotension, the information obtained from the 12-lead ECG can allow them to anticipate certain complications in advance. Should these complications present, a more effective treatment plan can be designed, one which considers the location of the infarction and the probable site of coronary artery occlusion.

Putting it to Use

The case-based approach to learning has recently gained much support. Following are several case studies designed to allow the reader to apply the five-step analysis to ECG interpretation. While some scenarios are real (except for patient biographic information) and others hypothetical, each is intended to provide the reader with the opportunity to apply many of the text's learning objectives. Included with each tracing is patient information and certain aspects of the clinical setting in which the tracing was obtained. Use this information, along with the card provided with the text, to follow the five-step analysis and formulate your interpretation and treatment plan.

CASE STUDY 1

It's your turn to staff triage in the emergency department. You expect to find a packed house, but you see only two patients in the waiting area. One patient is in for a suture removal and is being evaluated by the nurse whom you are relieving. The other is an elderly female patient sitting with her daughter.

The patient looks tired so you bring a wheelchair to her. "Please, have a seat here," you say. "Oh, I can walk," she replies. The patient's name is Mrs. Alberta Humphries. "What seems to be the trouble tonight, Mrs. Humphries?" "I'm having a little trouble breathing today and it didn't get better after I used my puffer. That scared my daughter and she wanted me to come and get checked out. I am breathing a little better now, though." "How long did your breathing trouble last and how many times did you use your puffer?" "Well, I say it started about 10:00 this morning" it's now 2:55 PM "and I used that puffer a lot today." "Is there anything else that's bothering you ma'am?" "No, not really. I guess I am pretty tired, but I usually take a little nap about this time."

The patient interview determines that Mrs. Humphries is 68 years old and has smoked for about 45 years. Her medical history includes COPD, angina, and hypertension, and she is overcoming a respiratory tract infection. When trying to ascertain if Mrs. Humphries has experienced any chest discomfort, she stated, "Yes, but that's not uncommon for me."

What is Mrs. Humphrie's underlying problem? The primary complaint of breathing difficulty could be attributed to her COPD, especially considering the recent respiratory tract infection. The patient secondarily complained of being "pretty tired." Any number of factors could account for her fatigue, including the recent illness. The complaint of chest pain was made only after specific questioning. In addition, the patient stated that she experiences some degree of chest pain on a regular basis. Given her medical history, this seems very possible.

During the initial triage of this patient, it is difficult to narrow the list of possible causes of these complaints, but myocardial infarction should be included in the list. Granted, these complaints are fairly common among elderly patients and are generally due to conditions less serious than myocardial infarction. However, when an elderly patient experiences a sudden onset of breathing difficulty, is tired, and admits to some chest pain, infarct must be considered a possibility.

Mrs. Humphries is taken directly to the treatment area because few patients are present in the emergency department. A 12-lead ECG machine is kept in the emergency department and an ECG is quickly obtained. That tracing is shown in Fig. 8-2.

Looking at the ECG, both you and the other nurse note the obvious ST segment elevation, suggestive of anteroseptal infarct. However, further inspection shows the presence of a left bundle branch block. Is the ST segment elevation due to an infarct or just simply the part of LBBB pattern? At this point, myocardial infarction is still just one of many possibilities, but you decide to notify the emergency department physician of that possibility. You find the physician reviewing the x-rays of another patient and advise her of Mrs. Humphrie's complaints and ECG. After looking at your 12-lead, she asks you to obtain a chest x-ray and lab work, including cardiac enzymes. She also asks you to check medical records for any old ECGs. You pass this information along to the patient's nurse and return to the triage area.

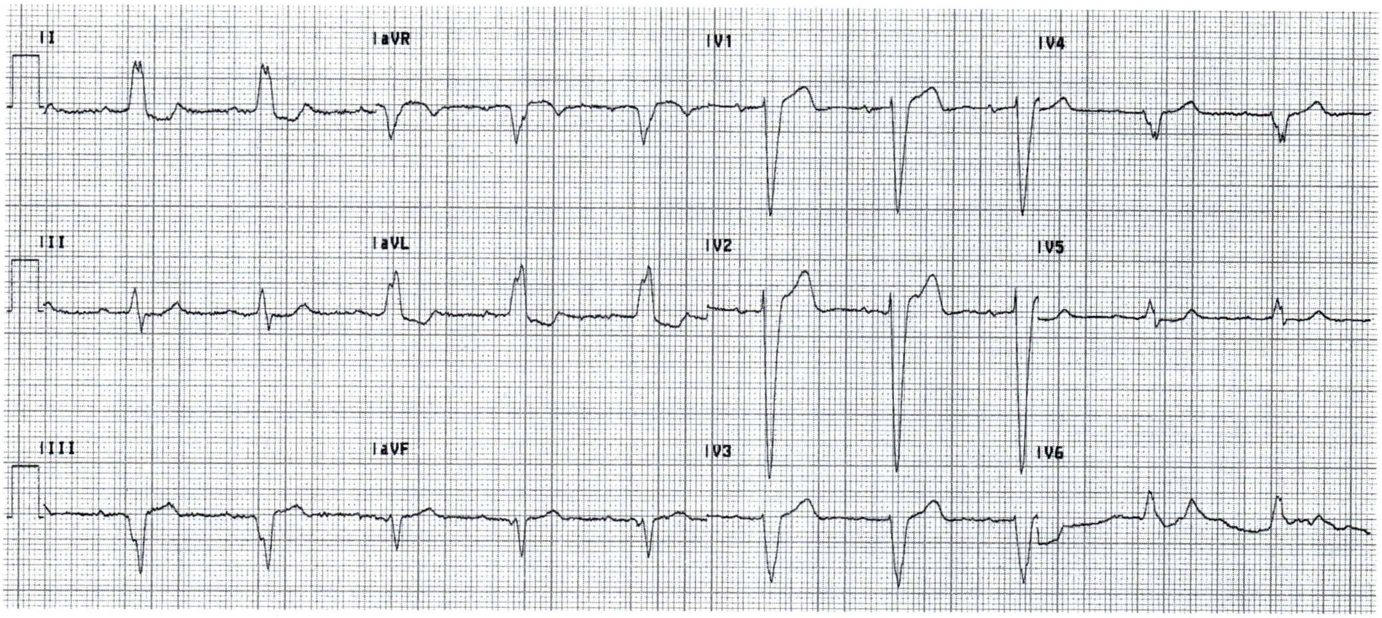

FIG. 8-2 Mrs. Humphries' 12-lead ECG.

It is important to remember that the ECG is not a lie detector test that can sort out infarcting patients from not infarcting patients. The ECG is an important tool that often helps recognize myocardial infarct, but only when used in the light of the patient's clinical presentation.

Occasionally, both the clinical presentation and the ECG are nonspecific. In such cases it may be the cardiac enzymes that provide the most definitive evidence. Thus, it is crucial to remember that even when myocardial infarction is present, the ECG does not always provide obvious evidence.

Later in your shift you decide to check on Mrs. Humphries. You find that she was admitted, but not for myocardial infarction. However, you were correct in being concerned that Mrs. Humphries may have been infarcting. Myocardial infarction was ruled out only after comparison with old tracings, serial ECGs, and the absence of cardiac enzymes. Had the results been different, your actions would have significantly reduced the time required to recognize and treat an infarcting patient.

CASE STUDY 2

While helping your partner transfer a patient from your ambulance stretcher to the ED's stretcher, the EMS dispatcher calls over the radio to find out if you can take another call. As your partner provides the ED staff with the pertinent information about his patient, you load your equipment onto the stretcher and approach the ambulance. You contact dispatch. "MED-7 available for call." "MED-7 respond to Franklin

Bridge. Man under the bridge complaining of chest pain." Since your partner ran the last call, you will be in charge of this one.

En route to the scene, the dispatcher provides you with some additional information. "Fire-rescue is on the scene and states that the patient is under the east side of the bridge. He is a 52-year-old male complaining of chest pain and dizziness." Arriving on the scene you see the patient reclining on the ground next to a bench and receiving oxygen from the basic life support crew. As you walk toward the patient you realize that he looks genuinely ill. The EMT informs you that the patient, Wally, was fishing when his chest began to hurt. "It didn't go away so he sat for a while but that didn't help at all," the EMT says. You are handed a piece of paper which reads "BP 108/palp, P 64, Resp 20." "Oh, yeah," the EMT adds, "he said he gets dizzy when he stands up."

"Wally, my name is Carl and I'm a paramedic. What seems to be the trouble today?" "Well, like I said, my chest hurts." "When did the pain start?" Wally is not wearing a watch. Before answering your question, he glances at the river. "It started just before high tide I guess." You ask him, "What time was that?" Wally gives you a look and answers, "About an hour after sunrise." It's 10:30 AM so you estimate that the pain started about 3 hours ago.

"How would you describe the pain?" you ask. "It's real bad," answers Wally. "On a 1 to 10 scale, 10 being the worst pain that you have ever had, how would you rate this pain?" Without hesitation Wally tells you that this is a 10. During the rest of your interview, you determine that the patient is complaining of a constant substernal chest pressure, without radiation; the onset was 3 hours ago while at rest; it is not associated with shortness of breath or nausea; and the patient has not done anything to attempt pain relief.

By this time your partner has applied the cardiac monitor and has an IV bag and tubing ready to go once you position the IV catheter. You glance at the monitor and see obvious ST segment elevation in lead II. Switching to diagnostic quality you obtain leads II and III. Gross ST segment elevation is noted in both of these leads. Your partner asks if you want him to administer nitroglycerin while you start the IV line. "Hold off on that for just a minute," you reply as you pick up the red electrode and place it in the V4R position. Recording a tracing in diagnostic quality again, you see obvious ST segment elevation. (The sample ECG is shown in Fig. 8-3.) "Let's not give the nitro until after I start the IV," you tell him. Glancing at the patient's neck you note distention of the jugular veins.

From the information provided, it seems probable that Wally is experiencing an infarction of the left ventricle's inferior wall and of the right ventricle. The clinical presentation strongly suggests the presence of AMI. The ECG seems to confirm the working diagnosis of infarct and allows for localization of the infarct. However, a quick check for any infarct imposters is appropriate.

The QRS complex determines that the complex is not wide. The presence of a QRS complex less than 120 ms in duration excludes bundle branch block and ventricular rhythms. (NOTE: Though the paramedics in this case did not, it is often helpful to measure the QRS complex in V1/MCL1 to more definitively rule out a wide QRS complex.) The standard chest leads were not provided so it was not possible to look for LVH. However, LVH is not a concern for two reasons. First, the ST segment is elevated in complexes which are upright, and the characteristic pattern of LVH calls for ST segment elevation in the leads with negative QRS complexes. Second, LVH generally produces changes in the chest leads and, to a much lesser extent, in the limb leads. Though pericarditis and early repolarization are still possibilities, given the patient's clinical presentation, infarct is far more likely. Therefore, the most logical conclusion is that

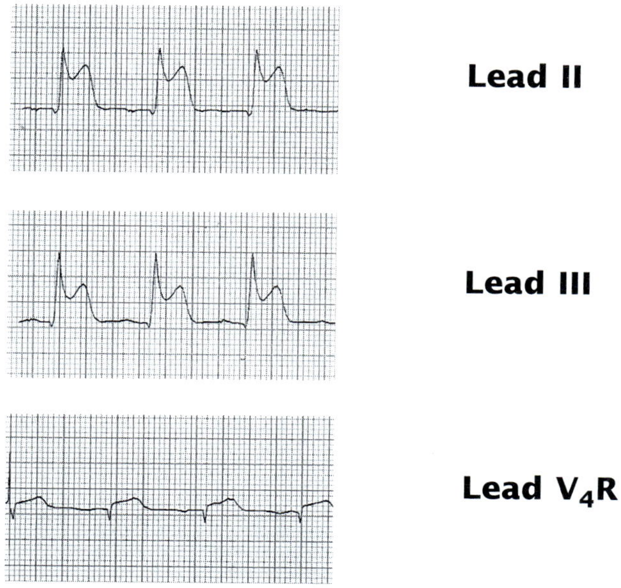

FIG. 8-3 The prehospital tracings obtained from a chest-pain patient.

the ST segment changes are due to infarct rather than some other condition. (It probably took longer to read this paragraph than it actually takes to consider the possibility of all five infarct impostors.)

"How long do you want me to wait before I give the nitro?" your partner asks. "Just hold on until I piggyback this second IV," you answer.

In the setting of right ventricular infarction, a reduction in preload can produce a significant reduction in blood pressure. Given the fact that the patient became dizzy upon standing, one must be concerned that this patient may be sensitive to changes in preload. Therefore, before administering nitroglycerin or morphine, it may be prudent to have a mechanism in place that can increase the preload if needed. The most simple means of accomplishing this is probably to have a bag of either normal saline or Ringer's lactate in place with a macro drip administration set. After the nitroglycerin is administered, monitor the patient's blood pressure and, if hypotension ensues, reposition the patient and administer fluids as needed.

Remember two points. First, it was not the inferior wall infarction that caused concern about the administration of nitroglycerin or morphine. The right ventricular infarction caused this concern. When there is no ECG or clinical evidence of RVI accompanying the inferior wall infarction, nitroglycerin and morphine are administered in their "usual" manner. Second, do not withhold nitroglycerin in situations in which it is not possible to quickly ascertain if an RVI is present. In other words, if you can't quickly determine whether or not an RVI exists, then it's probably safer to administer the nitroglycerin than it is to avoid it.

After the normal saline line has been established, your partner administers the nitroglycerin. You check Wally's blood pressure and record it as 80/52. Wally is still conscious, reclining against a bench, and you ask if he would like to lay down on your stretcher. While supine with his feet elevated, the patient's blood pressure is still low, so you opt to administer fluids and open the normal saline. Monitoring Wally's vital signs, you note that his blood pressure is above 100 mm Hg after 500 cc of fluids.

En route to the hospital, specific questions are asked of Wally to determine if he is a good candidate for thrombolytic therapy. His responses indicate that he is. The emergency department is then notified that a probable infarct patient is on the way and that no contraindications to thrombolytic therapy exist. Aspirin is administered and, as time permits, additional IV lines started and/or specific blood tubes filled.

Upon arrival at the emergency department, a team awaits to immediately review the data collected by the paramedic, reassess the patient, and administer thrombolytic therapy as appropriate. Wally receives thrombolytic therapy 16 minutes after his arrival at the hospital.

CASE STUDY 3

The local EMS agency has just brought a patient in and the charge nurse assigns her to one of your beds. When walking into the treatment room you look at the patient, a hyperventilating 22-year-old named Donna. The paramedics tells you that "she has been like this since we got to her. We've tried everything to calm her down but just can't do it."

When the paramedics encountered Donna, her hyperventilation was obvious. Her breathing difficulty was so severe that it was difficult for her to talk. When the paramedics asked if she was upset, Donna nodded yes. Carpal spasms were obvious and the paramedics' next question, "Are your hands tingling?" received another head nod. They also asked about chest pain and again received a nod.

After observing Donna for a few minutes, the paramedic began to feel that she was experiencing something more than just hyperventilation. Therefore, oxygen was administered at 6 liters/minute via a nasal cannula and an IV was established. The patient was taking no medications, and had no significant medical history other than being 5 months postpartum.

Since the paramedics were unsure of the underlying problem, they opted for a quick ride to the hospital. You have an uneasy feeling about Donna's situation and are doubtful that this is just simple hyperventilation, but are uncertain as to what the underlying problem is. Because of this uncertainty, you order some lab work, including a 12-lead ECG (Fig. 8-4), as permitted in the nurse's standing orders.

While hyperventilation itself can produce chest pain, one must consider other possibilities as well. At the crux of the issue is whether the anxiety produced the chest pain, or the chest pain produced the anxiety. The ECG sheds some light on this question.

Looking at the 12-lead, the pattern of extensive anterior infarction is obvious. Despite the patient's gender and her age, it seems that an acute myocardial infarction is the cause of her chest pain. This is an example of how the 12-lead ECG can help to identify infarct patients. A quick check shows no evidence of an infarct imposter. Given the probability of an infarct, the emergency department physician should be notified immediately.

Looking at Donna's 12-lead you recognize the probability of a very extensive anterior wall infarct. The on-duty physician examines her and

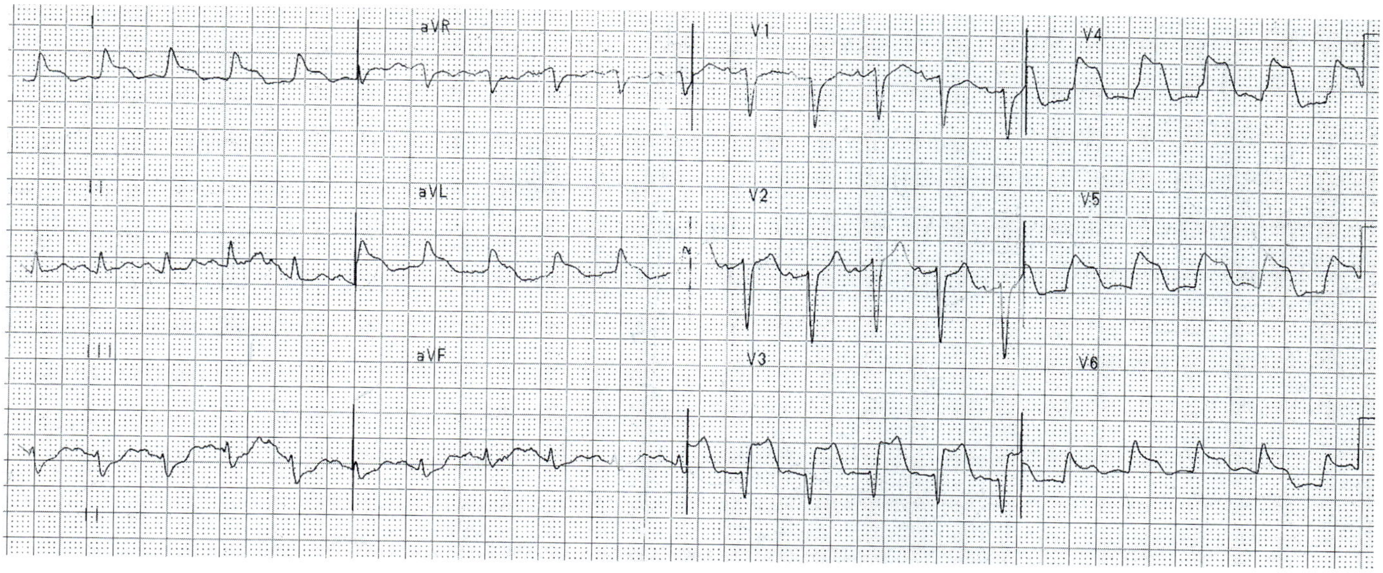

FIG. 8-4 The 12-lead obtained from a hyperventilating 24-year-old woman.

orders thrombolytic therapy and IV nitroglycerin for the patient. Are you cautious or concerned about this order?

No more than you would for any other patient. Remember, it is in the presence of a right ventricular infarct that you may become cautious about venodilators such as nitroglycerin, morphine, and furosemide. In this case, a proximal left coronary artery occlusion is suspected. Since the left coronary artery generally does not supply the right ventricle, the likelihood of a right ventricular infarct is very remote, and nitroglycerin can be administered with the routine precautions. In this setting, nitroglycerin can dilate the coronary arteries and slow the process of infarction.

The clot team draws blood, starts the additional IV lines, administers aspirin, and prepares heparin, as well as other ancillary agents. When the final preparations are complete, the thrombolytic agent is administered.

As the thrombolytic agent is administered, the patient must still be monitored. Remember, coronary reperfusion does not occur immediately upon the initiation of thrombolytic therapy. It may take anywhere from 30 minutes to over an hour for the occlusion to lyse and blood flow to return to the infarcting myocardium. It is difficult to determine the exact point of reperfusion, but a return of circulation is suspected when the ST segments begin to normalize and reperfusion arrhythmias develop.

CASE STUDY 4

You are sitting at the nurse's desk in the emergency department, waiting for a return phone call from the ICU concerning an admission. While waiting, you pick up a 12-lead lying on the desk.

Because the 12-lead was not attached to a patient's chart you have no clinical information available. By simply looking only at the 12-lead (Fig. 8-5), and blinded to any clinical information, what is your interpretation?

Indicative changes can be noted in many of the precordial leads. These changes suggest a possible anterolateral infarction. However, before that conclusion is drawn, one must evaluate for the possibility of an infarct imposter.

When the QRS duration is measured in several leads, including V1 and V2, the duration is consistently less than 120 ms. This duration excludes the possibility of both left bundle branch block and a ventricular rhythm. To assess for left ventricular hypertrophy, the depth of the largest S wave between V1 and V2 is added to the height of the tallest R wave between V5 and V6. The sum of the two deflections equals approximately 33 mm. While this does not exactly attain the 35 mm used to suspect LVH, it is very close, making it difficult to rule out LVH with a high degree of certainty.

Pericarditis is another possibility to consider. A close inspection of the tracing shows that leads II, III, and AVF also reveal some ST segment changes. The diffuse spreading of ST segment elevation may be suggestive of pericarditis. Furthermore, some J point notching can be discerned, also consistent with pericarditis.

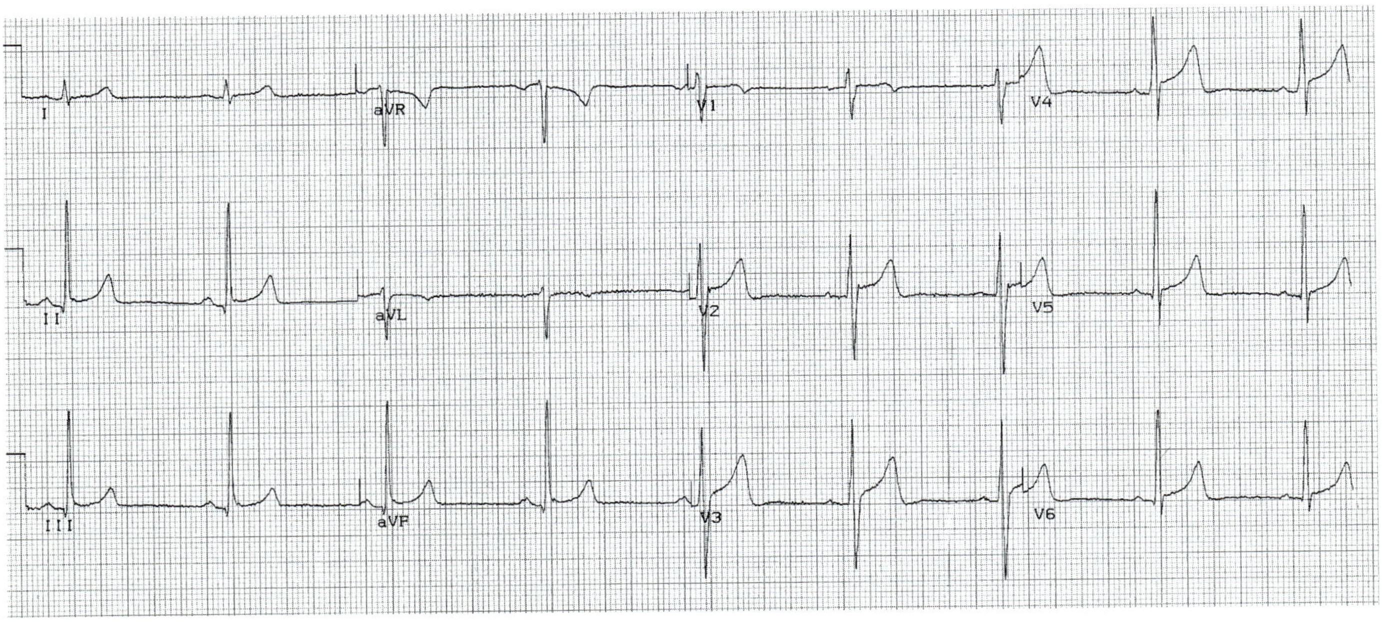

FIG. 8-5 An ECG found lying on the desk.

When early repolarization imitates infarct, it usually does so by producing tall, pointed T waves and ST segment elevation in the chest leads. That pattern is noted, so early repolarization must also be considered a possible cause of the noted changes.

Possible explanations for the ST segment elevation include anterolateral infarction, left ventricular hypertrophy, pericarditis, and early repolarization. The obvious question is how to differentiate between these alternatives. Remember, the intent is not to rule out infarct, but to quickly identify it when it is present. Cardiologists experience similiar situations every day when overreading ECGs.

In the hospital, the 12-lead is first interpreted by the physician that ordered it. The physician is aware of the clinical presentation and can easily integrate the patient's clinical presentation. However, each day, all of the 12-leads ordered in a hospital are read a second time (overread) by a cardiologist. When these tracings are overread, the cardiologist is often blinded to the patient's clinical presentation. The cardiologist's interpretation is derived strictly from the tracing itself. A frequent comment made during the overreading is, "clinical correlation advised." In other words, without clinical information even cardiologists cannot always differentiate between potential interpretations. To illustrate this point, let's see how the interpretation can differ with varying clinical presentations.

If you were to learn that this was the ECG of a 52-year-old man complaining of squeezing chest pain, then acute infarction would be your conclusion. Early repolarization could produce these changes and would be likely if this was found to be the resting ECG of a healthy, asymptomatic young black male. However, what if this tracing was obtained from a postcardiac surgery patient complaining of sharp chest pain with radiation to the trapezius area? In that setting, pericarditis is a distinct possibility. In fact, a closer look shows ST segment changes in leads II, III, and AVF, and this spreading of ST segment changes further suggests pericarditis.

The interpretation changed greatly with the clinical presentation. Remember that the patient's clinical presentation must always be integrated into the final interpretation. (This ECG was taken from an asymptomatic, young, black male, and is an example of early repolarization.)

CASE STUDY 5

Just after one of the patients in your care in the emergency department is admitted to the floor, the change nurse directs a chest pain patient into the room. You begin to assess the patient as you go about the task of administering oxygen and starting an IV. The patient is a 62-year-old man named J.T. Henderson and he appears to be in marked distress. Mr. Henderson relays a description of a tightness in his chest that started just after he awoke at 6:30 this morning. The tightness quickly became very painful and he decided to go back to bed and rest. However, after an hour of rest he felt no better and called his office to tell them that he was taking a sick day. After much urging from his wife, Mr. Henderson

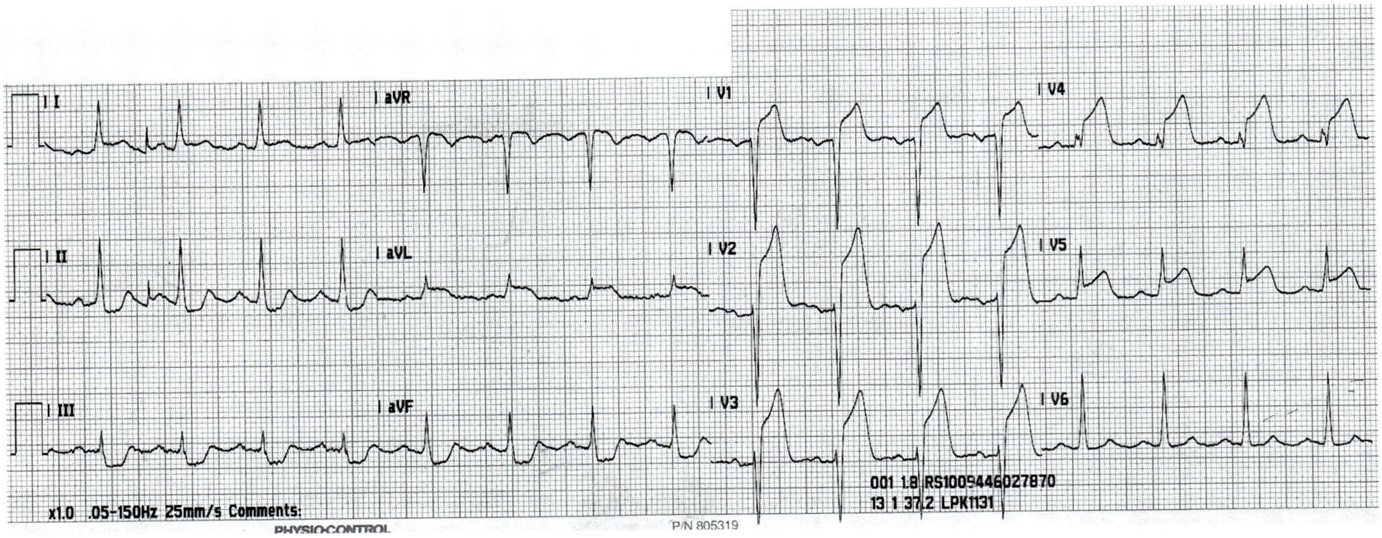

FIG. 8-6 Mr. Henderson's 12-lead ECG.

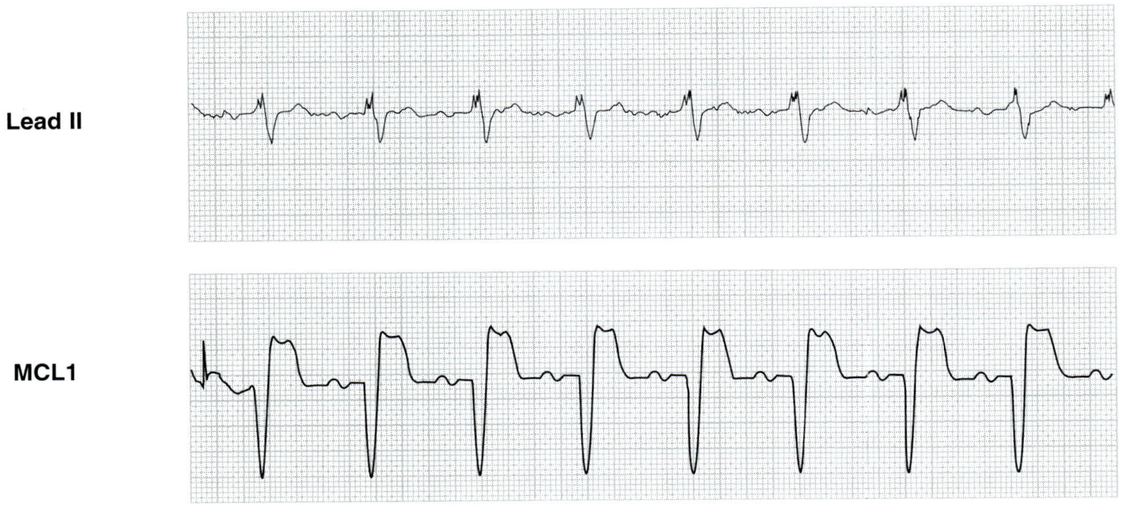

FIG. 8-7 A change in rhythm prompted the leads to be obtained.

allowed her to drive him to the hospital, arriving there at approximately 10:00 AM. As you continue to talk with Mr. Henderson, you wheel in the 12-lead cart and obtain the 12-lead ECG shown in Fig. 8-6.

The ECG clearly shows evidence of an anteroseptal infarct in progress. Therefore, the emergency department physician should be notified immediately. Specific questions designed to determine if the patient is a good candidate for thrombolytic therapy should have been prepared in advance and should be asked of the patient.

It is 10:20 AM and Mr. Henderson was seen by the on-duty physician who has ordered thrombolytic therapy. As you and your co-workers are preparing to administer the medication, someone points out a change on the monitor. A tracing is run (shown in Fig. 8-7) and handed to you. Noted is the onset of a first degree AV block with a wide

QRS complex. You instruct a coworker to prepare the external pacemaker for standby pacing. "But this is just a first degree block," he responds.

The combination of an AV block with a wide QRS complex in the presence of an anteroseptal infarct (left coronary artery occlusion) is cause for concern. This suggests an infranodal location of the AV block, probably in the bundle branches.

Infranodal AV block produced by myocardial infarction carries with it several concerns. It is a more serious block, probably caused by tissue loss or serious tissue injury. Also, there is a significant possibility that the block will progress into complete heart block. If this occurs, a subsidiary ventricular pacemaker may be all that stands between this patient and asystole. Atropine will likely not do much to improve this condition and a pacemaker will be required. Given this combination of factors, it is often a good idea to prepare the pacemaker for standby pacing before the ventricular rate slows.

In addition to AV block management, remember that you have just witnessed the onset of a new bundle branch block. A myocardial infarction that produces a bundle branch block also produces a large amount of tissue death. The extensive tissue loss results in a high incidence of pump failure and a mortality rate of about 50%.

9

OBJECTIVE

- Gain familiarity with the variety of ECG manifestations produced by myocardial infarction.

Practice ECGs

CHAPTER 9

Before the emergency cardiac care provider can confidently integrate 12-lead interpretation into the clinical setting, one must have ample opportunity to practice the skill. Because this factor is so important, 50 additional 12-lead ECGs with interpretation are included in this chapter. A collection of this size represents years of clinical practice for many emergency cardiac care providers.

All of the tracings included in this chapter were obtained from patients diagnosed with acute myocardial infarction. In fact, every tracing was the first 12-lead ECG obtained during the acute myocardial infarction. Interpretations for all 50 tracings are available at the end of this chapter. Good luck!

Format

The manner in which the interpretations are presented resembles the way in which emergency cardiac care providers should interpret the 12-lead — one lead at time.

The information obtained from each lead is presented in a particular order. First, the tracing quality is assessed. If baseline wander or artifact are present to any significant degree, that observation is noted. If the presence of either of these two conditions interferes with the assessment of any lead, a modifier such as "possible" or "apparent" is used. Second, each lead is examined for the presence of a Q wave and/or poor R wave progression. When a Q wave is present, the duration is expressed in milliseconds. Next, the ST segment is assessed for the presence of elevation or depression. When ST segment elevation is noted, it is expressed in millimeters. Last, the T wave is examined for any changes in orientation, shape, and size.

Each lead is assessed for:

- Baseline artifact and wander.
- Q waves and/or R wave progression.
- ST segment changes.
- T wave changes.

This information is displayed in table form with the location of infarct at the bottom of the table. Certain abbreviations are used throughout the interpretations and they are collected here for your review.

$>$	Greater than
$\geq$	Greater than or equal to
$<$	Less than
$\leq$	Less than or equal to
mm	millimeter
ms	millisecond

Example 9–1 shows how the information is formatted in this chapter.

Example

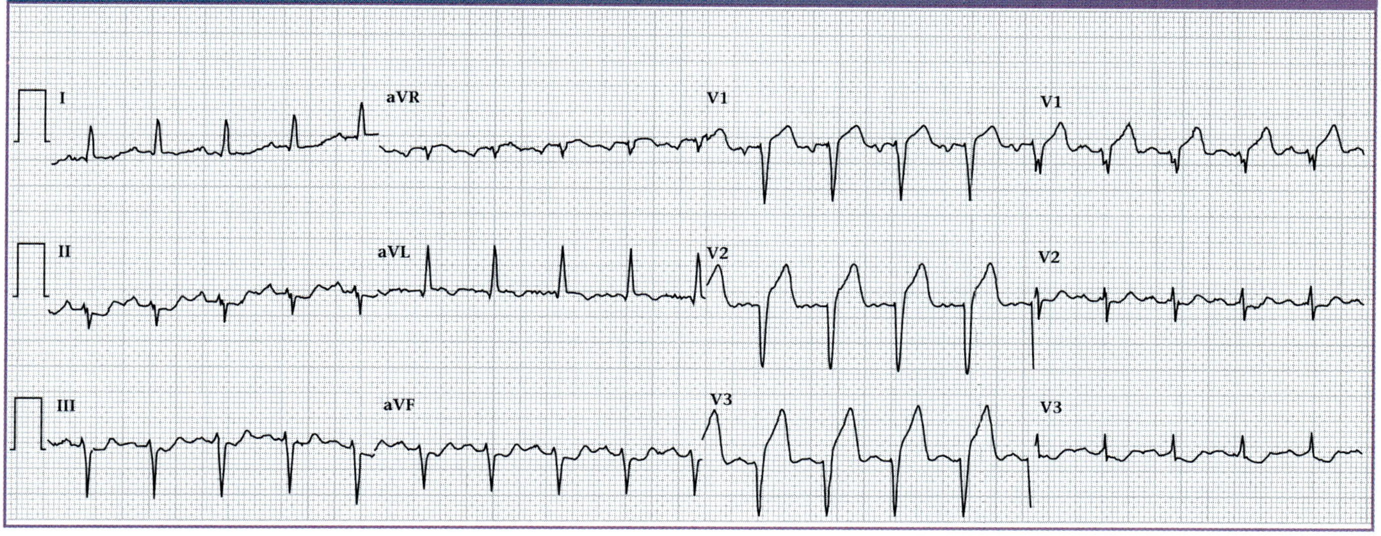

Interpretation / Example

I

II

III

AVL

AVF

V1

V2

V3

V4

V5

V6

Example: Interpretation

I	Baseline wander. No indicative changes noted.
II	ST segment depression ≤ 1 mm.
III	ST segment depression ≤ 1 mm.
AVL	Q wave < 40 ms. Inverted T wave.
AVF	ST segment depression ≥ 1 mm.
V1	ST segment elevation > 1 mm.
V2	Poor R wave progression. ST segment elevation > 1 mm.
V3	Poor R wave progression. ST segment elevation > 1 mm.
V4	Poor R wave progression. ST segment elevation > 1 mm.
V5	Poor R wave progression. ST segment depression ≥ 1 mm.
V6	ST segment depresion ≥ 1 mm.

Comments:
Anteroseptal infarction.

Before you begin

Please note that the interpretation of each lead and tracing includes only the material discussed in this text. Therefore, experienced electrocardiographers will note the presence of some conditions or findings that are not listed in the interpretation.

Fig 9-1

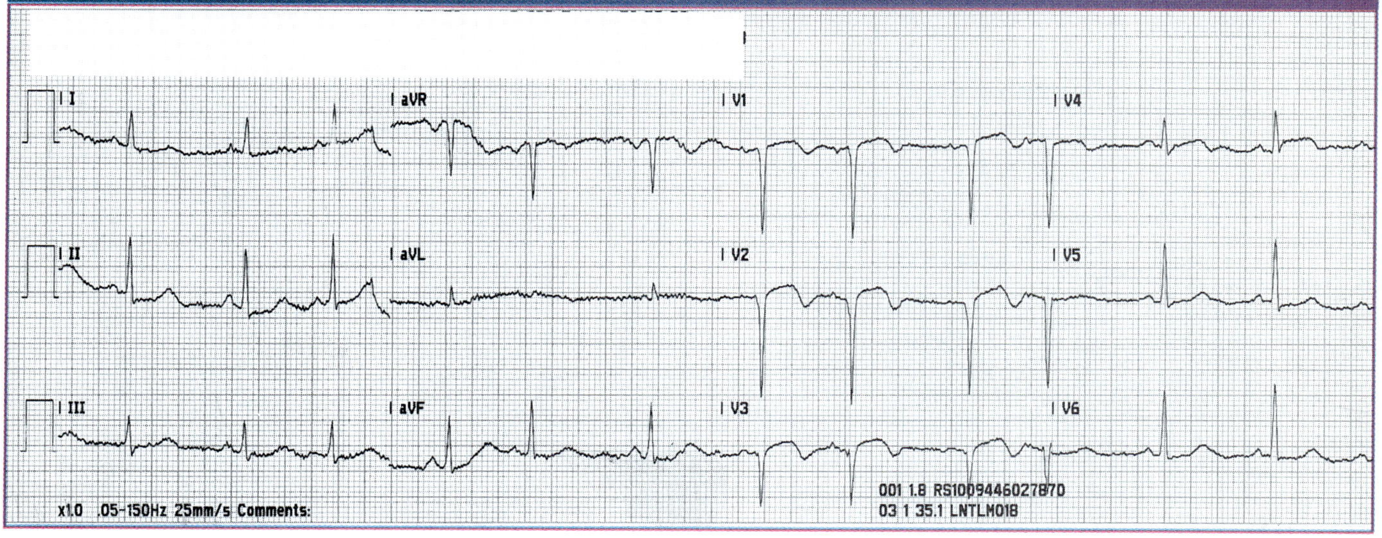

Interpretation /9-1

I

II

III

AVL

AVF

V1

V2

V3

V4

V5

V6

Fig 9-1: Interpretation

I	Baseline artifact. No other changes noted.
II	Baseline wander and artifact. ST segment analysis difficult.
III	Baseline artifact. No other changes noted.
AVL	Low voltage. No other changes noted.
AVF	No changes noted.
V1	Elevated ST segment elevation.
V2	Q wave. Elevated ST segment > 1 mm. Inverted T wave.
V3	Q wave. Elevated ST segment > 1 mm. Inverted T wave.
V4	Baseline wander. Possible ST segment elevation.
V5	No changes noted.
V6	No changes noted.

Comments:
Anteroseptal infarction.

Fig 9-2

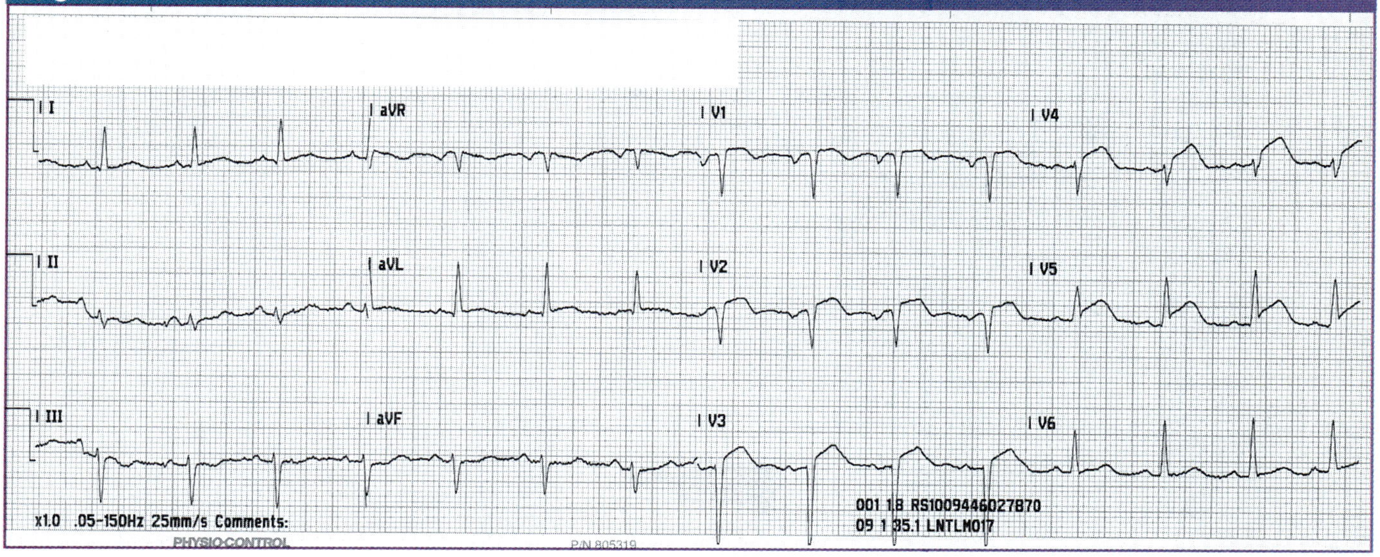

Interpretation /9-2

I

II

III

AVL

AVF

V1

V2

V3

V4

V5

V6

Fig 9-2: Interpretation

I	Narrow Q wave. Slight ST segment elevation (possibly due to baseline wander).
II	Baseline wander. No other changes noted.
III	No changes noted.
AVL	Narrow Q wave. Slight ST segment elevation.
AVF	No changes noted.
V1	ST segment elevation.
V2	Q wave. ST segment elevation.
V3	Poor R wave progression. ST segment elevation.
V4	Poor R wave progression. ST segment elevation.
V5	ST segment elevation.
V6	No changes noted.

Comments:
Anteroseptal infarct, lateral wall extension.

Fig 9-3

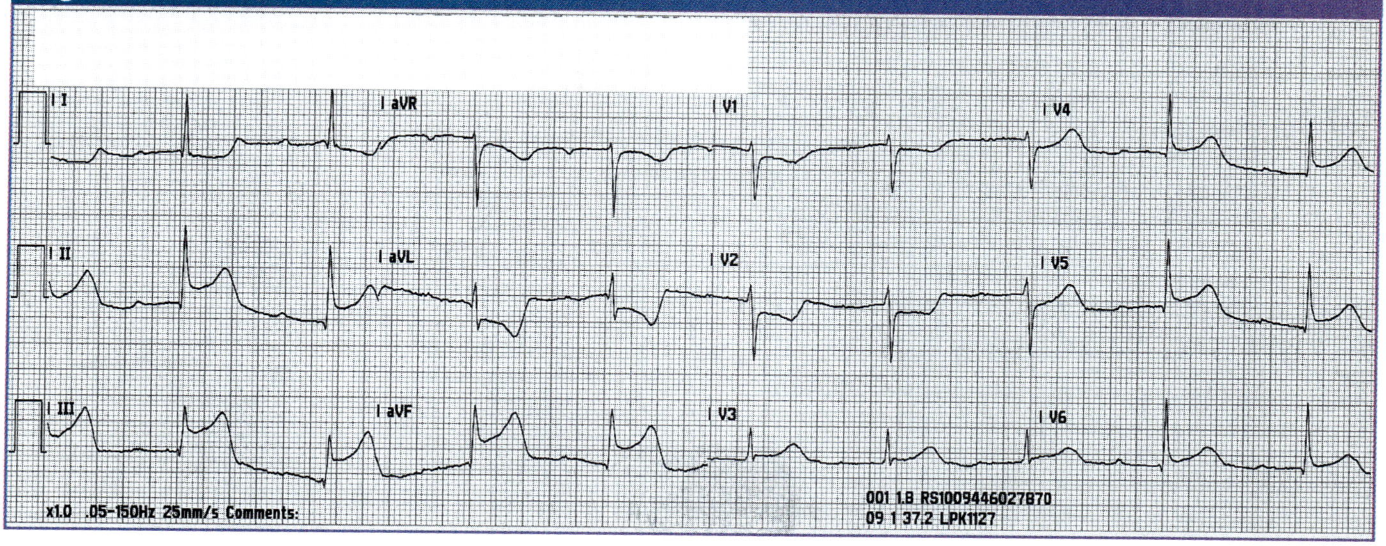

Interpretation /9-3

I

II

III

AVL

AVF

V1

V2

V3

V4

V5

V6

Fig 9-3: Interpretation

I	Narrow Q wave. Slight ST segment depression.
II	Narrow Q wave. ST segment elevation > 1 mm.
III	ST segment elevation. Tall/peaked T wave.
AVL	Narrow Q wave. ST segment elevation > 1 mm.
AVF	Narrow Q wave. ST segment elevation > 1 mm.
V1	Slight ST segment depression.
V2	ST segment depression.
V3	Slight ST segment elevation.
V4	Narrow Q wave. ST segment elevation ≥ 1 mm.
V5	Narrow Q wave. ST segment elevation > 1 mm.
V6	Narrow Q wave. ST segment elevation >1 mm.

Comments:
Inferior wall infarction. Lateral wall extension.

Fig 9-4

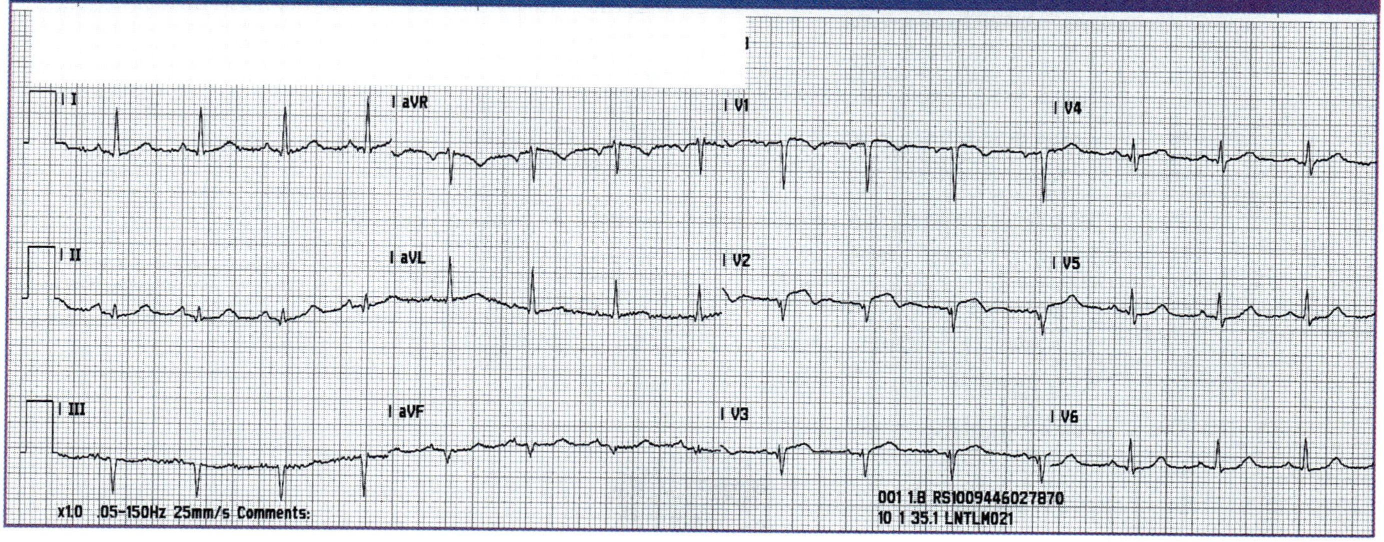

Interpretation /9-4

I

II

III

AVL

AVF

V1

V2

V3

V4

V5

V6

Fig 9-4: Interpretation

I	Narrow Q wave. No other changes noted.
II	Q wave < 40 ms. Low voltage. No other changes noted.
III	Q wave > 40 ms. No other changes noted.
AVL	Baseline artifact. No other changes noted
AVF	Q wave > 40 ms. No other changes noted.
V1	Minimal R wave. Slight ST segment elevation.
V2	Q wave. ST segment elevation > 1 mm. T wave inversion.
V3	Q wave < 40 ms. ST segment elevation ≥ 1 mm
V4	No changes noted.
V5	No changes noted.
V6	No changes noted.

Comments:
Anteroseptal infarct. Previous inferior wall infarction.

Fig 9-5

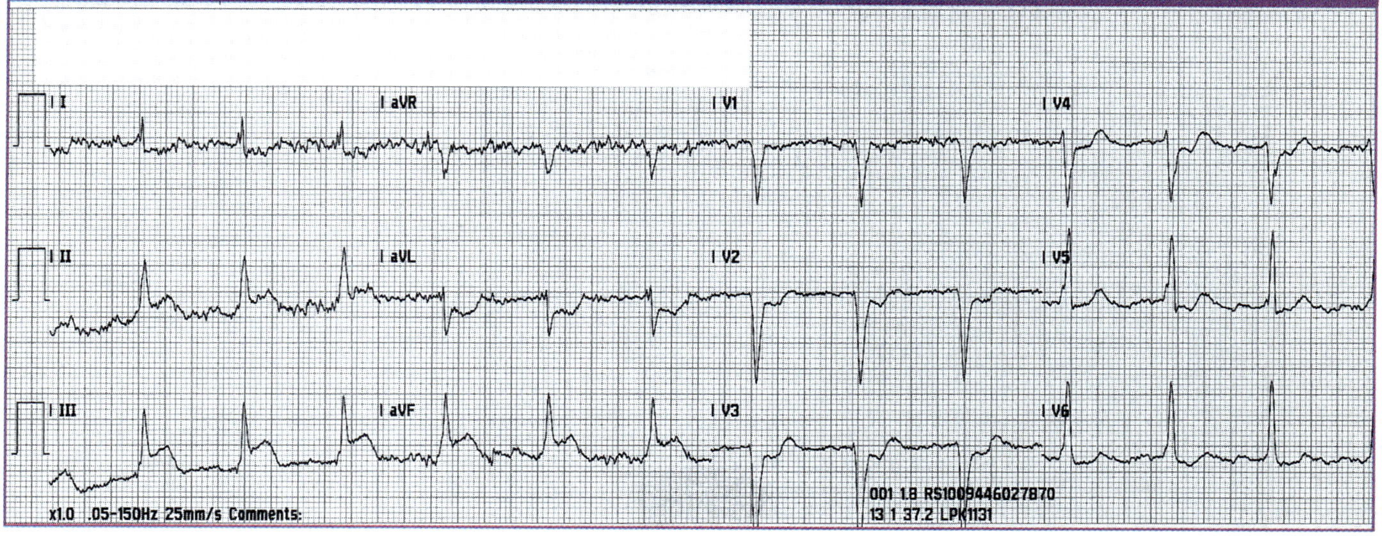

Interpretation /9-5

I

II

III

AVL

AVF

V1

V2

V3

V4

V5

V6

Fig 9-5: Interpretation

I	Baseline artifact. Possible ST segment depression.
II	Baseline artifact. ST segment elevation > 1 mm.
III	ST segment elevation > 1 mm.
AVL	Baseline artifact. ST segment depression.
AVF	Baseline artifact. ST segment elevation > 1 mm.
V1	Baseline artifact. Difficult to assess ST segment.
V2	Q wave > 40 ms. ST segment depression.
V3	Q wave > 40 ms. ST segment depression.
V4	Poor R wave progression. ST segment depression.
V5	Baseline artifact. Possible ST segment depression.
V6	Baseline artifact. Possible ST segment depression.

Comments:
Inferior infarction. Suspect previous anteroseptal infarction. ST segment depression in V leads due either to reciprocal changes or posterior infarction.

Fig 9-6

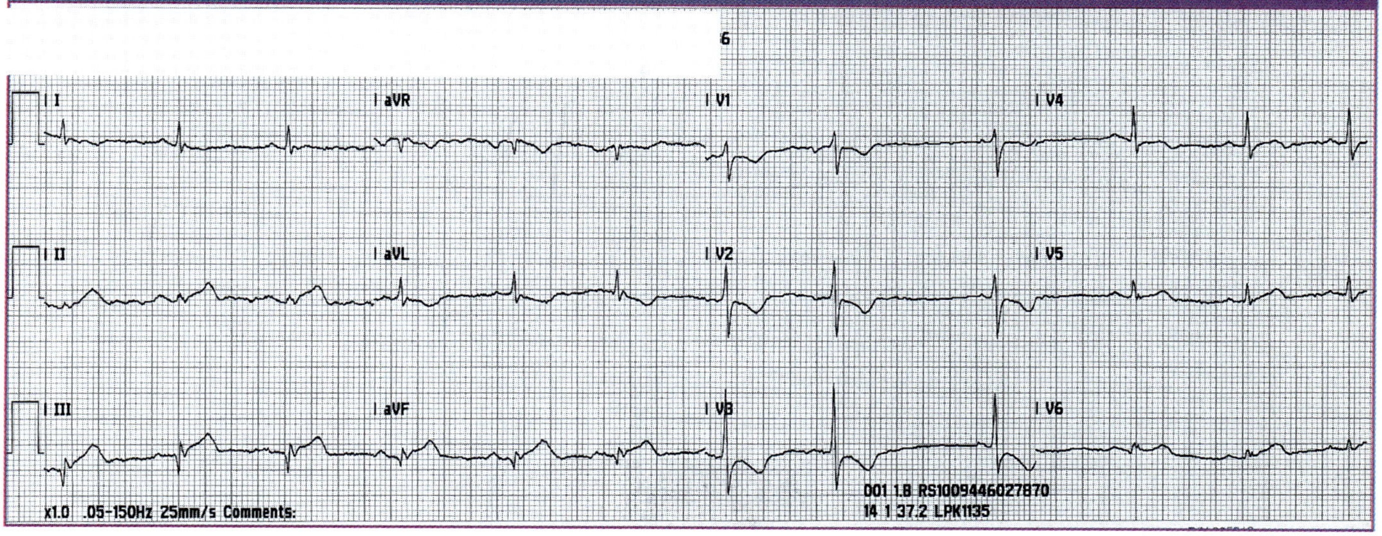

Interpretation /9-6

I

II

III

AVL

AVF

V1

V2

V3

V4

V5

V6

Fig 9-6: Interpretation

I	No changes noted.
II	Low voltage. ST segment elevation ≥ 1 mm.
III	Q wave ≥ 40 ms. ST segment elevation > 1 mm.
AVL	Inverted T wave.
AVF	Q wave ≥ 40 ms. ST segment elevation ≥ 1 mm.
V1	Slight ST segment depression. No other changes noted.
V2	Slight ST segment depression. Tall R wave. Inverted T wave.
V3	Slight ST segment depression. Tall R wave. Inverted T wave.
V4	Slight ST segment depression. Inverted T wave.
V5	Low voltage.
V6	Low voltage. Difficult to assess.

Comments:
Inferior infarction. Possible posterior infarction (tall R waves in V1 and V2).

Fig 9-7

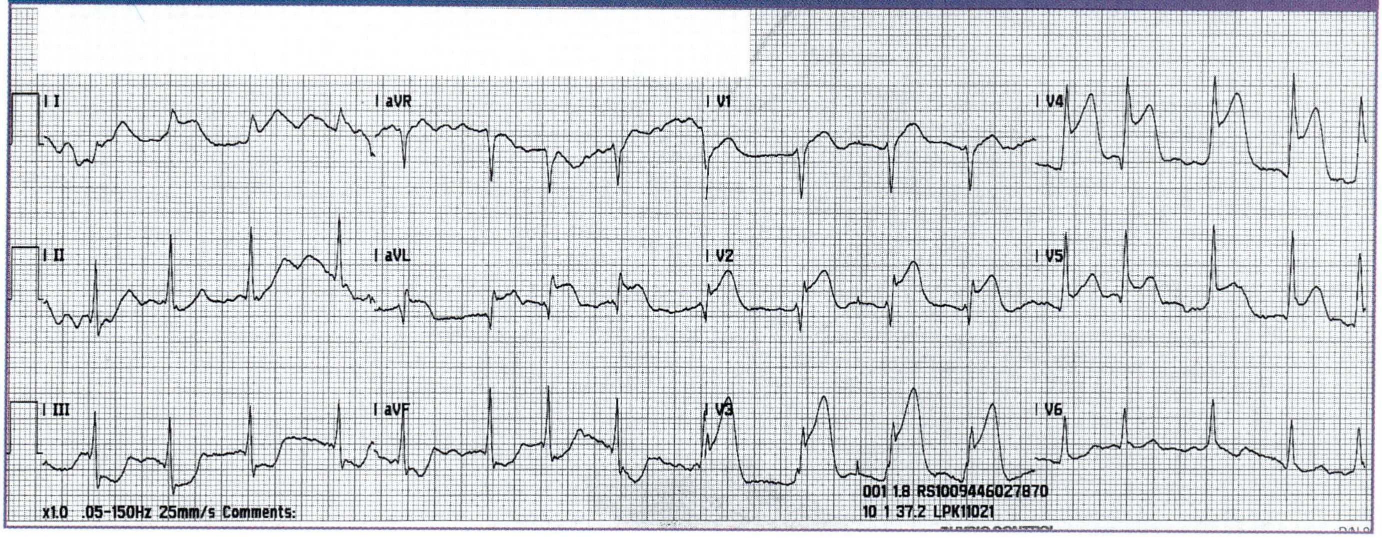

Interpretation /9-7

I

II

III

AVL

AVF

V1

V2

V3

V4

V5

V6

Fig 9-7: Interpretation

I	Wandering baseline. ST segment elevation > 1 mm.
II	Wandering baseline. Apparent ST segment depression.
III	ST segment depression.
AVL	Q wave ≥ 40 ms. ST segment elevation ≥ 1 mm.
AVF	ST segment depression.
V1	Baseline wander. ST segment elevation ≥ 1 mm.
V2	Poor R wave progression. ST segment elevation. Peaked T wave.
V3	ST segment elevation > 1 mm. Tall/peaked T wave.
V4	ST segment elevation > 1 mm. Tall/peaked T wave.
V5	ST segment elevation > 1 mm.
V6	Baseline wander. No other changes noted.

Comments:
Anteroseptal infarction. Lateral extension. Reciprocal changes noted.

Fig 9-8

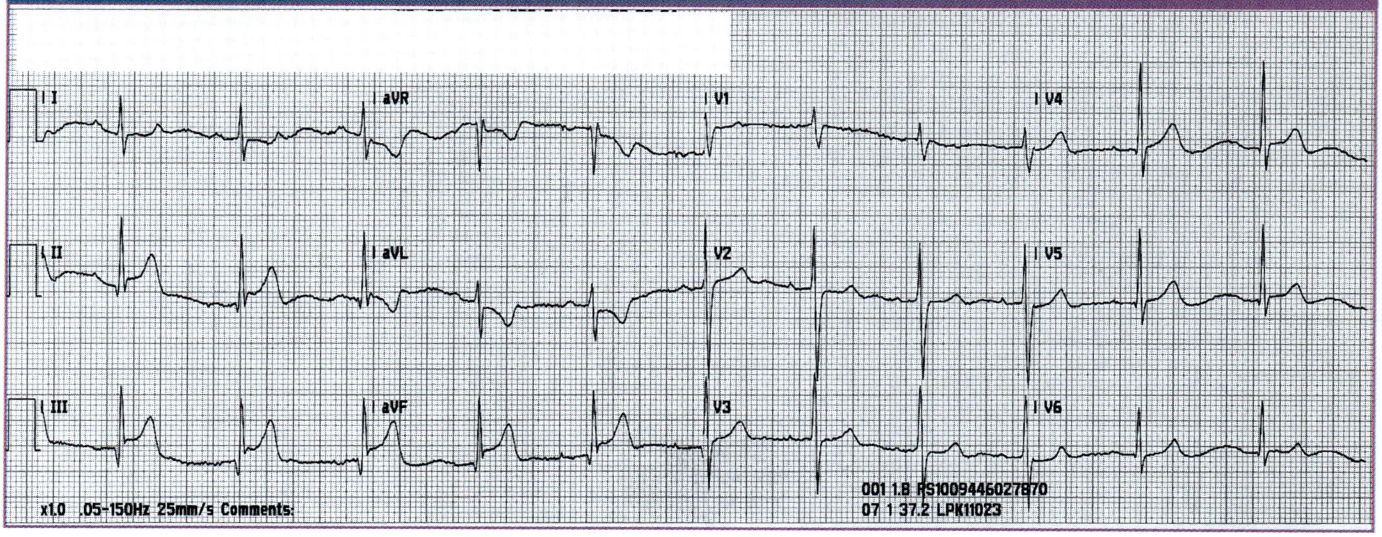

Interpretation /9-8

I

II

III

AVL

AVF

V1

V2

V3

V4

V5

V6

Fig 9-8: Interpretation

I	**Wandering baseline. No other changes noted.**
II	**Q wave ≥ 40 ms. ST segment elevation > 1 mm. Tall peaked T wave.**
III	**Q wave ≥ 40 ms. ST segment elevation > 1 mm. Tall peaked T wave.**
AVL	**ST segment depression. Inverted T wave.**
AVF	**Q wave ≥ 40 ms. ST segment elevation > 1 mm. Tall peaked T wave.**
V1	**Prominent R wave.**
V2	**Tall R wave.**
V3	**Tall R wave.**
V4	**Slight ST segment elevation < 1 mm.**
V5	**Slight ST segment elevation <1 mm.**
V6	**No changes noted.**

Comments:
Inferior infarction. Possible posterior infarct (tall R waves in V1-V3).

Fig 9-9

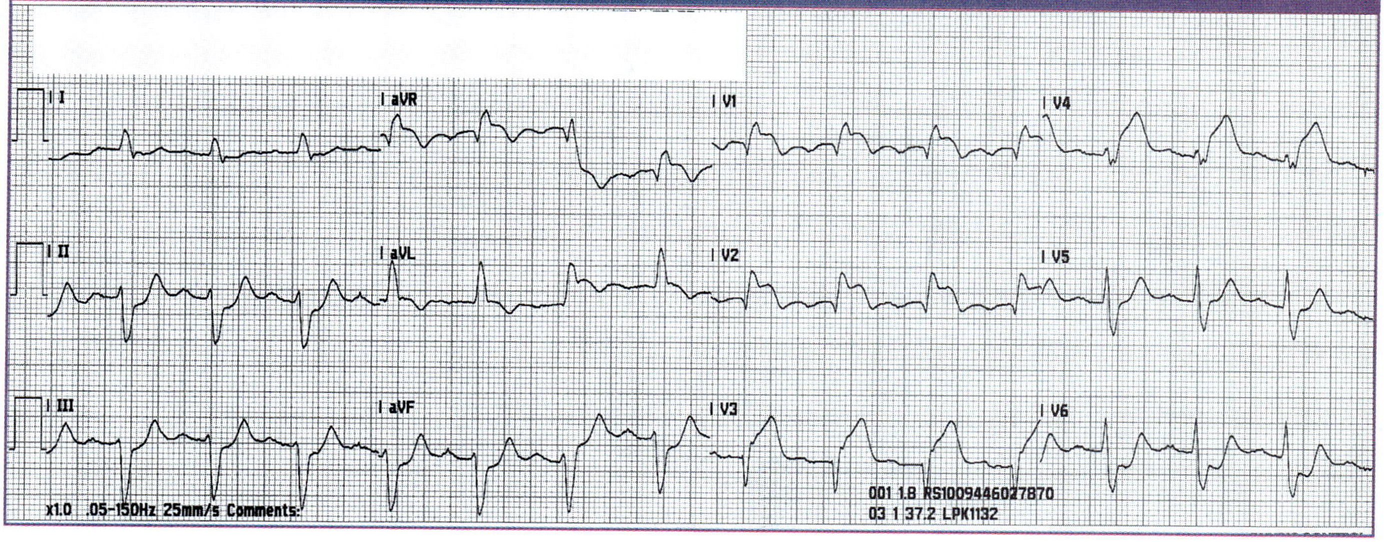

Interpretation /9-9

I

II

III

AVL

AVF

V1

V2

V3

V4

V5

V6

Fig 9-9: Interpretation

I	Slight ST segment depression. No other changes noted.
II	ST segment depression.
III	ST segment depression.
AVL	Inverted T wave.
AVF	ST segment depression.
V1	Q wave > 40 ms. ST segment elevation > 1 mm.
V2	Q wave > 40 ms. ST segment elevation > 1 mm.
V3	Q wave > 40 ms. ST segment elevation > 1 mm. Tall/peaked T wave.
V4	Poor R wave progression. ST segment elevation > 1 mm. Tall/peaked T wave.
V5	Poor R wave progression.
V6	ST segment depression.

Comments:
Anteroseptal infarct. Right bundle branch block.

Fig 9-10

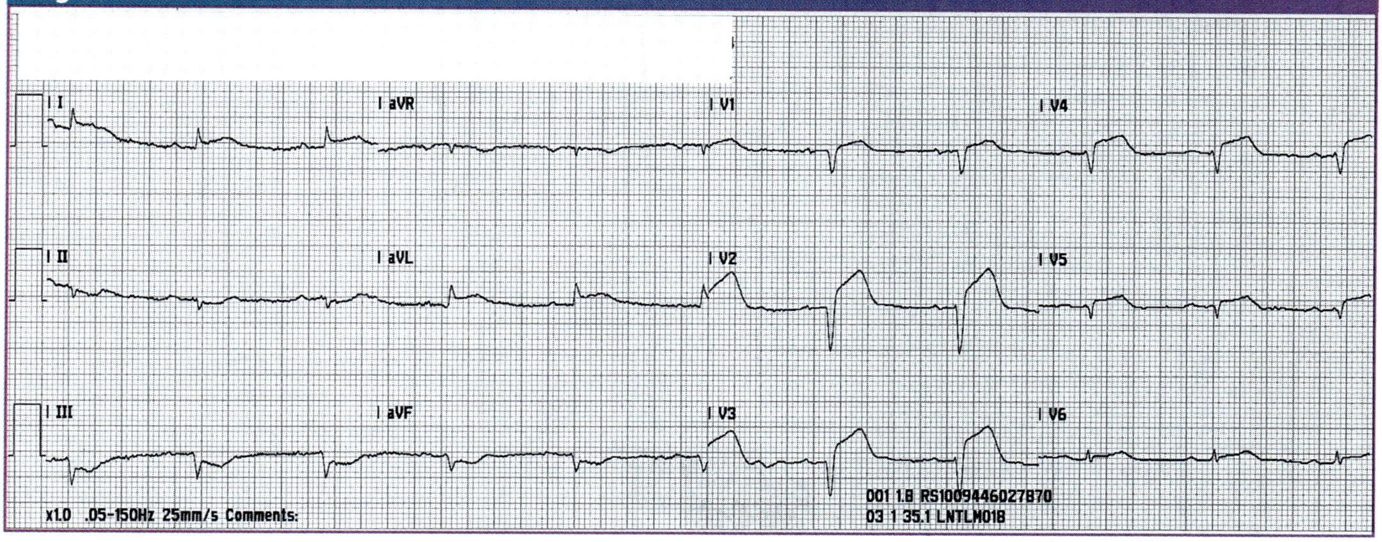

Interpretation /9-10

I

II

III

AVL

AVF

V1

V2

V3

V4

V5

V6

Fig 9-10: Interpretation

I	Low voltage. Baseline wander. Apparent ST segment elevation ≥ 1 mm.
II	Low voltage. Q wave > 40 ms.
III	Low voltage. Q wave > 40 ms vs. rS complex.
AVL	Low voltage. ST segment elevation > 1 mm.
AVF	Low voltage. Q wave > 40 ms vs. rS complex.
V1	Q wave. ST segment elevation ≥ 1 mm.
V2	Poor R wave progession. ST segment elevation > 1 mm.
V3	Poor R wave progression. ST segment elevation > 1 mm.
V4	Low voltage. Poor R wave progression. ST segment elevation > 1 mm.
V5	Low voltage. Poor R wave progression. ST segment elevation ≥ 1 mm.
V6	Low voltage. ST segment elevation < 1 mm.

Comments:
Extensive anterior infarct. Reciprocal changes. Possible previous inferior infarct.

Fig 9-11

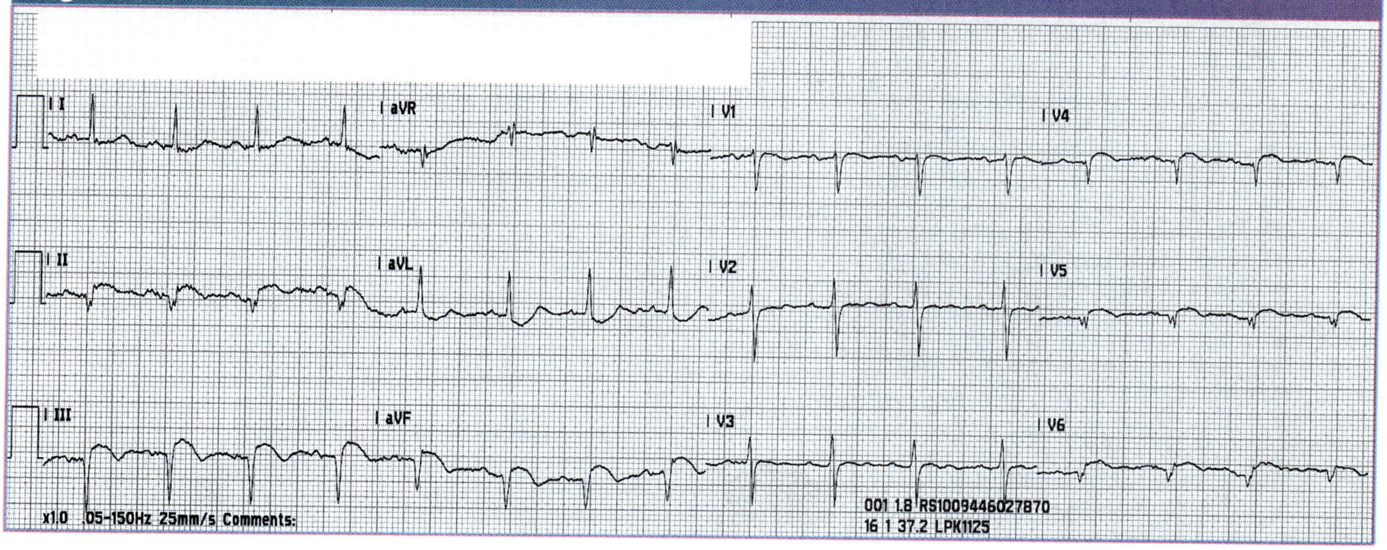

Interpretation /9-11

I

II

III

AVL

AVF

V1

V2

V3

V4

V5

V6

Fig 9-11: Interpretation

I	ST segment depression.
II	Q wave > 40 ms. ST segment elevation > 1 mm. Inverted T wave.
III	Q wave > 40 ms. ST segment elevation > 1 mm. Inverted T wave.
AVL	ST segment depression.
AVF	Q wave > 40 ms. ST segment elevation > 1 mm. Inverted T wave.
V1	ST segment elevation ≥ 1 mm.
V2	ST segment elevation ≤ 1 mm.
V3	Poor R wave progression.
V4	Low voltage. Q wave > 40 ms. ST segment elevation > 1 mm.
V5	Low voltage. Q wave > 40 ms. ST segment elevation ≥ 1 mm.
V6	Low voltage. Q wave > 40 ms. ST segment elevation > 1 mm.

Comments:

Inferolateral infarct. Possible right ventricular infarction (ST segment elevation greater in V1 than V2).

Fig 9-12

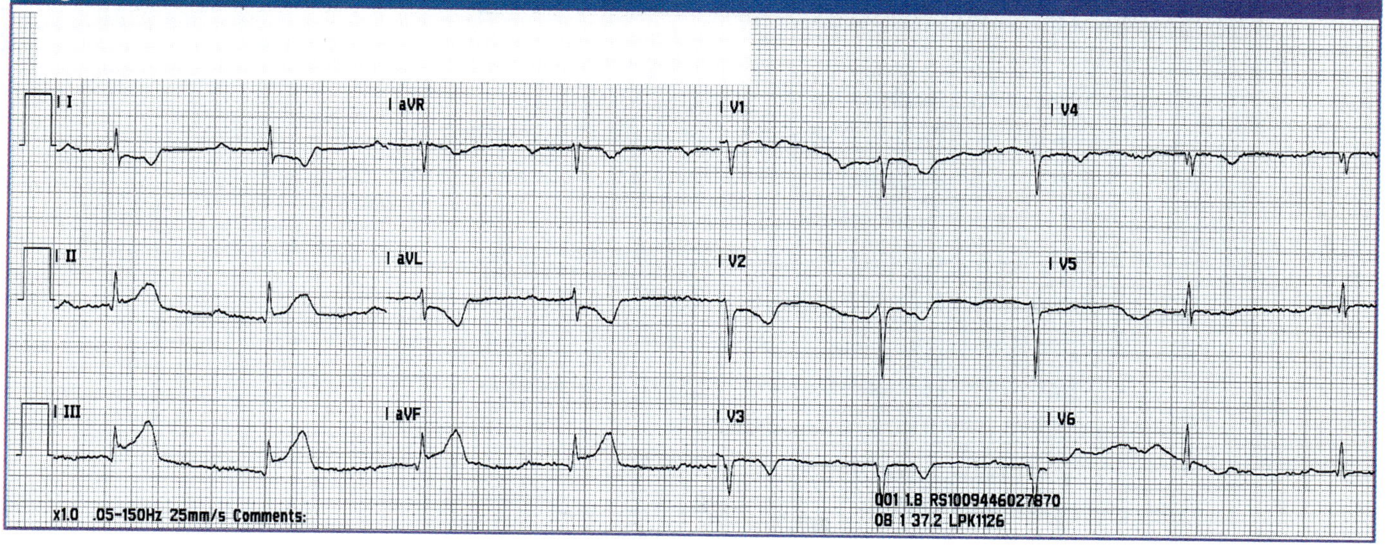

Interpretation /9-12

I

II

III

AVL

AVF

V1

V2

V3

V4

V5

V6

Fig 9-12: Interpretation

I	ST segment depression. Inverted T wave.
II	Q wave approaching 40 ms. ST segment elevation ≥ 1 mm.
III	Q wave approaching 40 ms. ST segment elevation > 1 mm. Tall/peaked T wave.
AVL	ST segment depression. Inverted T wave.
AVF	Q wave approaching 40 ms. ST segment elevation > 1 mm. Tall/peaked T wave.
V1	Baseline wander. No changes noted.
V2	Poor R wave progression. ST segment depression. T wave inversion.
V3	Poor R wave progression. ST segment depression. T wave inversion.
V4	Q wave < 40 ms. T wave inversion.
V5	Flattened T wave.
V6	Flattened T wave.

Comments:
Inferior infarct. Possible posterior wall infarct. Possible previous anteroseptal infarct (poor R wave progression).

Fig 9-13

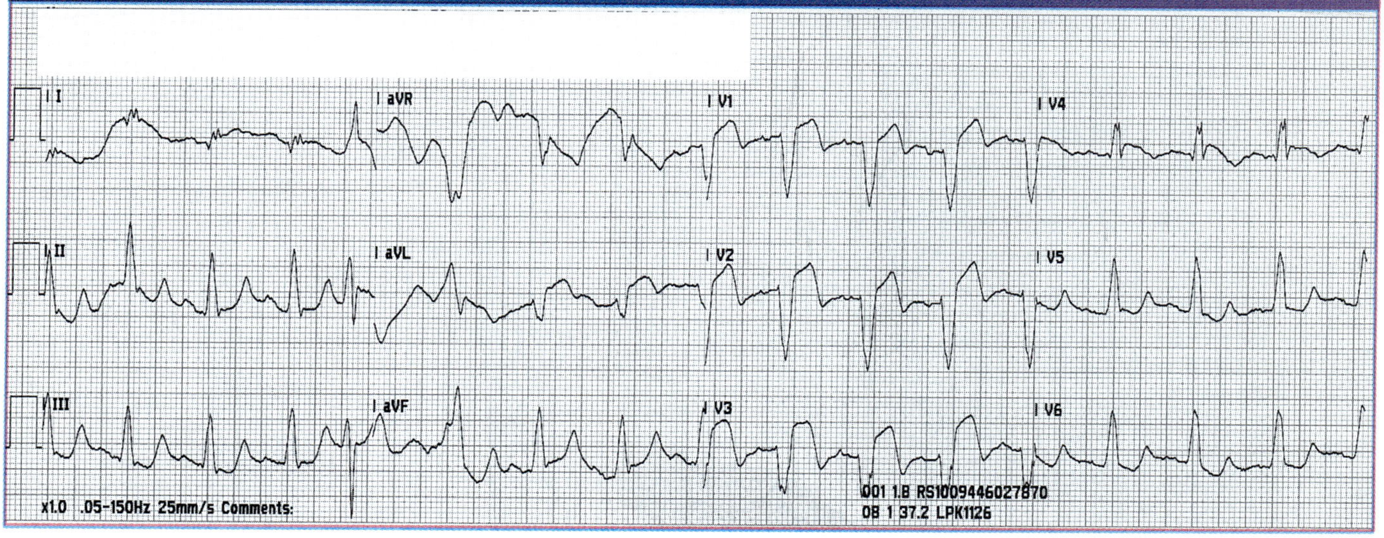

Interpretation /9-13

I

II

III

AVL

AVF

V1

V2

V3

V4

V5

V6

Fig 9-13: Interpretation

I	**Wandering baseline. Q wave ≥ 40 ms.**
II	**Wandering baseline. Peaked T wave.**
III	**Wandering baseline. Peaked T wave.**
AVL	**Wandering baseline. Apparent ST segment elevation > 1 mm.**
AVF	**Baseline wander. Peaked T wave. Further assessment difficult.**
V1	**ST segment elevation > 1 mm.**
V2	**Poor R wave progression. ST segment elevation > 1 mm. Inverted T wave (terminal force).**
V3	**Poor R wave progression. ST segment elevation > 1 mm. Inverted T wave (terminal force).**
V4	**ST segment elevation > 1 mm. Inverted T wave.**
V5	**Possible ST segment depression. T wave not oppositely directed from QRS.**
V6	**ST segment depression. T wave not oppositely directed from QRS.**

Comments:

Anteroseptal infarct. Left bundle branch block. Note how the T waves were not oppositely deflected from the QRS complex as is expected in bundle branch block.

Fig 9-14

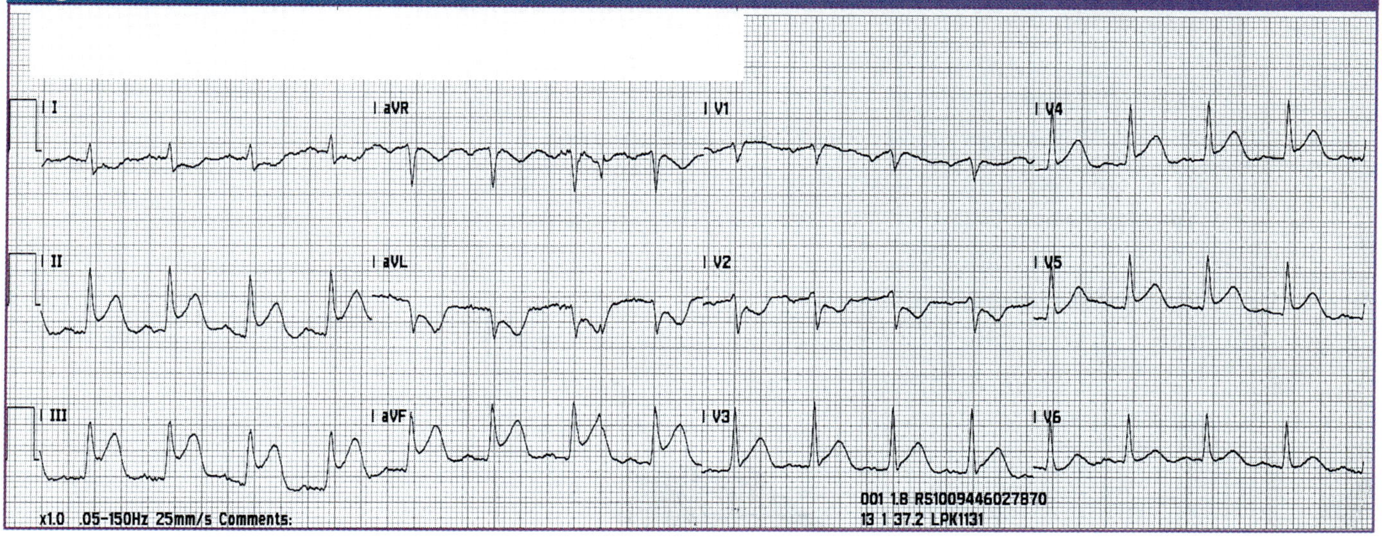

Interpretation /9-14

I

II

III

AVL

AVF

V1

V2

V3

V4

V5

V6

Fig 9-14: Interpretation

I	ST segment depression > 1 mm.
II	ST segment depression > 1 mm. T wave peaked.
III	ST segment elevation > 1 mm. T wave tall/peaked.
AVL	Q wave > 40 ms. ST segment depression > 1 mm. Inverted T wave.
AVF	ST segment elevation ≥ 1 mm. T wave tall/peaked.
V1	No indicative changes noted.
V2	ST segment depression > 1 mm. Inverted T wave.
V3	ST segment elevation ≥ 1 mm. T wave peaked.
V4	ST segment elevation > 1 mm. T wave peaked.
V5	ST segment elevation ≥ 1 mm. T wave peaked.
V6	No indicative changes noted.

Comments:
Inferio-Apical infarction.

Fig 9-15

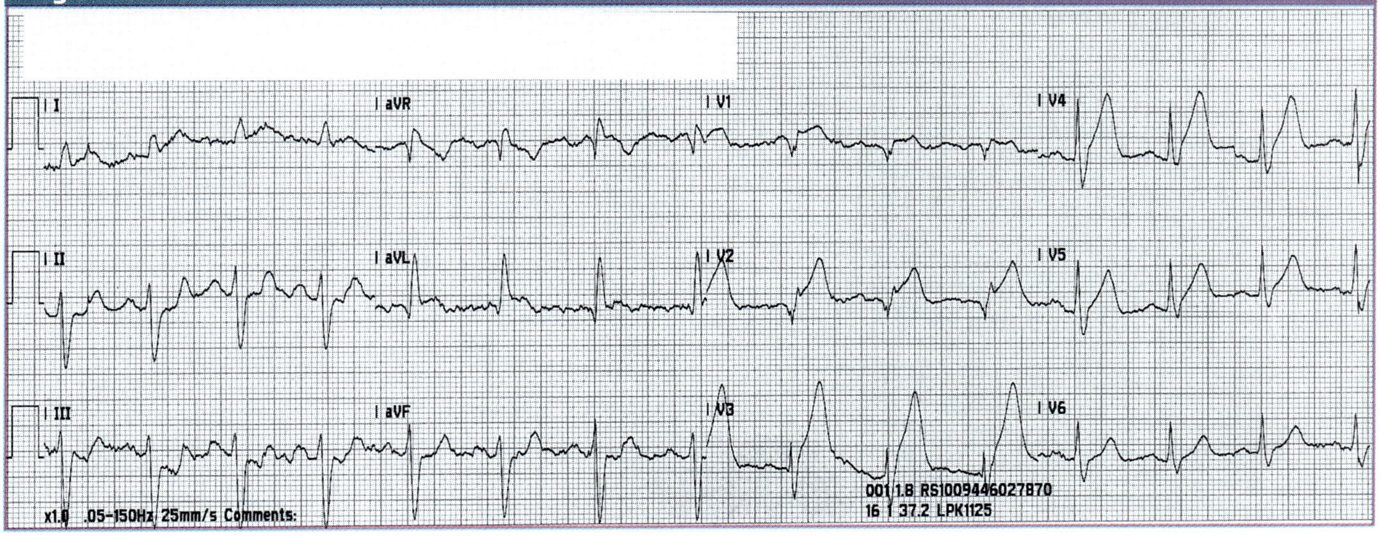

Interpretation /9-15

I

II

III

AVL

AVF

V1

V2

V3

V4

V5

V6

Fig 9-15: Interpretation

I	**Baseline wander and artifact. Further interpretation difficult.**
II	**Baseline wander. No indicative changes noted.**
III	**Baseline wander and artifact. No indicative changes noted.**
AVL	**Baseline artifact. Q wave ≥ 40 ms. Difficult to assess ST segment elevation due to artifact.**
AVF	**No indicative changes noted.**
V1	**No initial R wave. ST segment elevation.**
V2	**Q wave > 40 ms. ST segment elevation. Tall/peaked T wave.**
V3	**Q wave < 40 ms. ST segment elevation. Tall/peaked T wave.**
V4	**ST segment elevation. Tall/peaked T wave.**
V5	**ST segment elevation. Tall/peaked T wave.**
V6	**No indicative changes.**

Comments:
Anteroseptal infarct; extension into lateral wall. Right bundle branch block.

Fig 9-16

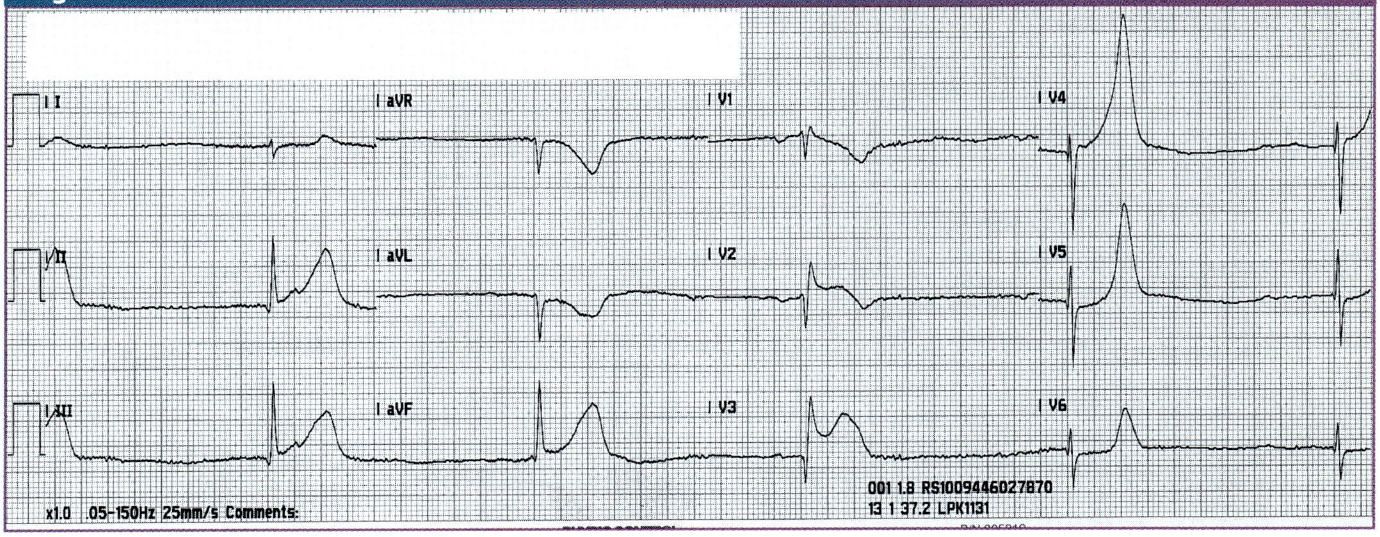

Interpretation /9-16

I

II

III

AVL

AVF

V1

V2

V3

V4

V5

V6

Fig 9-16: Interpretation

I	**No indicative changes.**
II	**Q wave ≥ 40 ms. ST segment elevation > 1 mm. Tall/ peaked T wave.**
III	**Q wave ≥ 40 ms. ST segment elevation > 1 mm. Tall/ peaked T wave.**
AVL	**ST segment depression. Inverted T wave.**
AVF	**Q wave < 40 ms. ST segment elevation > 1 mm. Tall/ peaked T wave.**
V1	**No indicative changes noted.**
V2	**Poor R wave progression. ST segment elevation > 1 mm. Inverted T wave (terminal force).**
V3	**Q wave > 40 ms. ST segment elevation > 1 mm. Tall T wave.**
V4	**Q wave < 40 ms. Apparent ST segment elevation ≥ 1 mm. Tall/peaked T wave.**
V5	**Q wave < 40 ms. Tall/peaked T wave.**
V6	**Q wave < 40 ms. Tall/peaked T wave.**

Comments:

Inferior infarct extending to the apex (boundary of the anterior wall and the inferior wall). RSR' pattern in V1, QRS duration < 120 ms, therefore no BBB is present. This is often referred to as incomplete BBB.

Fig 9-17

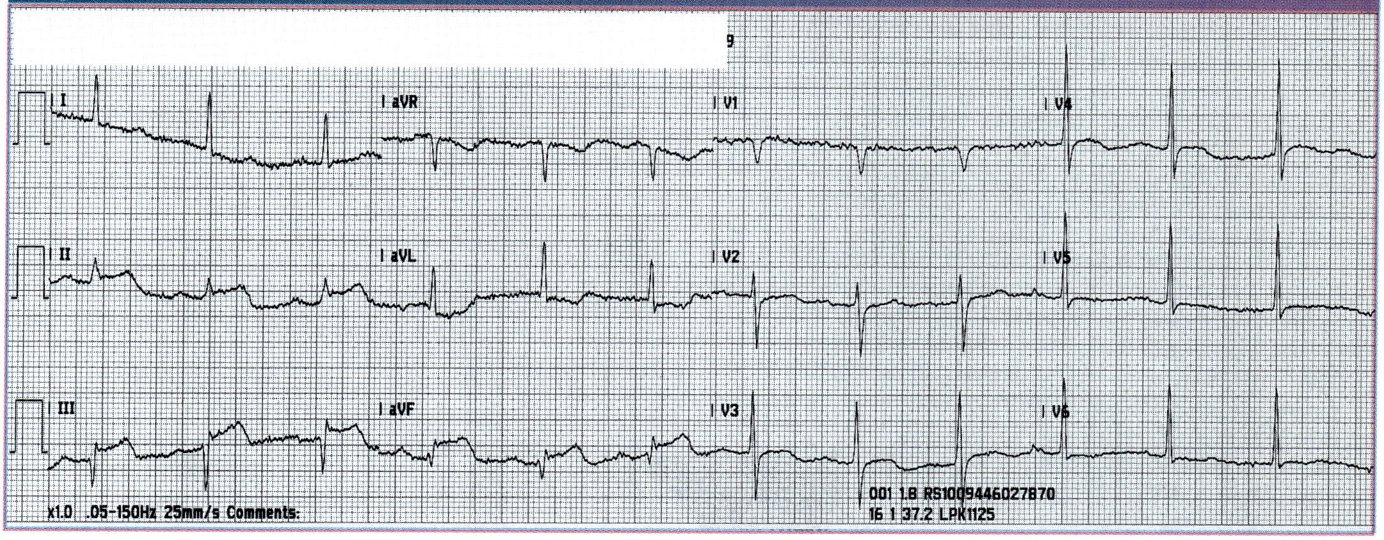

Interpretation /9-17

I

II

III

AVL

AVF

V1

V2

V3

V4

V5

V6

Fig 9-17: Interpretation

I	Baseline wander and artifact. No indicative changes noted.
II	Baseline wander and artifact. ST segment elevation > 1 mm.
III	Baseline wander and artifact. Q Wave ≥ 40 ms (initial R wave vs. artifact). ST segment elevation > 1 mm.
AVL	Baseline wander and artifact ST segment depression.
AVF	Baseline wander and artifact. Q Wave ≥ 40 ms (initial R wave vs. artifact). ST segment elevation > 1 mm.
V1	Baseline artifact. No indicative changes noted.
V2	No indicative changes noted.
V3	No indicative changes noted. Inverted T wave (terminal force).
V4	No indicative changes noted. Inverted T wave (terminal force).
V5	No indicative changes noted. Flattened T wave.
V6	No indicative changes noted. Flattened T wave.

Comments:
Inferior infarct. Possible posterior involvement.

Fig 9-18

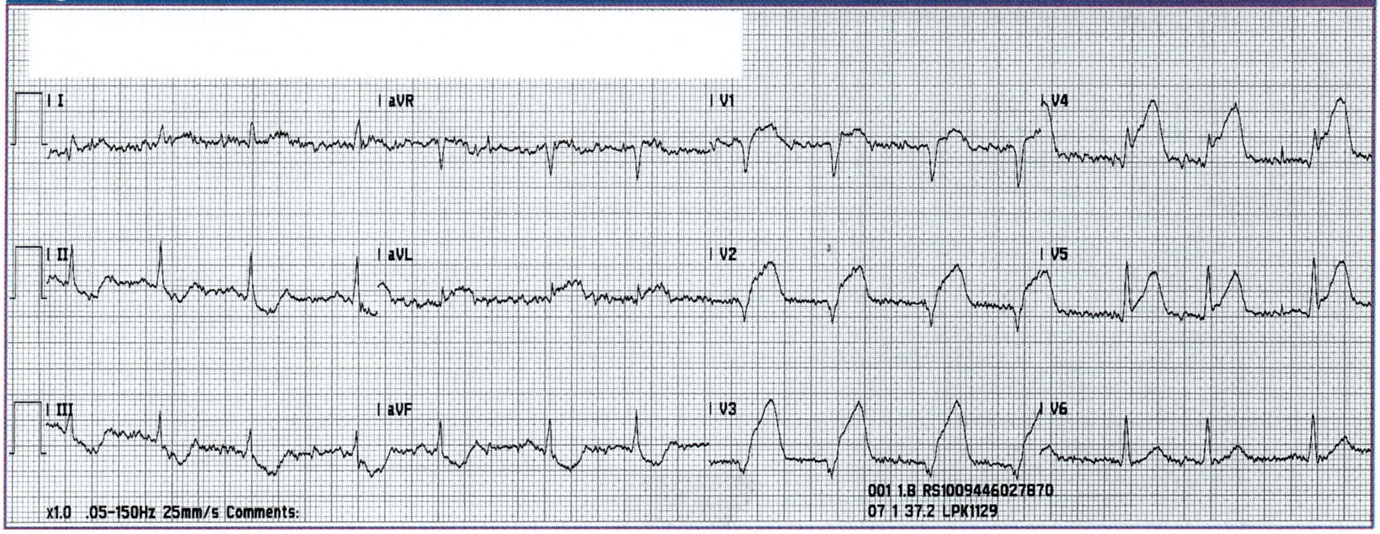

Interpretation /9-18

I

II

III

AVL

AVF

V1

V2

V3

V4

V5

V6

Fig 9-18: Interpretation

I	Baseline artifact. Unable to assess ST segment.
II	Baseline artifact. ST segment depression.
III	Baseline artifact. ST segment depression.
AVL	Baseline artifact. Apparent ST segment elevation > 1 mm.
AVF	Baseline artifact. ST segment depression.
V1	No initial R wave. ST segment elevation > 1 mm.
V2	Q wave > 40 ms. ST segment elevation > 1 mm. Tall T wave.
V3	Q wave > 40 ms. ST segment elevation > 1 mm. Tall/peaked T wave.
V4	Baseline artifact. Q wave ≥ 40 ms. ST segment elevation > 1 mm. Tall/peaked T wave.
V5	Baseline artifact. ST segment elevation ≥ 1 mm.
V6	Baseline artifact. No indicative changes noted.

Comments:
Anteroseptal infarct with lateral extension.

Fig 9-19

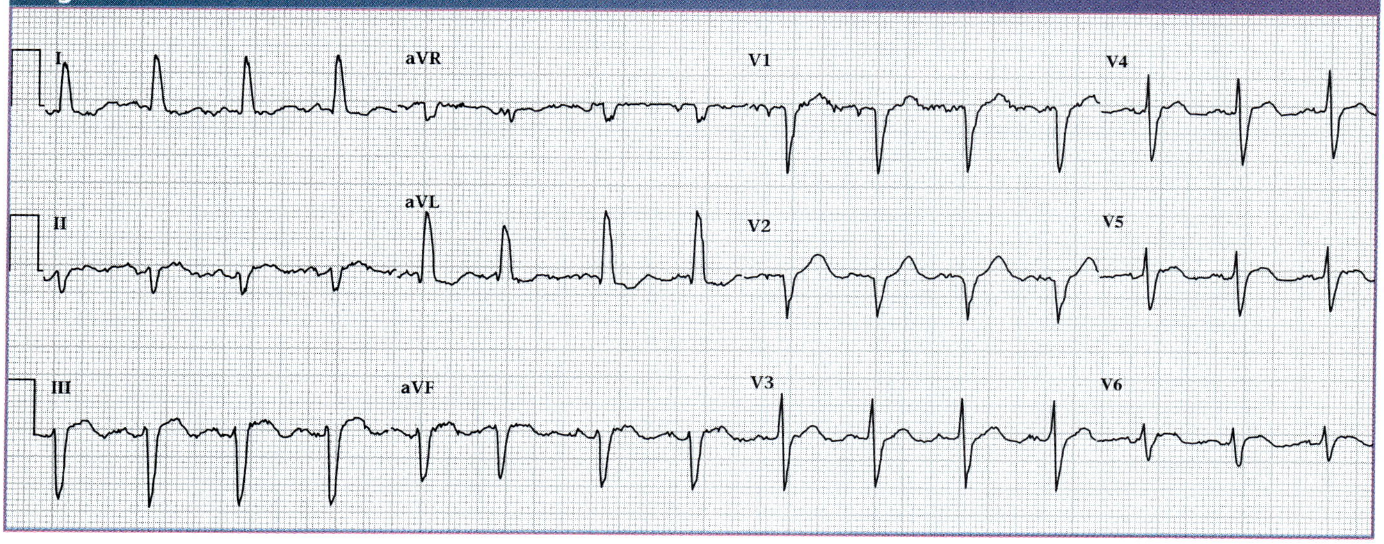

Interpretation /9-19

I

II

III

AVL

AVF

V1

V2

V3

V4

V5

V6

Fig 9-19: Interpretation

I	Q wave < 40 ms. No indicative changes noted.
II	Slight ST segment elevation (coving noted).
III	ST segment elevation ≥ 1 mm.
AVL	Q wave < 40 ms. ST segment depression.
AVF	ST segment elevation ≥ 1 mm.
V1	No indicative changes.
V2	Q wave > 40 ms.
V3	Poor R wave progression.
V4	Poor R wave progression. Inverted T wave (terminal force).
V5	Poor R wave progression. Inverted T wave (terminal force).
V6	Poor R wave progression.

Comments:
Left bundle branch block pattern. Inferior infarct. Possible previous anterior infarct.

Fig 9-20

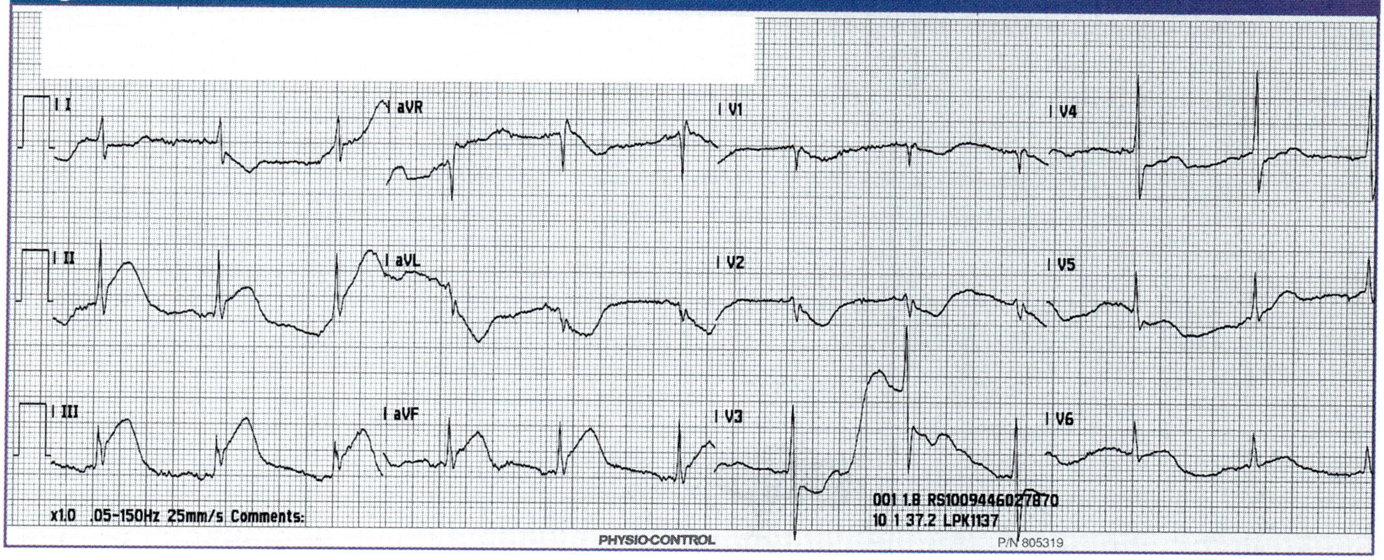

Interpretation /9-20

I

II

III

AVL

AVF

V1

V2

V3

V4

V5

V6

Fig 9-20: Interpretation

I	Baseline wander. Possible ST segment depression.
II	Baseline wander. ST segment elevation > 1 mm.
III	ST segment elevation > 1 mm. Tall/peaked T wave.
AVL	ST segment depression. Inverted T wave.
AVF	ST segment elevation. Tall Peaked T wave.
V1	Baseline wander. Possible ST segment depression.
V2	Poor R wave progression. ST segment depression. Inverted T wave.
V3	Tall R wave. ST segment depression.
V4	ST segment depression.
V5	Baseline wander. Difficult to assess ST segment.
V6	Baseline wander. Difficult to assess ST segment.

Comments:
Inferior infarct. Possible posterior infarct. Possible previous septal infarct.

Fig 9-21

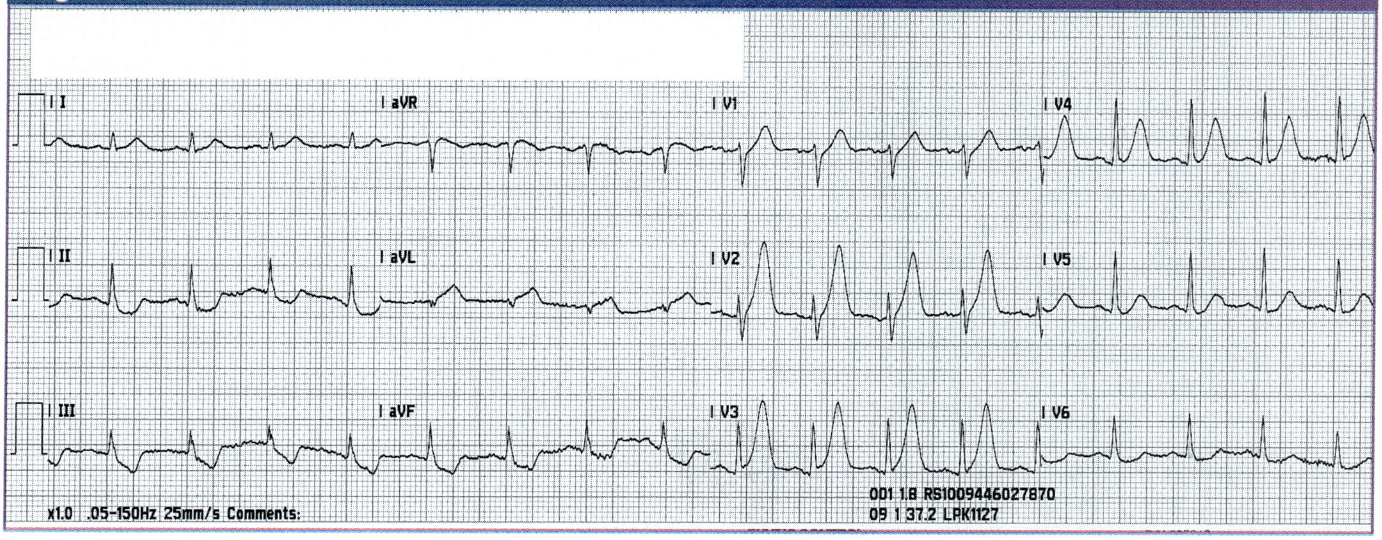

Interpretation /9-21

I

II

III

AVL

AVF

V1

V2

V3

V4

V5

V6

Fig 9-21: Interpretation

I	No indicative changes noted.
II	ST segment depression.
III	ST segment depression. T wave inversion.
AVL	Low voltage. ST segment elevation ≥ 1 mm.
AVF	ST segment depression. Inverted T wave.
V1	T wave slightly peaked. No other indicative changes noted.
V2	ST segment elevation ≥ 1 mm. Tall/peaked T wave.
V3	ST segment elevation ≥ 1 mm. Tall/peaked T wave.
V4	Tall /peaked T wave.
V5	Slight ST segment depression. No indicative changes noted.
V6	Slight ST segment depression. No indicative changes noted.

Comments:
Anteroseptal infarct with possible lateral extension. Reciprocal changes.

Fig 9-22

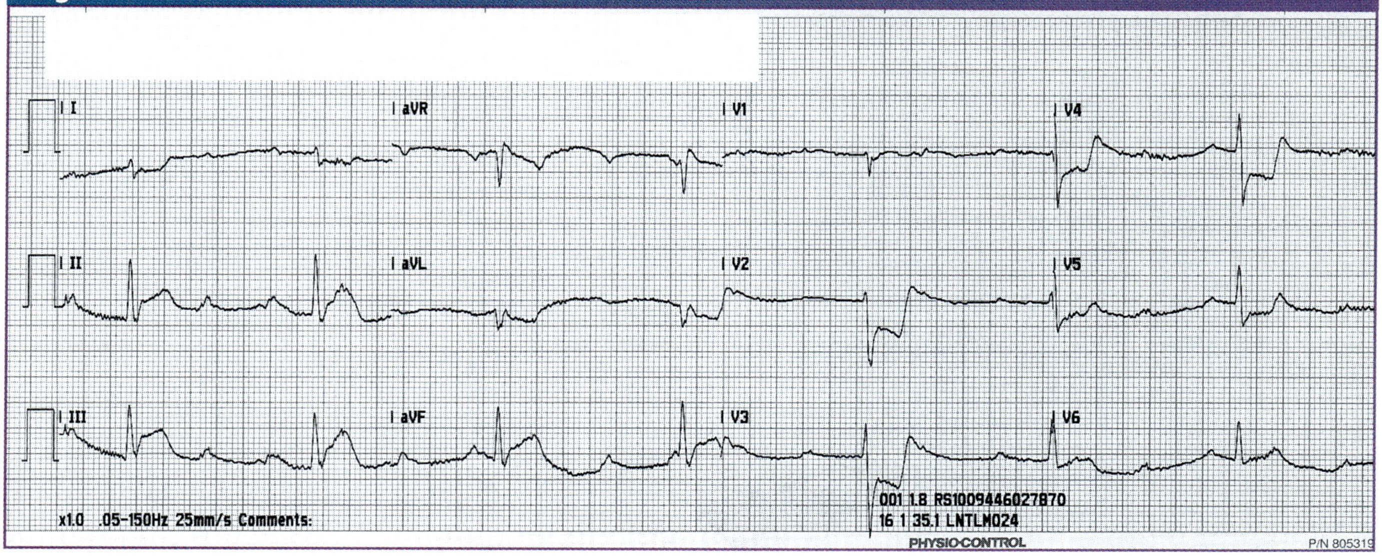

Interpretation /9-22

I

II

III

AVL

AVF

V1

V2

V3

V4

V5

V6

Fig 9-22: Interpretation

I	Baseline wander. ST segment depression.
II	Baseline wander. Apparent ST segment elevation ≥ 1 mm.
III	Baseline wander. Apparent ST segment elevation > 1 mm.
AVL	ST segment depression.
AVF	ST segment elevation ≥ 1 mm.
V1	No indicative changes noted.
V2	ST segment depression.
V3	ST segment depression.
V4	Poor R wave progression. ST segment depression.
V5	ST segment depression.
V6	No indicative changes noted.

Comments:

Inferior infarct. Possible posterior infarct. Note: Third degree AV block present with escape rhythm present. QRS complex width appraches 120 ms but ST segment elevation is not likely produced by a ventricular rhythm because T waves are not oppositely directed from QRS.

Fig 9-23

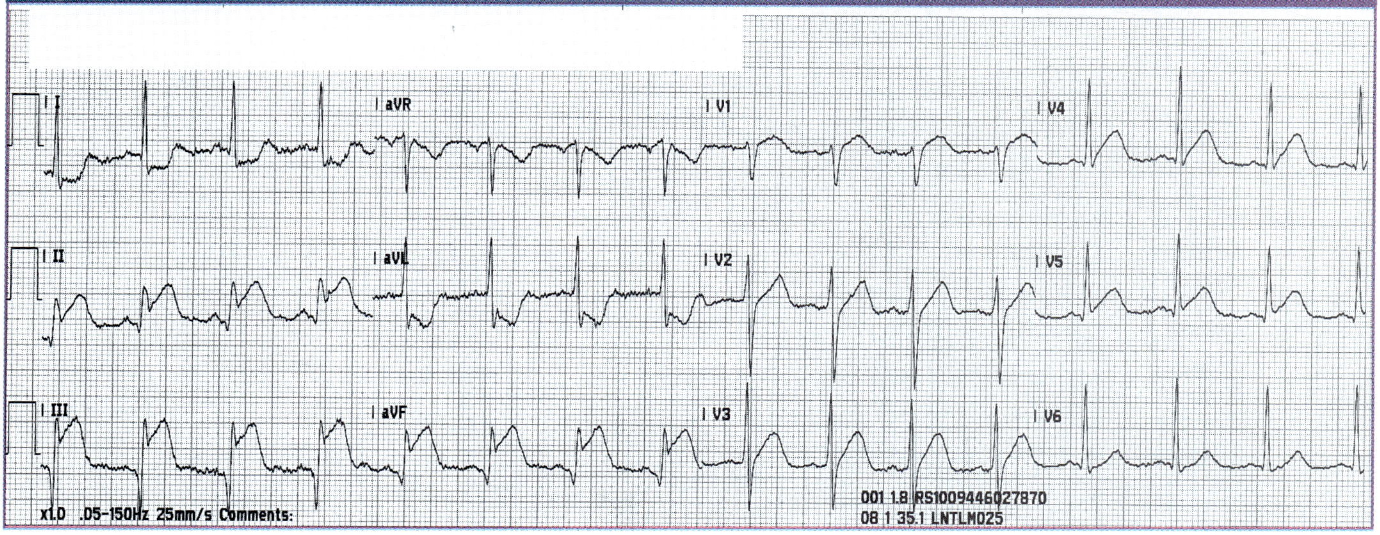

Interpretation /9-23

I

II

III

AVL

AVF

V1

V2

V3

V4

V5

V6

Fig 9-23: Interpretation

I	Baseline artifact. ST segment depression.
II	Q wave ≤ 40 ms. ST segment elevation > 1 mm. Tall/peaked T wave.
III	Q wave > 40 ms. ST segment elevation > 1 mm. Tall/peaked T wave.
AVL	ST segment depression.
AVF	Q wave > 40 ms. ST segment elevation. Tall/peaked T wave.
V1	ST segment elevation ≥ 1 mm.
V2	Tall R wave. Peaked T wave.
V3	Tall R wave. ST segment elevation > 1 mm.
V4	Tall R wave. ST segment elevation > 1 mm.
V5	Q wave < 40 ms. ST segment elevation > 1 mm.
V6	No indicative changes noted.

Comments:
Inferior infarct. Possible right ventricular infarction (ST elevation in V1 > V2). Possible posterior infarct (tall R waves in early precordial leads). Possible apical infarct (coving V3 and V4).

Fig 9-24

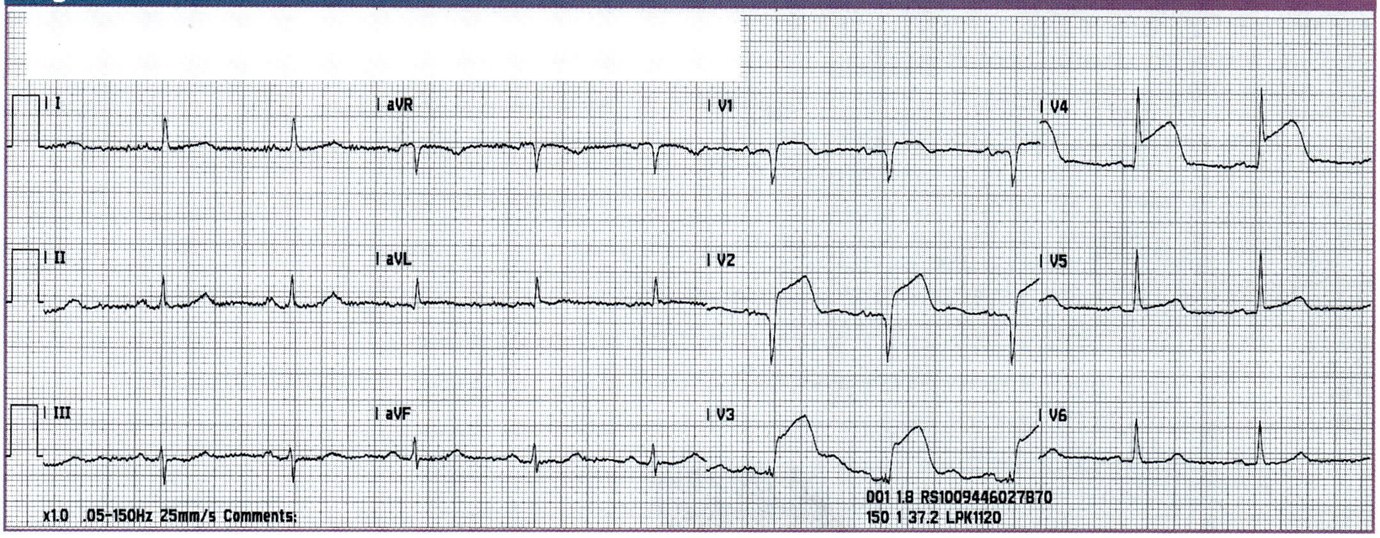

Interpretation /9-24

I

II

III

AVL

AVF

V1

V2

V3

V4

V5

V6

Fig 9-24: Interpretation

I	No indicative changes noted.
II	No indicative changes noted.
III	No indicative changes noted.
AVL	Q wave < 40 ms. Slight ST segment elevation (well < 1 mm). Flat T wave.
AVF	No indicative changes noted.
V1	No initial R wave. ST segment elevation > 1 mm.
V2	Q wave > 40 ms. ST segment elevation > 1 mm. Tall/peaked T wave.
V3	Poor R wave progression. ST segment elevation > 1 mm. Tall/peaked T wave.
V4	ST segment elevation > 1 mm. Tall /peaked T wave.
V5	ST segment elevation ≥ 1 mm.
V6	No indicative changes noted.

Comments:
Anteroseptal infarct. Slight lateral extension (changes in V5).

Fig 9-25

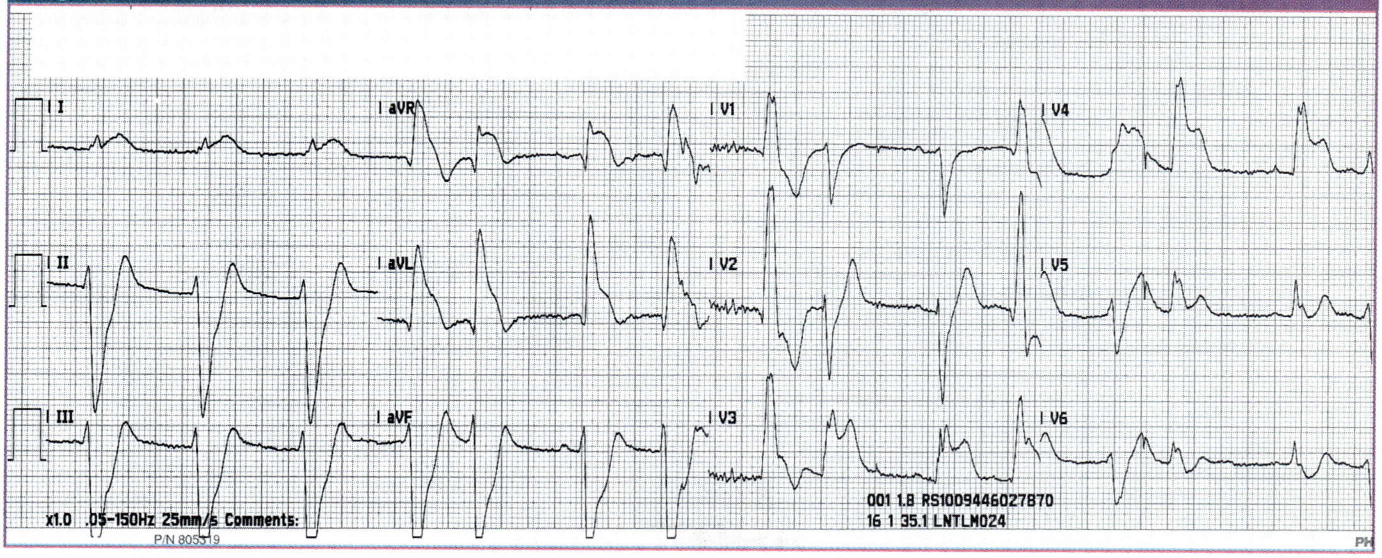

Interpretation /9-25

I

II

III

AVL

AVF

V1

V2

V3

V4

V5

V6

Fig 9-25: Interpretation

I	Low voltage. ST segment elevation ≥ 1 mm.
II	St segment depression. Peaked T wave.
III	ST segment depression. Peaked T wave.
AVL	Q wave ≥ 40 ms. ST segment elevated > 1 mm. Inverted T wave.
AVF	ST segment depression. Peaked T wave.
V1	No indicative changes noted.
V2	ST segment depression. Peaked T wave.
V3	ST segment elevation > 1 mm. Tall/peaked T wave.
V4	ST segment elevation. Peaked T wave.
V5	Peaked T wave.
V6	ST segment depression.

Comments:
Anterolateral infarct. (Some beats ectopic, others used for interpretation.) Left bundle branch block present, but not cause of ST segment elevation in V3 and V4 (T wave not oppositely directed from QRS).

Fig 9-26

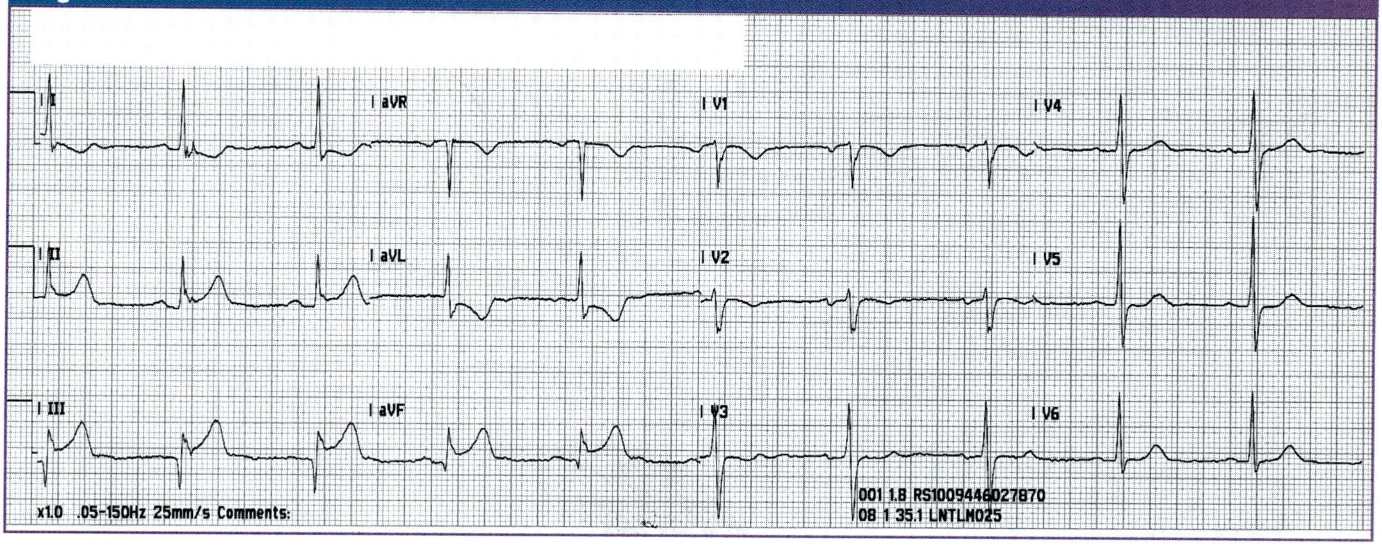

Interpretation /9-26

I

II

III

AVL

AVF

V1

V2

V3

V4

V5

V6

Fig 9-26: Interpretation

I	ST segment depression.
II	ST segment elevation > 1 mm. Peaked T wave
III	Q wave ≥ 40 ms. ST segment elevation > 1 mm. Tall/ peaked T wave.
AVL	ST segment depression. Inverted T wave.
AVF	Q wave ≥ 40 ms. ST segment elevation > 1 mm. Peaked T wave.
V1	No indicative changes.
V2	Inverted T wave. No other indicative changes.
V3	Rapid increase in R wave height from V2. No indicative changes noted.
V4	No indicative changes noted.
V5	No indicative changes noted.
V6	No indicative changes noted.

Comments:
Inferior infarct.

Fig 9-27

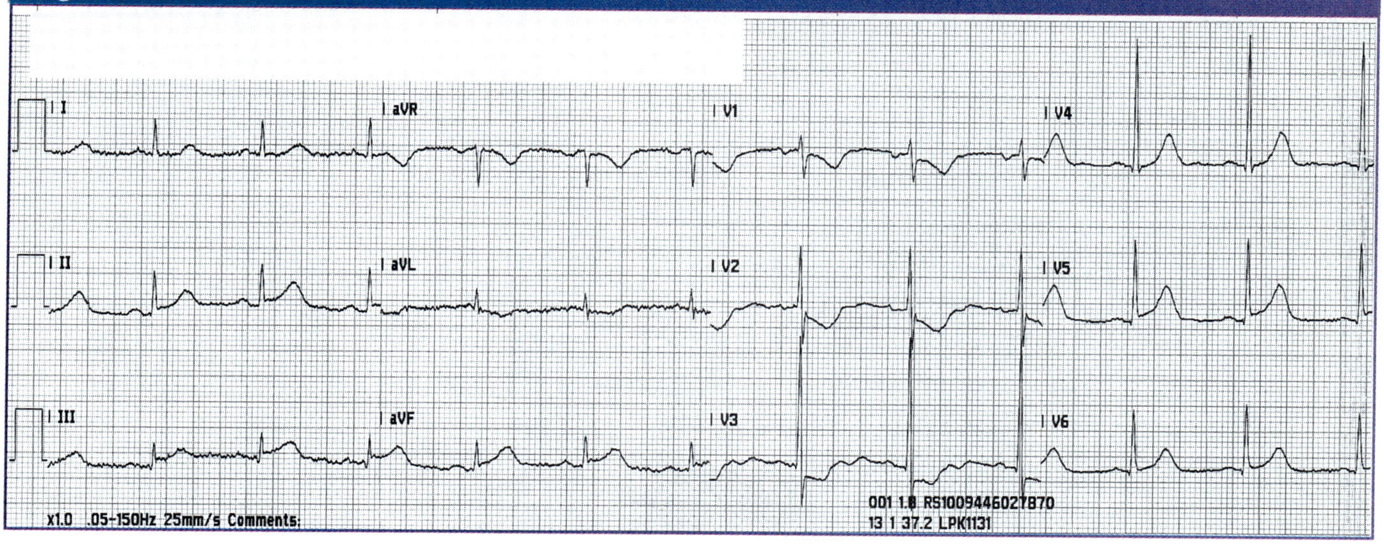

Interpretation /9-27

I

II

III

AVL

AVF

V1

V2

V3

V4

V5

V6

Fig 9-27: Interpretation

I	Baseline artifact. No indicative changes noted.
II	ST segment elevation ≥ 1 mm.
III	Q wave approaching 40 ms. ST segment elevation ≥ 1 mm.
AVL	No indicative changes.
AVF	ST segment elevation ≥ 1 mm.
V1	ST segment depression.
V2	Tall R wave. ST segment depression. Inverted T wave.
V3	Tall R wave. ST segment depression. Inverted T wave.
V4	Tall R wave. Peaked T wave.
V5	ST segment elevation ≥ 1 mm. Peaked T wave.
V6	ST segment elevation < 1 mm.

Comments:
Inferior infarct with suspected lateral extension. Possible posterior infarct.

Fig 9-28

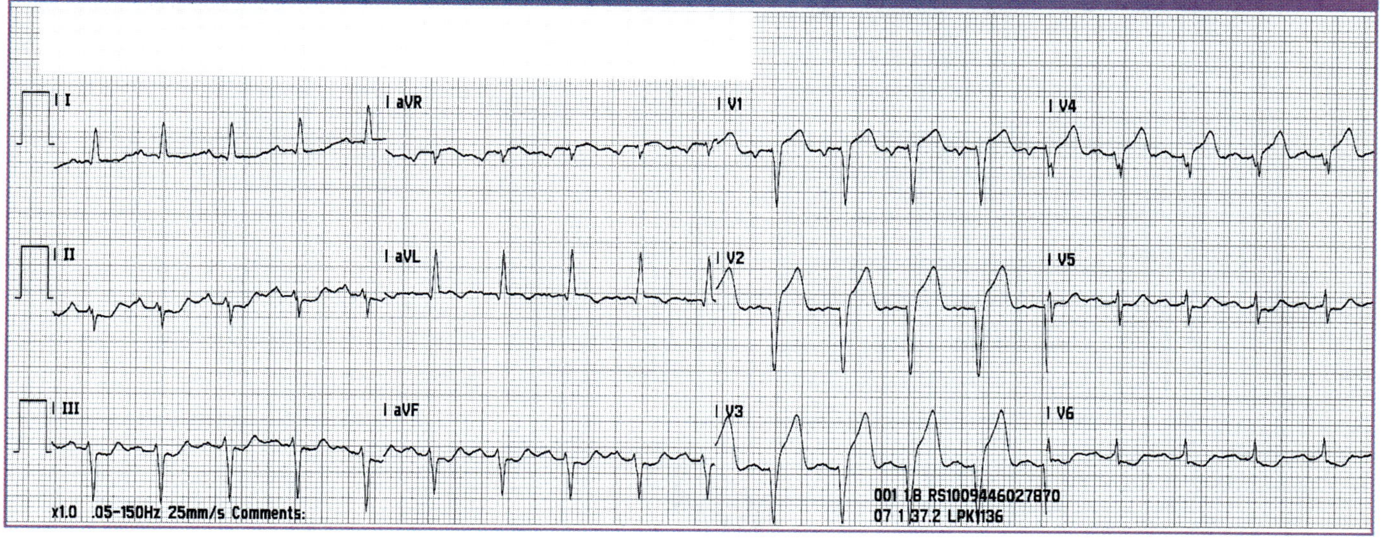

Interpretation /9-28

I

II

III

AVL

AVF

V1

V2

V3

V4

V5

V6

Fig 9-28: Interpretation

I	Q wave < 40 ms.
II	ST segment depression.
III	ST segment depression.
AVL	Q wave ≤ 40 ms.
AVF	ST segment depression.
V1	ST segment elevation > 1 mm.
V2	Poor R wave progression. ST segment elevation > 1 mm. Tall/peaked T wave
V3	Poor R wave progression. ST segment elevation > 1 mm. Tall/peaked T wave.
V4	Poor R wave progression. ST segment elevation > 1 mm. Peaked T wave.
V5	Low voltage. Poor R wave progression. ST segment depression.
V6	Low voltage. ST segment depression.

Comments:
Anteroseptal infarct. Reciprocal changes noted.

Fig 9-29

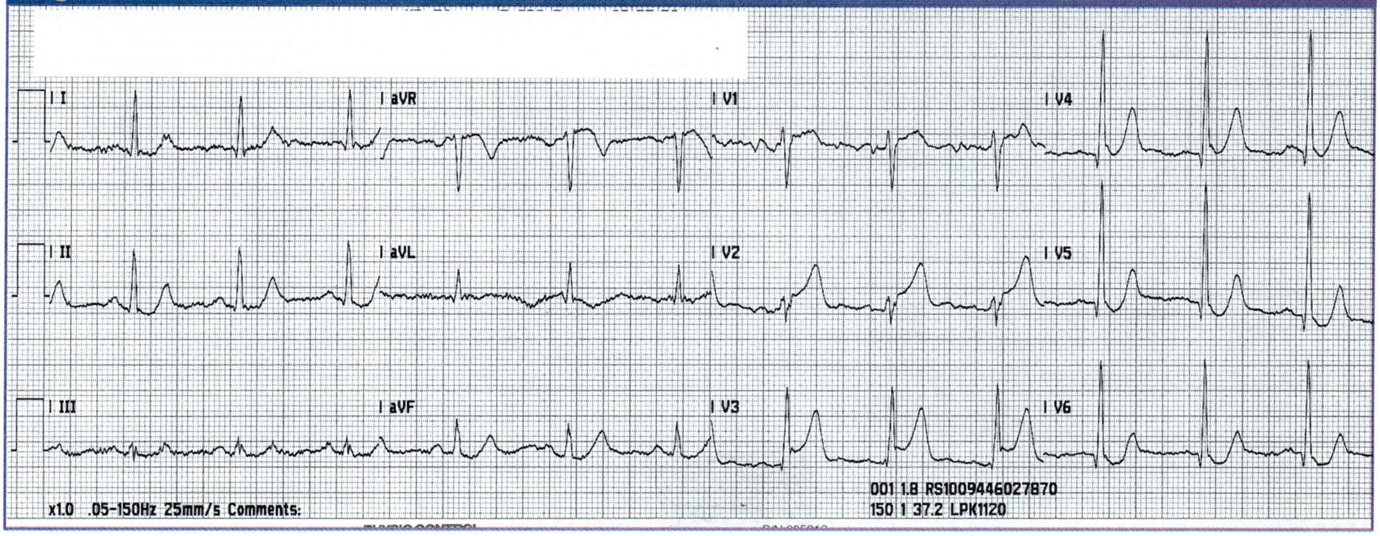

Interpretation /9-29

I

II

III

AVL

AVF

V1

V2

V3

V4

V5

V6

Fig 9-29: Interpretation

I	**Baseline artifact. No indicative changes noted.**
II	**Baseline artifact. Peaked T wave.**
III	**Baseline artifact. Further description difficult.**
AVL	**Baseline artifact. Apparent inverted T wave.**
AVF	**Peaked T wave.**
V1	**Baseline artifact. ST segment elevation > 1 mm.**
V2	**ST segment elevation > 1 mm. Tall/peaked T wave.**
V3	**Q wave < 40 ms. Tall R wave. ST segment elevation > 1 mm. Tall/peaked T wave.**
V4	**Q wave approaching 40 ms. Tall/peaked T wave.**
V5	**Q wave ≥ 40 ms. ST segment depression. Peaked T wave.**
V6	**Q wave ≥ 40 ms. ST segment depression. Peaked T wave.**

Comments:
Anteroseptal infarct. Possible previous lateral infarct. Nearing voltage criteria for LVH. Pattern similar to early repolarization.

Fig 9-30

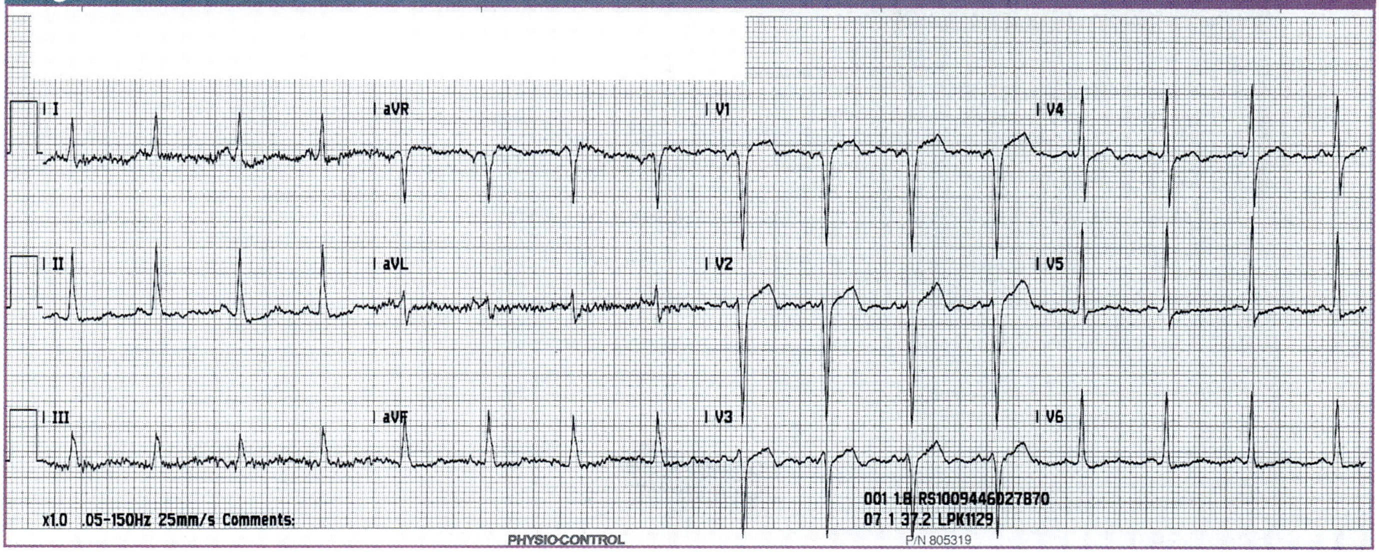

Interpretation /9-30

I

II

III

AVL

AVF

V1

V2

V3

V4

V5

V6

Fig 9-30: Interpretation

I	Baseline artifact. No further description possible.
II	Baseline artifact. No indicative changes noted.
III	Baseline artifact. No indicative changes noted.
AVL	Baseline artifact. No further description possible.
AVF	Baseline artifact. No indicative changes noted.
V1	Baseline artifact. ST segment elevation ≥ 1 mm.
V2	Poor R wave progression. ST segment elevation ≥ 1 mm.
V3	Poor R wave progression. T wave inversion (terminal force).
V4	Inverted T wave (terminal force).
V5	Flat T wave. No indicative changes noted.
V6	Flat T wave. No indicative changes noted.

Comments:
Septal infarct. Meets voltage criteria for LVH.

Fig 9-31

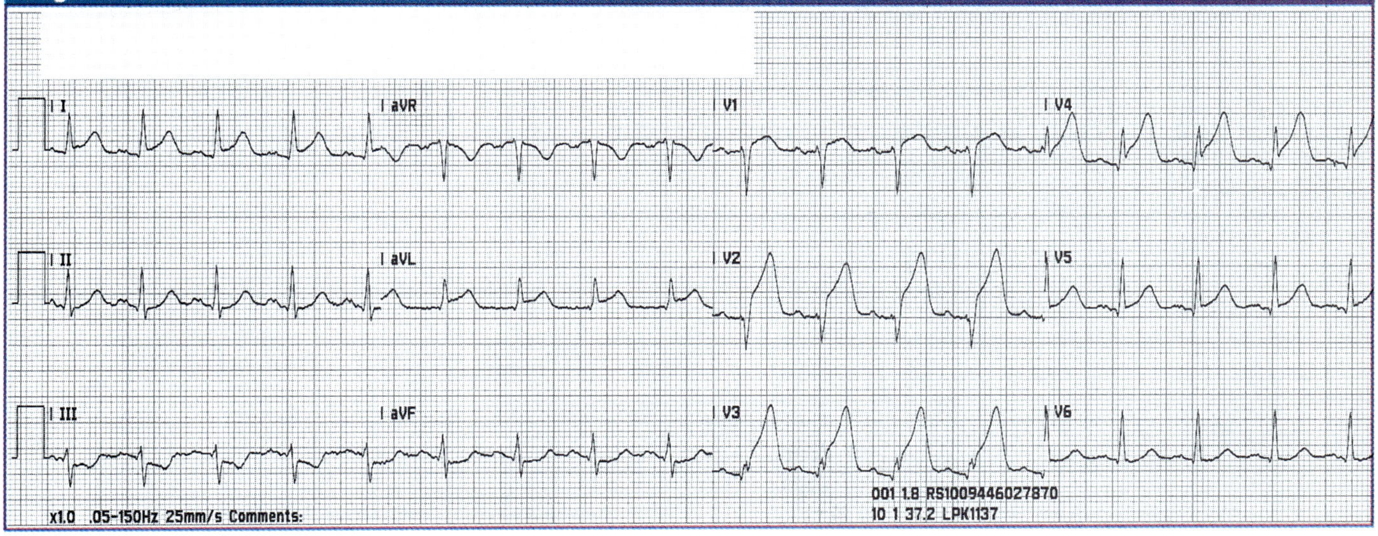

Interpretation /9-31

I

II

III

AVL

AVF

V1

V2

V3

V4

V5

V6

Fig 9-31: Interpretation

I	ST segment elevation ≥ 1 mm.
II	Slight ST segment depression.
III	ST segment depression. Inverted T wave.
AVL	Q wave < 40 ms. ST segment elevation > 1 mm.
AVF	ST segment depression.
V1	ST segment elevation > 1 mm.
V2	R wave regression. ST segment elevation > 1 mm. Tall/peaked T wave.
V3	Q wave < 40 ms. ST segment elevation > 1 mm. Tall/peaked T wave.
V4	Q wave < 40 ms. ST segment elevation > 1 mm. Tall/peaked T wave.
V5	Slight ST segment elevation < 1 mm.
V6	No indicative changes noted.

Comments:
Anteroseptal infarct. Reciprocal changes present.

Fig 9-32

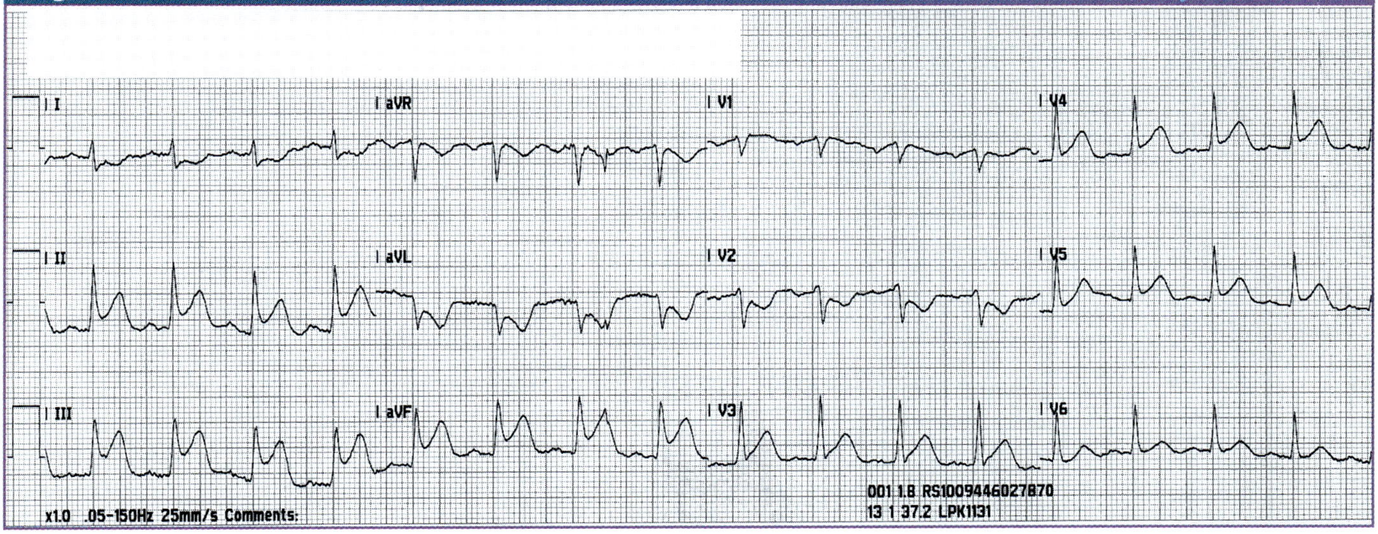

Interpretation /9-32

I

II

III

AVL

AVF

V1

V2

V3

V4

V5

V6

Fig 9-32: Interpretation

I	ST segment depression.
II	ST segment elevation > 1 mm. Peaked T wave.
III	ST segment elevation > 1 mm. Peaked T wave.
AVL	Q wave > 40 ms. ST segment depression. Inverted T wave.
AVF	ST segment elevation > 1 mm. Peaked T wave.
V1	No indicative changes noted.
V2	Minimal R wave. ST segment depression. T wave inversion.
V3	Early transition. ST segment elevation ≥ 1 mm. Peaked T wave.
V4	ST segment elevation > 1 mm. Peaked T wave.
V5	ST segment elevation ≥ 1 mm.
V6	No indicative changes noted.

Comments:
Inferior infarct with extension to apical region.

Fig 9-33

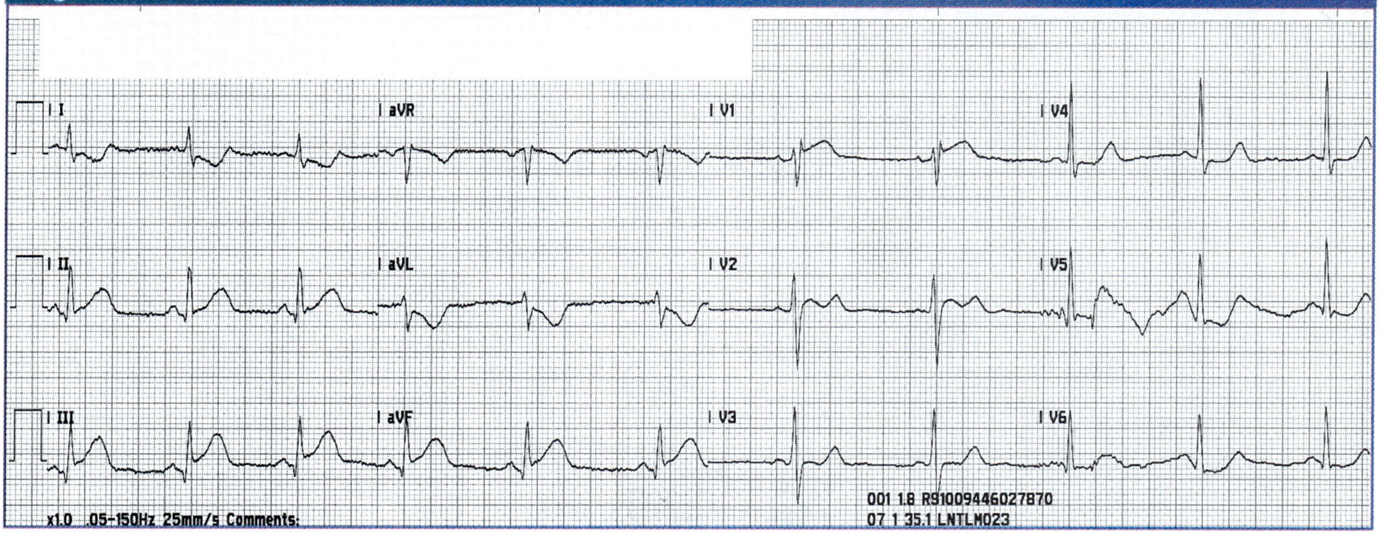

Interpretation /9-33

I

II

III

AVL

AVF

V1

V2

V3

V4

V5

V6

Fig 9-33: Interpretation

I	ST segment depression. Inverted T wave.
II	Q wave < 40 ms. ST segment elevation approaching 1 mm.
III	Q wave ≥ 40 ms. ST segment elevation > 1 mm.
AVL	ST segment depression. Inverted T wave.
AVF	Q wave < 40 ms. ST segment elevation ≥ 1 mm.
V1	ST segment elevation > 1 mm. Upright T wave.
V2	ST segment elevation ≥ 1 mm.
V3	Tall R wave.
V4	Tall R wave.
V5	Baseline wander. Possible ST segment depression.
V6	Baseline wander. Possible ST segment depression.

Comments:
Inferior infarct. Possible right ventricular infarct (ST segment elevation > in V1 than V2). Possible posterior infarction (early transition).

Fig 9-34

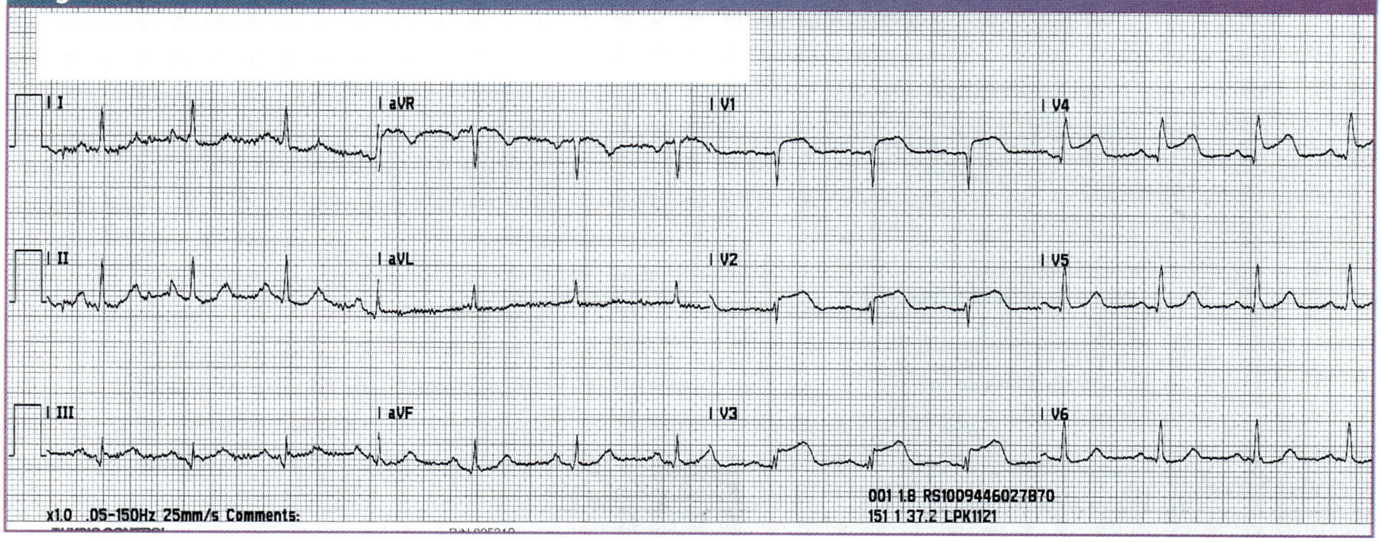

Interpretation /9-34

I

II

III

AVL

AVF

V1

V2

V3

V4

V5

V6

Fig 9-34: Interpretation

I	Baseline wander and artifact.
II	Baseline artifact (Q wave present?) ST segment depression.
III	Baseline artifact. Q wave > 40 ms (artifact vs. small initial R wave).
AVL	Baseline artifact. Flattened T wave.
AVF	Q wave ≥ 40 ms.
V1	No initial R wave. ST segment elevation > 1 mm.
V2	ST segment elevation > 1 mm.
V3	Poor R wave progression. ST segment elevation > 1 mm.
V4	Q wave < 40 ms. ST segment elevation > 1 mm.
V5	Q wave < 40 ms.
V6	No indicative changes noted.

Comments:

Anteroseptal infarct. Possible previous inferior infarct.

Fig 9-35

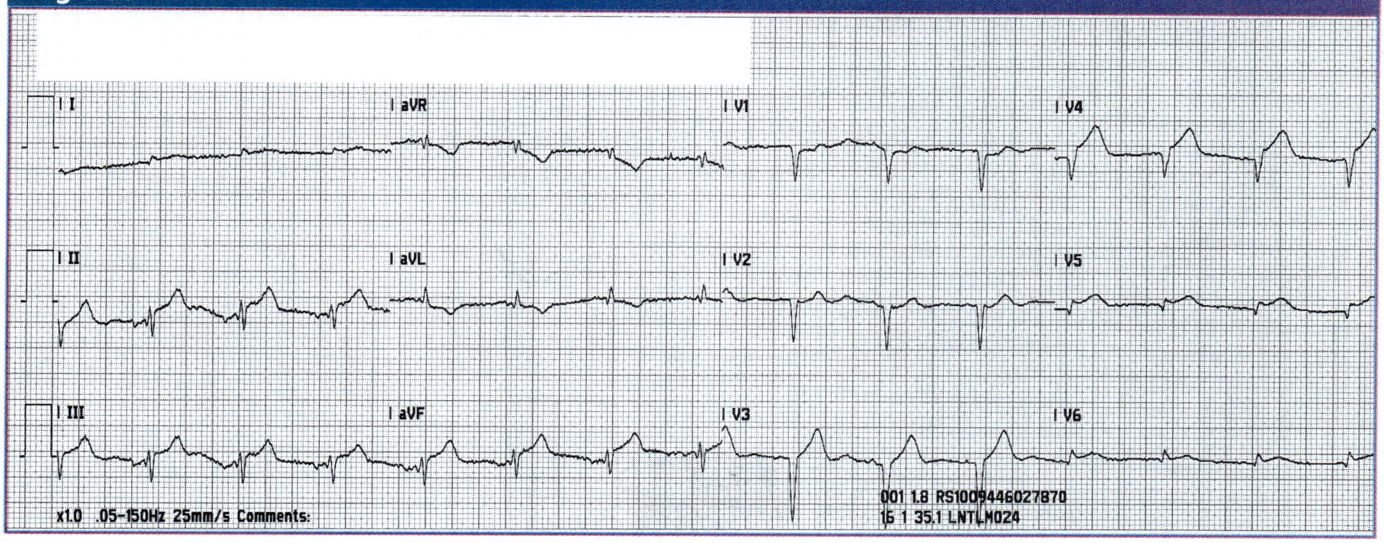

Interpretation /9-35

I

II

III

AVL

AVF

V1

V2

V3

V4

V5

V6

Fig 9-35: Interpretation

I	Low amplitude. Baseline wander. Difficult to assess.
II	ST segment elevation > 1 mm. Peaked T wave.
III	ST segment elevation ≥ 1 mm. Peaked T wave.
AVL	Inverted T wave.
AVF	ST segment elevation > 1 mm. Peaked T wave.
V1	ST segment depression. Upright T wave.
V2	Q wave > 40 ms.
V3	Q wave > 40 ms. Peaked T wave.
V4	Q wave > 40 ms. Peaked T waves. ST segment elevation > 1 mm.
V5	ST segment elevation ≥ 1 mm.
V6	Slight ST segment elevation.

Comments:
Low voltage throughout tracing. Inferior infarct, lateral extension.

Fig 9-36

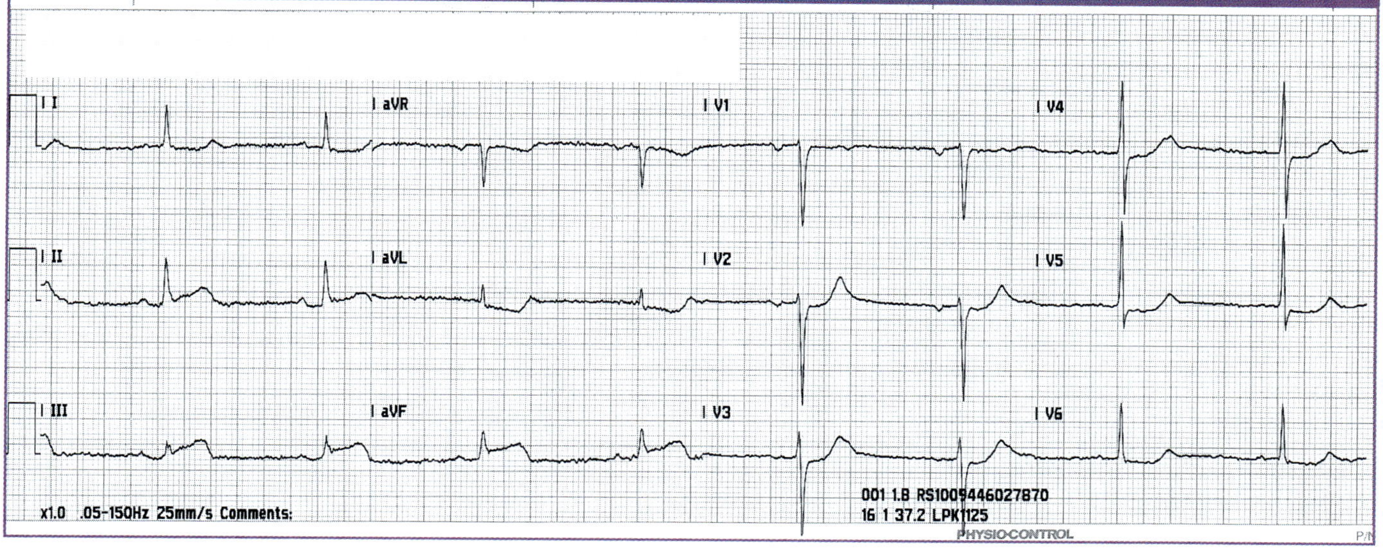

Interpretation /9-36

I

II

III

AVL

AVF

V1

V2

V3

V4

V5

V6

Fig 9-36: Interpretation

I	No indicative changes.
II	ST segment elevation > 1 mm.
III	ST segment elevation > 1 mm.
AVL	Low voltage. ST segment depression.
AVF	ST segment elevation > 1 mm.
V1	No indicative changes.
V2	ST segment depression. Minimal R wave progression.
V3	ST segment depression. Minimal R wave progression.
V4	ST segment depression.
V5	ST segment depression.
V6	ST segment depression.

Comments:

Inferior infarct.

Fig 9-37

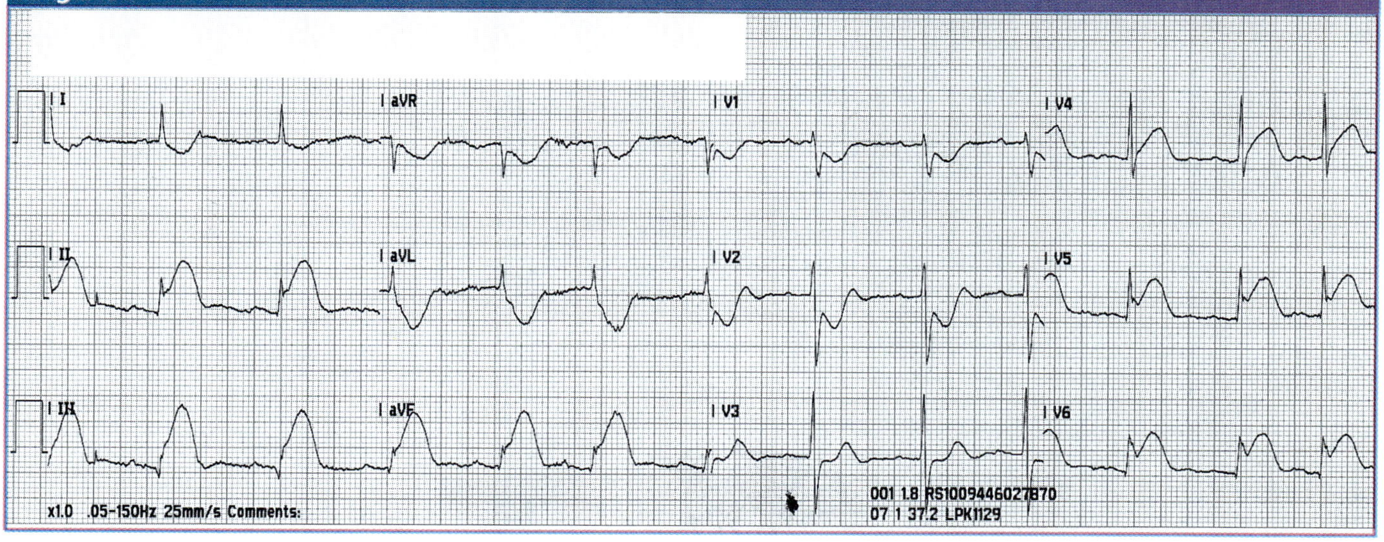

Interpretation /9-37

I

II

III

AVL

AVF

V1

V2

V3

V4

V5

V6

Fig 9-37: Interpretation

I	ST segment depression ≥ 1 mm.
II	ST segment elevation > 1 mm. Tall T wave.
III	Q wave > 40 ms. ST segment elevation > 1 mm.
AVL	ST segment depression. T wave inversion.
AVF	Q wave < 40 ms. ST segment elevation > 1 mm.
V1	ST segment depression > 1 mm.
V2	ST segment depression > 1 mm.
V3	No indicative changes.
V4	ST segment elevation > 1 mm.
V5	ST segment elevation > 1 mm. T wave tall/peaked.
V6	ST segment elevation > 1 mm. T wave tall/peaked.

Comments:
Inferior infarct with lateral extension. Possible posterior infarct.

Fig 9-38

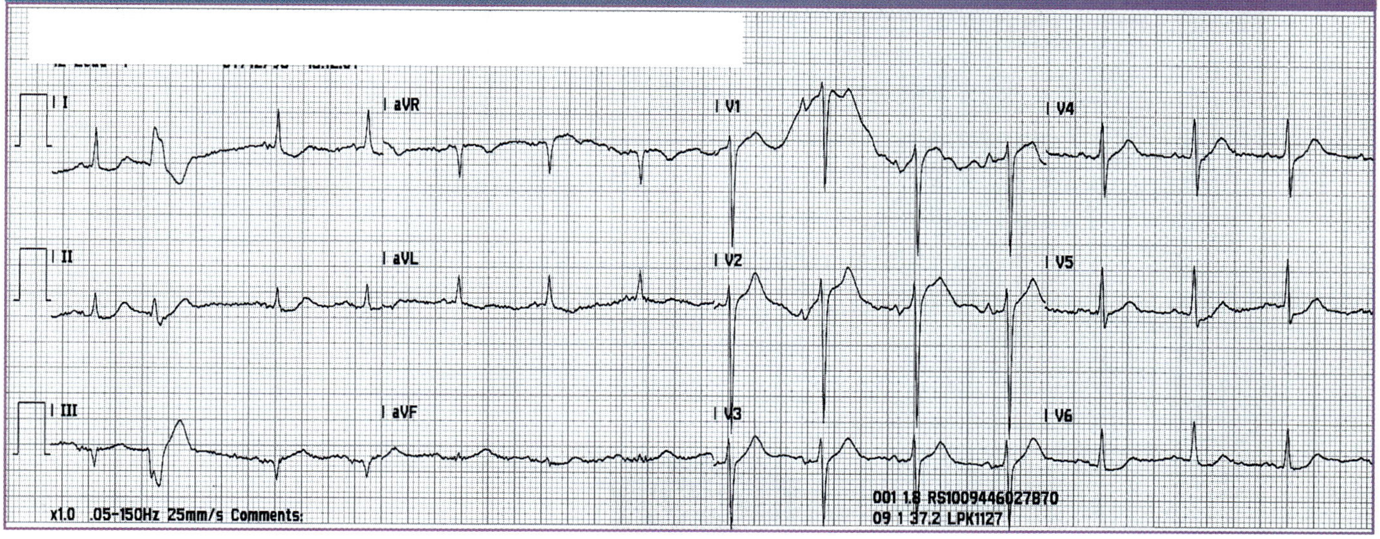

Interpretation /9-38

I

II

III

AVL

AVF

V1

V2

V3

V4

V5

V6

Fig 9-38: Interpretation

I	ST segment depression.
II	ST segment depression.
III	Q wave > 40 ms.
AVL	Slight ST segment depression.
AVF	Low voltage. Difficult to assess.
V1	Baseline wander. Apparent ST segment elevation ≥ 1 mm.
V2	ST segment elevation > 1 mm.
V3	Poor R wave progression.
V4	ST segment depression.
V5	ST segment depression.
V6	Slight ST segment depression.

Comments:

Septal infarct. Reciprocal changes noted. Possible previous inferior wall infarct (Q in lead 3)?

Fig 9-39

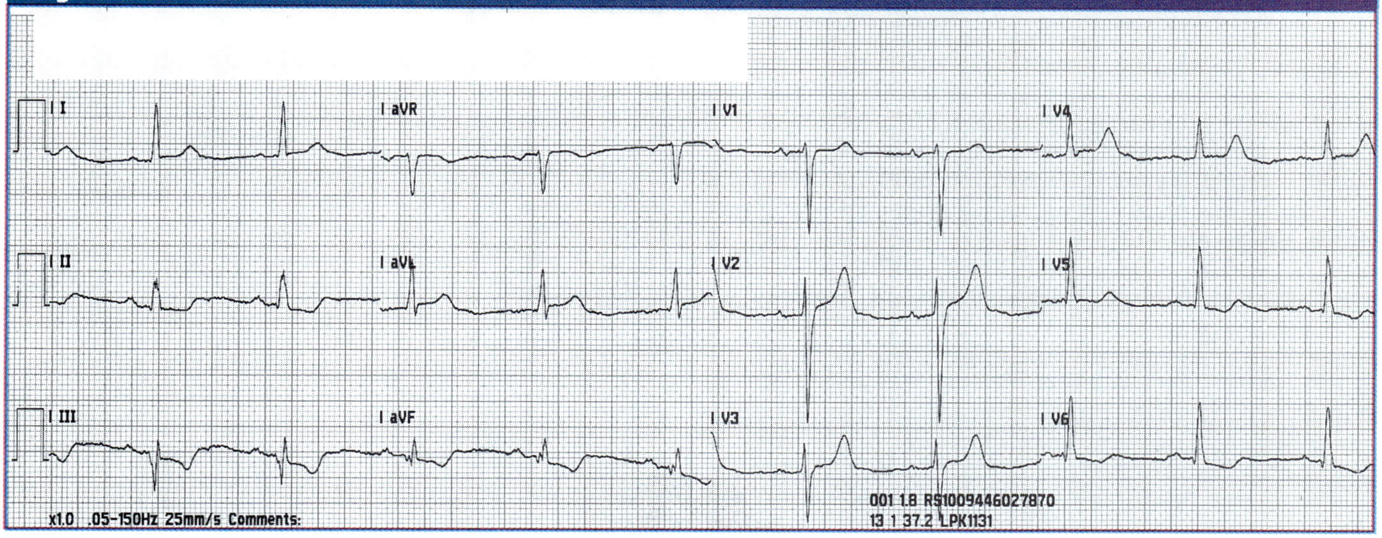

Interpretation /9-39

I

II

III

AVL

AVF

V1

V2

V3

V4

V5

V6

Fig 9-39: Interpretation

I	Baseline wander. ST segment elevated ≤ 1 mm.
II	Q wave < 40 ms. ST segment depression.
III	Q wave > 40 ms. ST segment depression. T wave inversion.
AVL	ST segment elevation ≥ 1 mm.
AVF	Q wave approaching 40 ms. ST segment depression. T wave inversion.
V1	No indicative changes noted.
V2	ST segment elevation > 1 mm. Tall/peaked T wave.
V3	Poor wave progression. ST segment ≥ 1 mm. Peaked T wave.
V4	ST segment elevation ≤ 1 mm. Peaked T wave.
V5	ST segment depression.
V6	ST segment depression.

Comments:
Anteroseptal infarction, changes also noted in one lateral lead. Possible previous inferior infarct. Possible posterior infarct.

Fig 9-40

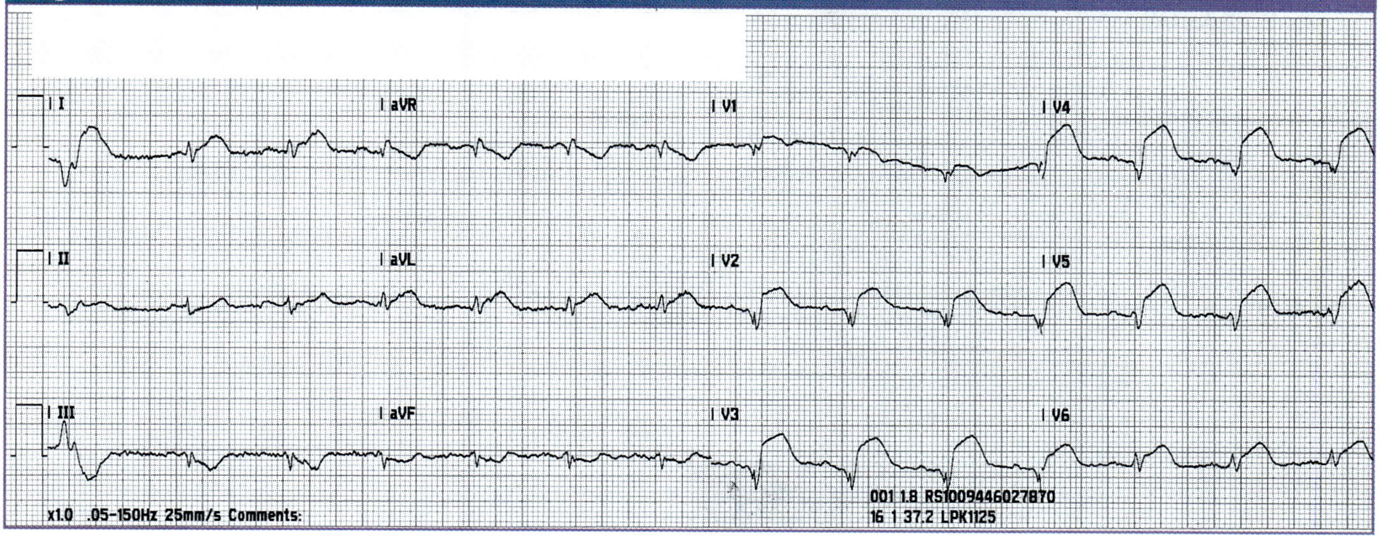

Interpretation /9-40

I

II

III

AVL

AVF

V1

V2

V3

V4

V5

V6

Fig 9-40: Interpretation

I	Low voltage. Baseline artifact. ST segment elevation > 1 mm.
II	Low voltage. ST segment depression.
III	Low voltage. Baseline artifact. Possible Q wave (artifact?). ST segment depression. T wave inversion.
AVL	Low voltage. ST segment elevation > 1 mm.
AVF	Low voltage. Baseline artifact. ST segment depression. T wave inversion.
V1	Baseline wander. No initial R wave. Possible ST segment elevation ≥ 1 mm.
V2	Q wave > 40 ms. ST segment elevation > 1 mm.
V3	Q wave > 40 ms. ST segment elevation > 1 mm. Tall T wave.
V4	Q wave. ST segment elevation > 1 mm. Tall T wave.
V5	Poor R wave progression. ST segment elevation > 1 mm. Tall T wave.
V6	ST segment elevation > 1 mm.

Comments:
Extensive anterior infarct. Reciprocal changes. Low voltage over entire tracing.

Fig 9-41

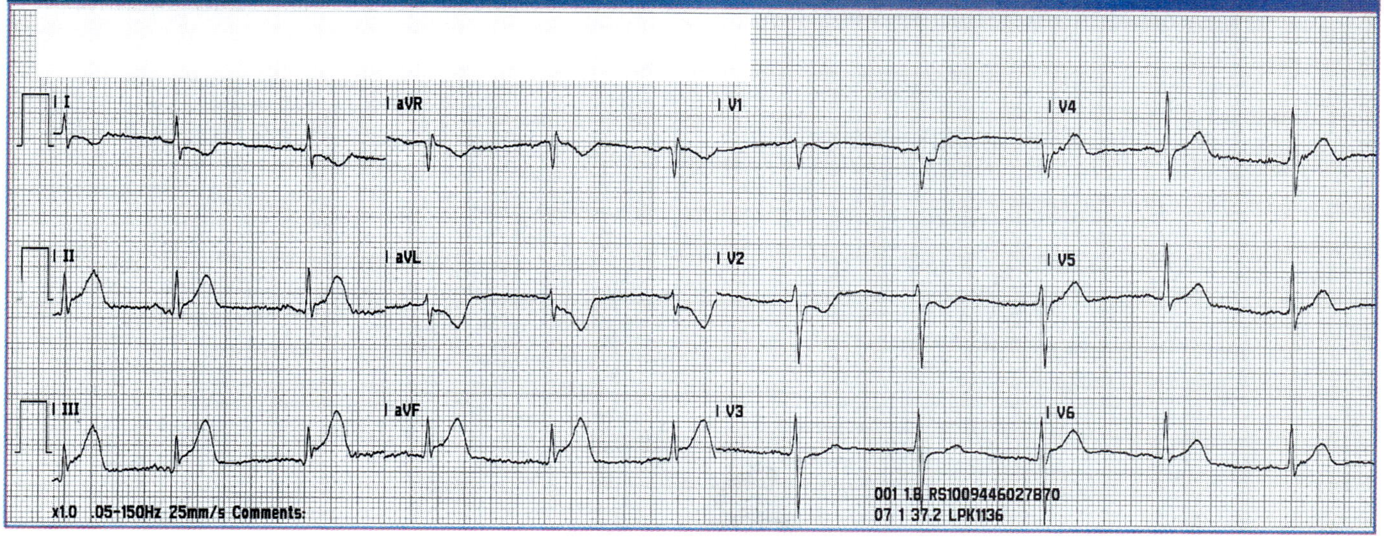

Interpretation /9-41

I

II

III

AVL

AVF

V1

V2

V3

V4

V5

V6

Fig 9-41: Interpretation

I	ST segment depression. T wave inversion.
II	ST segment elevation ≥ 1 mm. Tall/peaked T wave.
III	Q wave ≤ 40 ms. ST segment elevation > 1 mm. Tall/peaked T wave.
AVL	ST segment depression. T wave inversion.
AVF	ST segment elevation > 1 mm. Tall T wave.
V1	ST segment depression.
V2	ST segment depression. Inverted T wave.
V3	ST segment depression.
V4	Baseline wander. Apparent ST segment depression.
V5	Baseline wander. No indicative changes noted.
V6	Baseline wander. No indicative changes noted.

Comments:
Inferior wall infarct. Possible posterior infarct. Reciprocal changes.

Fig 9-42

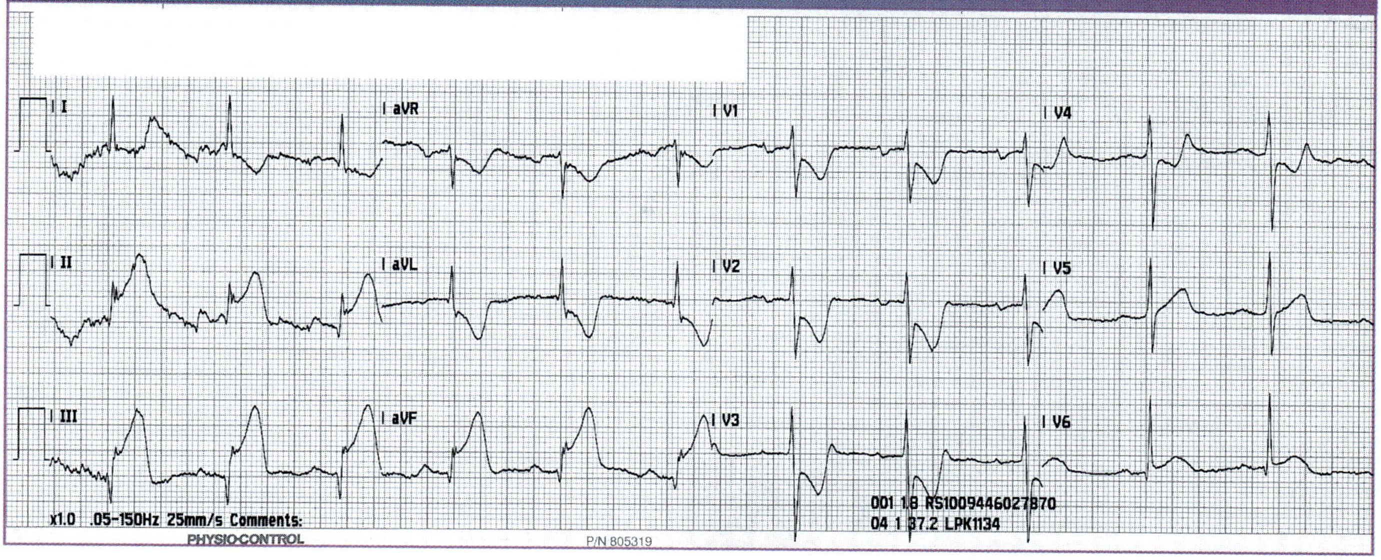

Interpretation /9-42

I

II

III

AVL

AVF

V1

V2

V3

V4

V5

V6

Fig 9-42: Interpretation

I	Baseline artifact. ST segment depression. Inverted T wave.
II	Baseline artifact. Q wave ≤ 40 ms. ST segment elevation > 1 mm. Tall/peaked T wave.
III	Q wave ≥ 40 ms. ST segment elevation > 1 mm.
AVL	Q wave < 40 ms. ST segment depression.
AVF	Q wave ≥ 40 ms. ST segment elevation. Tall/peaked T wave.
V1	ST segment depression.
V2	ST segment depression. Inverted T wave.
V3	ST segment depression. Inverted T wave.
V4	Poor R wave progression. ST segment depression.
V5	Poor R wave progression. ST segment elevation ≥ 1 mm.
V6	Q wave < 40 ms. ST segment elevation ≥ 1 mm.

Comments:
Inferior infarct with lateral extension. Possible posterior infarct.

Fig 9-43

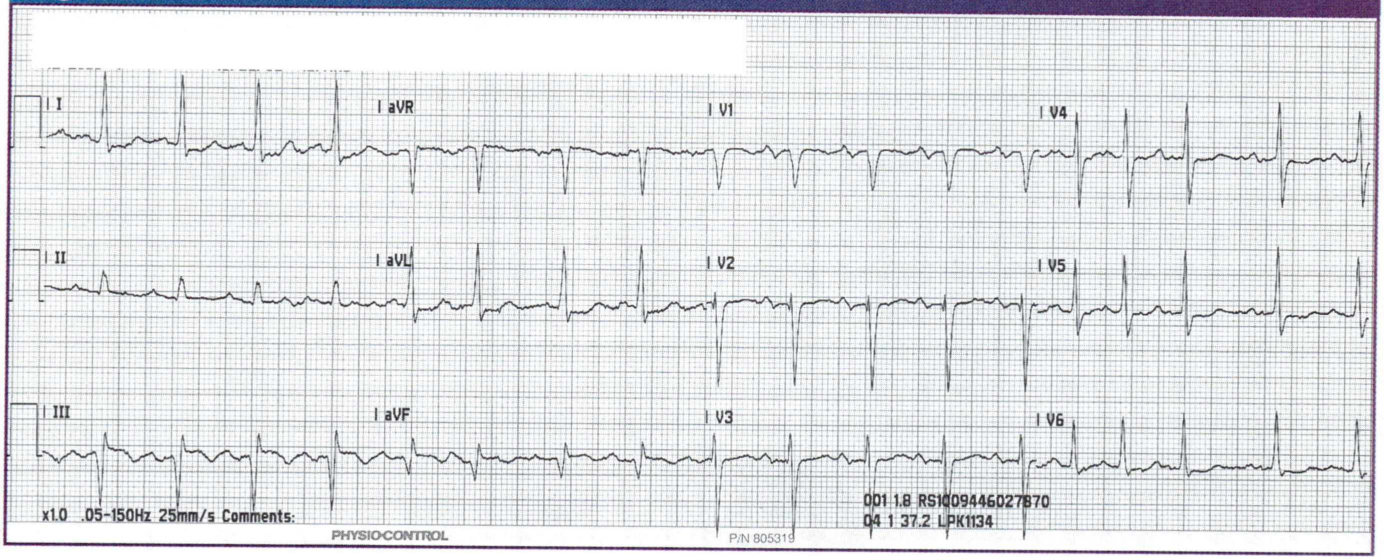

Interpretation /9-43

I

II

III

AVL

AVF

V1

V2

V3

V4

V5

V6

Fig 9-43: Interpretation

I	ST segment depression.
II	Low voltage. Q wave < 40 ms.
III	ST segment elevation ≥ 1 mm. Inverted T wave.
AVL	ST segment depression.
AVF	Q wave > 40 ms. ST segment elevation approaching 1 mm. T wave inversion.
V1	No initial R wave.
V2	Q wave < 40 ms. Biphasic T wave.
V3	Poor R wave progression. Biphasic T wave.
V4	No indicative changes noted.
V5	No indicative changes noted.
V6	No indicative changes noted.

Comments:
Inferior infarct. Possible previous anterior infarct.

Fig 9-44

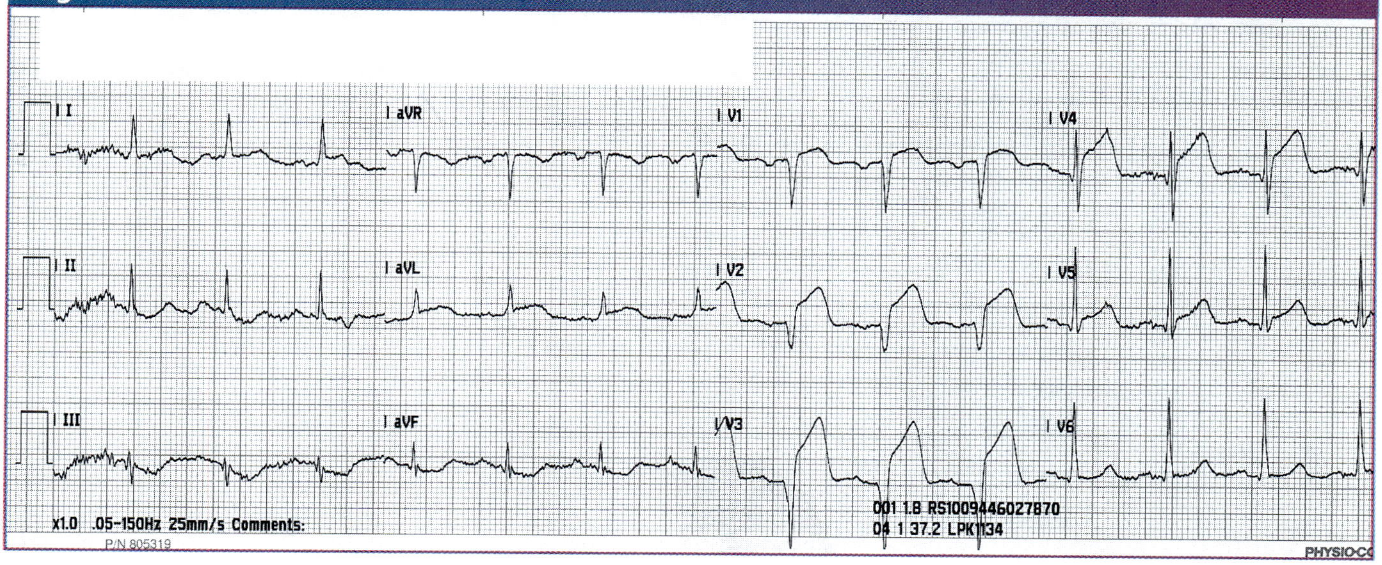

Interpretation /9-44

I

II

III

AVL

AVF

V1

V2

V3

V4

V5

V6

Fig 9-44: Interpretation

I	Baseline artifact.
II	Baseline artifact. ST segment depression.
III	Baseline wander and artifact. ST segment depression.
AVL	ST segment elevation > 1 mm.
AVF	Baseline artifact. ST segment depression.
V1	ST segment elevation > 1 mm.
V2	Q wave > 40 ms (or minimal R wave). ST segment elevation > 1 mm. Tall T wave.
V3	Q wave > 40 ms. ST segment elevation > 1 mm. Tall/peaked T wave.
V4	Q wave ≤ 40 ms. ST segment elevation > 1 mm. Tall/peaked T wave.
V5	Q wave < 40 ms. ST segment elevation.
V6	Q wave < 40 ms.

Comments:
Extensive anterior infarct. Reciprocal changes present.

Fig 9-45

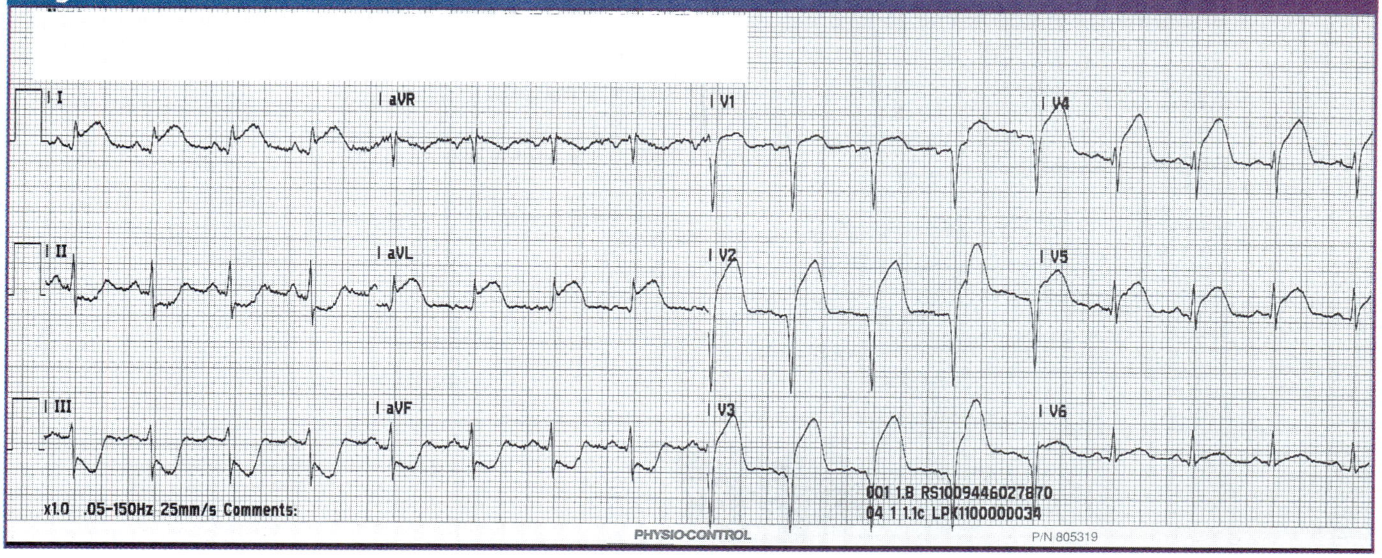

Interpretation /9-45

I

II

III

AVL

AVF

V1

V2

V3

V4

V5

V6

Fig 9-45: Interpretation

I	Q wave < 40 ms. ST segment elevation > 1 mm. Tall T wave.
II	ST segment depression.
III	ST segment depression.
AVL	Q wave ≤ 40 ms. ST segment elevation > 1 mm. Tall T wave.
AVF	ST segment depression.
V1	No initial R wave. ST segment elevation ≥ 1 mm.
V2	Q wave > 40 ms. ST segment elevation > 1 mm. Tall/ peaked T wave.
V3	Q wave > 40 ms. ST segment elevation > 1 mm. Tall Peaked T wave.
V4	Poor R wave progression. ST segment elevation > 1 mm. Tall/peaked T wave.
V5	ST segment elevation > 1 mm. Tall T wave.
V6	Slight ST segment elevation < 1 mm.

Comments:

Extensive anterior infarct. Reciprocal changes present.

Fig 9-46

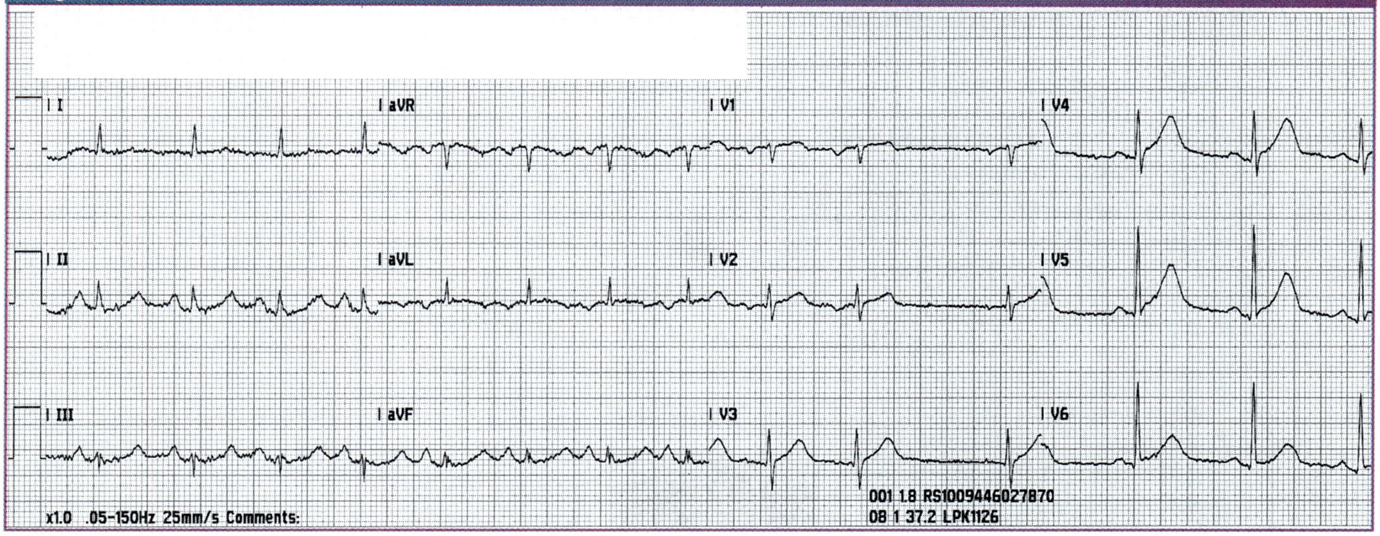

Interpretation /9-46

I

II

III

AVL

AVF

V1

V2

V3

V4

V5

V6

Fig 9-46: Interpretation

I	Baseline artifact. Flat T wave
II	Low voltage. Baseline artifact. Peaked T wave.
III	Low voltage. Baseline artifact. Peaked T wave.
AVL	Baseline artifact. Inverted T wave.
AVF	Low voltage.
V1	ST segment elevation < 1 mm.
V2	ST segment elevation < 1 mm.
V3	ST segment elevation > 1 mm.
V4	ST segment elevation > 1 mm. Tall/peaked T wave.
V5	Q wave < 40 ms. ST segment elevation ≤ 1 mm. Tall/ peaked T wave.
V6	Q wave < 40 ms.

Comments:
Anterior infarct.

Fig 9-47

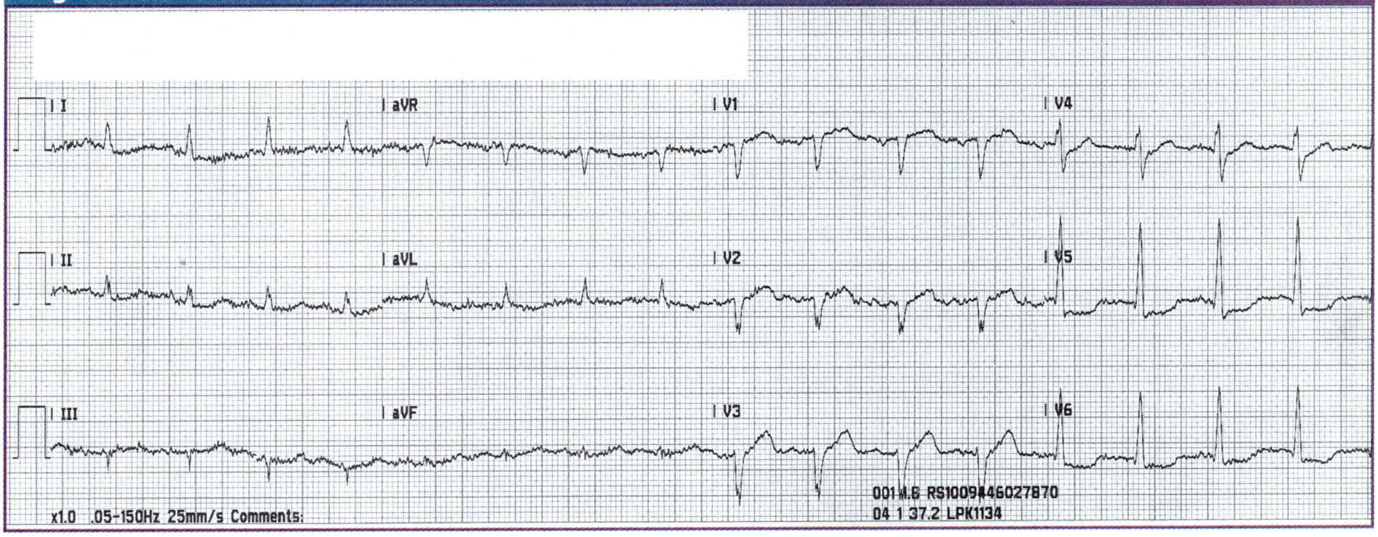

Interpretation /9-47

I

II

III

AVL

AVF

V1

V2

V3

V4

V5

V6

Fig 9-47: Interpretation

I	Slight ST segment depression
II	Low voltage. Slight ST segment depression
III	Baseline artifact. Possible Q wave > 40 ms (initial R wave vs. artifact).
AVL	Baseline artifact.
AVF	Low voltage. Baseline artifact. No evaluation possible.
V1	No intial R wave. ST segment elevation.
V2	Baseline artifact. Q wave > 40 ms. ST segment elevation ≥ 40 ms.
V3	Poor R wave progression. ST segment elevation ≥ 40 ms.
V4	Poor R wave progression
V5	ST segment depression.
V6	ST segment depression.

Comments:
Anteroseptal infarct.

Fig 9-48

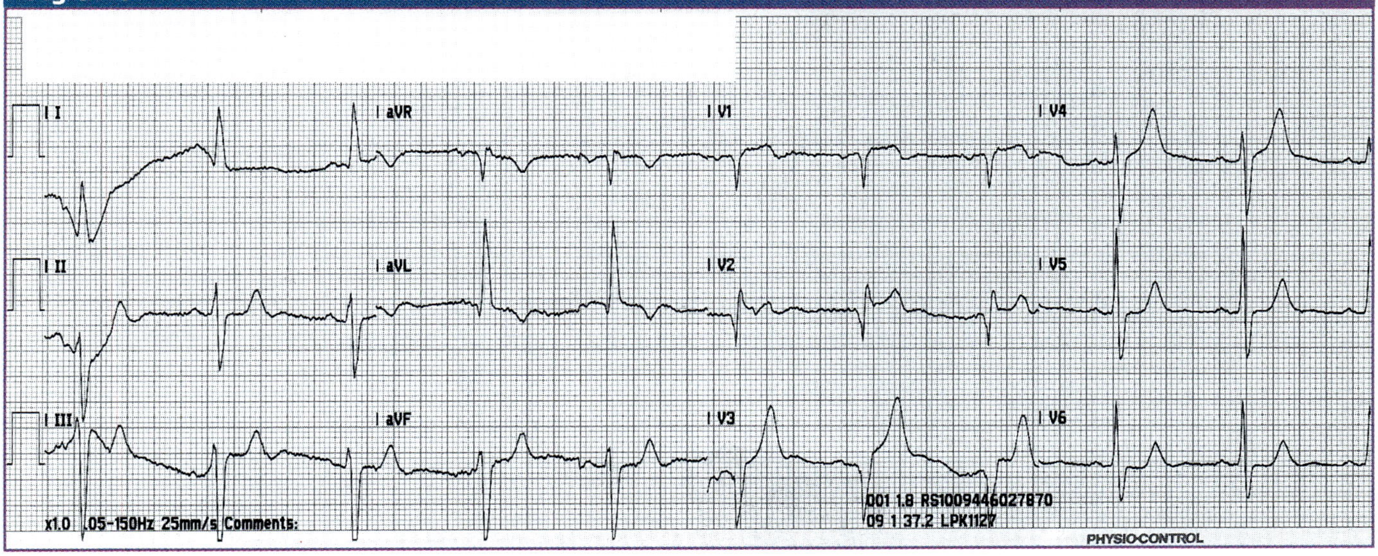

Interpretation /9-48

I

II

III

AVL

AVF

V1

V2

V3

V4

V5

V6

Fig 9-48: Interpretation

I	Baseline wander. Difficult to assess ST segment.
II	Baseline wander. Peaked T wave.
III	Baseline wander. Peaked T wave.
AVL	Q wave ≥ 40 ms. Inverted T wave.
AVF	Baseline wander. Peaked T wave.
V1	No initial R wave. ST segment elevation > 1 mm.
V2	Q wave > 40 ms. ST segment elevation > 1 mm. Peaked T wave.
V3	Q wave > 40 ms. ST segment elevation > 1 mm. Tall/peaked T wave.
V4	ST segment elevation ≥ 1 mm. Tall/peaked T wave.
V5	Peaked T wave
V6	Peaked T wave.

Comments:
Anteroseptal infarct, possible lateral extension (Q in AVL).

Fig 9-49

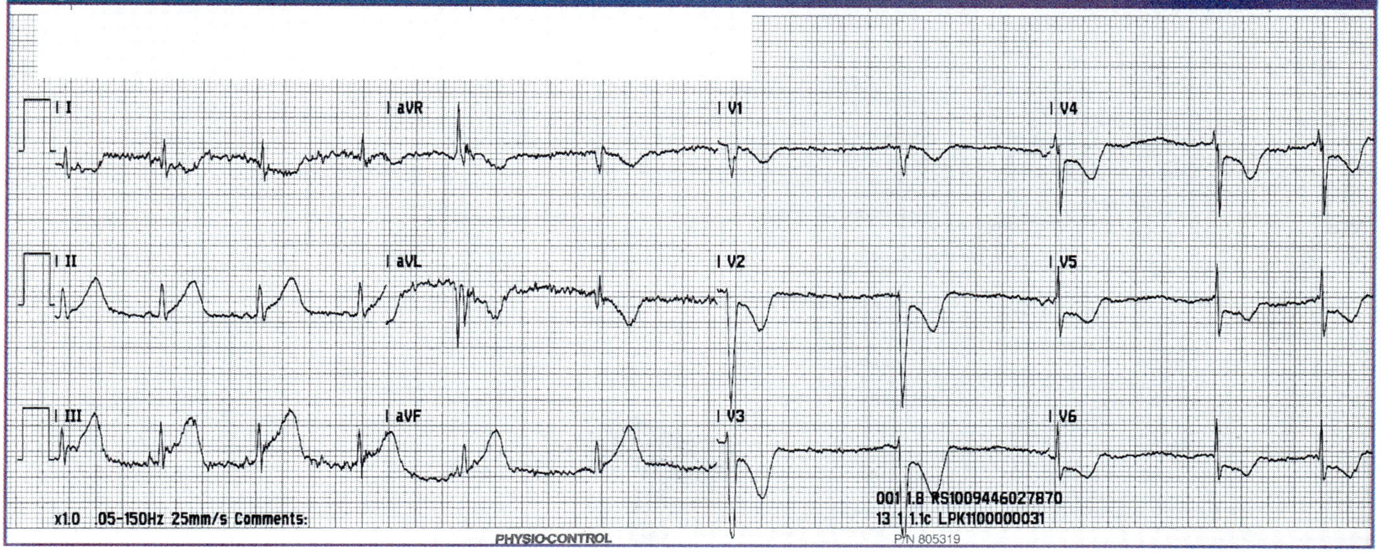

Interpretation /9-49

I

II

III

AVL

AVF

V1

V2

V3

V4

V5

V6

Fig 9-49: Interpretation

I	Baseline artifact. ST segment depression.
II	ST segment elevation > 1 mm. Tall/peaked T wave.
III	ST segment elevation > 1 mm. Tall/peaked T wave.
AVL	Baseline artifact. ST segment depression. Inverted T wave.
AVF	ST segment elevation > 1 mm. Tall/peaked T wave.
V1	No initial R wave.
V2	Poor R wave progression. ST segment depression. Inverted T wave.
V3	Poor R wave progression. ST segment depression. Inverted T wave.
V4	Poor R wave progression. ST segment depression. Inverted T wave.
V5	Poor R wave progression. ST segment depression. Inverted T wave.
V6	Poor R wave progression. ST segment depression. Inverted T wave.

Comments:
Inferior infarct. Reciprocal changes. Possible posterior infarct.

Fig 9-50

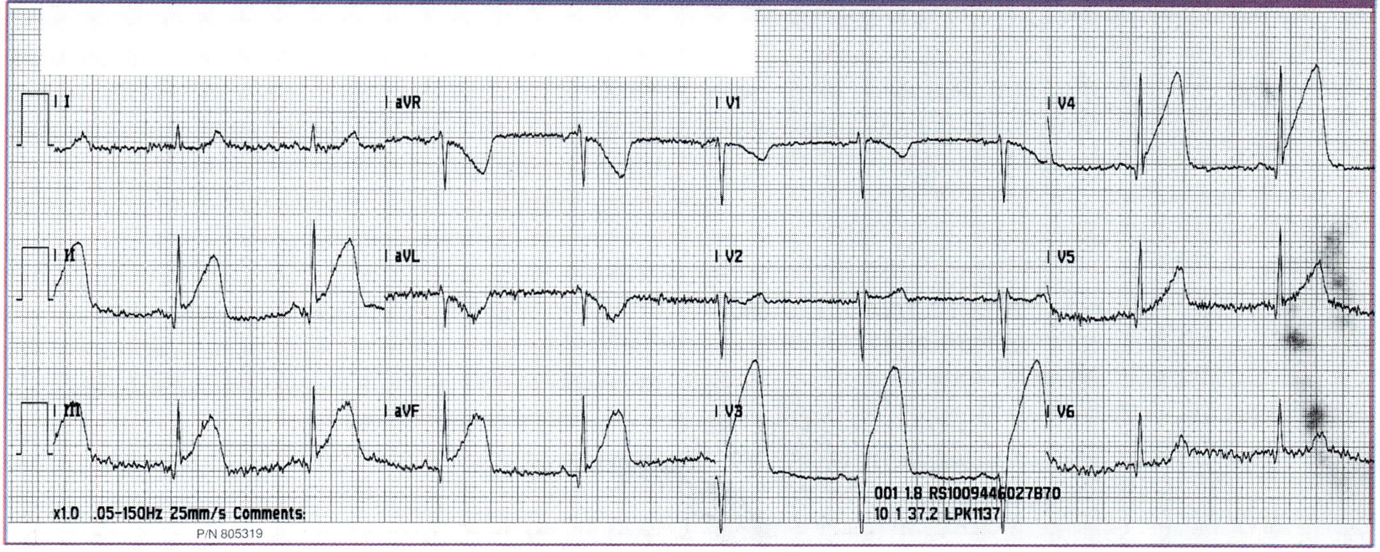

Interpretation /9-50

I

II

III

AVL

AVF

V1

V2

V3

V4

V5

V6

Fig 9-50: Interpretation

I	Baseline artifact.
II	Baseline artifact. Q wave ≤ 40 ms. ST segment elevation > 1 mm. Tall/peaked T wave.
III	Baseline artifact. Q wave ≤ 40 ms. ST segment elevation > 1 mm. Tall/peaked T wave.
AVL	Baseline artifact. ST segment depression. Inverted T wave.
AVF	Baseline artifact. Q wave ≤ 40 ms. ST segment elevation > 1 mm. Tall/peaked T wave.
V1	No indicative changes noted.
V2	Poor R wave progression.
V3	Poor R wave progression. ST segment elevation > 1 mm. Tall/peaked T wave.
V4	Q wave < 40 ms. ST segment elevation. Tall/peaked T wave.
V5	Baseline artifact. Q wave < 40 ms. Tall/peaked T wave.
V6	Baseline artifact. Q wave ≤ 40 ms.

Comments:
Inferoapical infarct.

Appendix A

Infarct Recognition Criteria

Throughout this text, ST segment elevation of 1 mm or more, in two contiguous leads, has been the only criteria used for infarct recognition. However, another set of criteria may be used, one that applies a more stringent requirement for ST segment elevation. In this alternate means of infarct recognition, at least 2 mm of ST segment elevation is required in the precordial leads before infarct is suspected. Each method has its advantage: The 1 mm threshold for ST segment elevation favors sensitivity, and the 2 mm criteria favors specificity.

Not only is there a difference in the amount of elevation required for infarct recognition, there is some difference of opinion as to where the ST segment should be measured. Some authorities simply measure elevation at the J-point, others look for elevation 40 ms after the J-point, while still others measure ST segment elevation 60 ms after the J-point.

Experienced electrocardiographers may not depend so much on the exact mms of ST segment elevation or worry about the precise point at which the ST segment should be measured. They may recognize infarct by the shape of the ST segment. It seems that myocardial infarction tends to produce an upwardly convex ST segment (see Fig. A-1). This upward convexity is referred to as coving and is noted in the leads directed towards the infarct site.

The reason that the objective criteria for ST segment elevation are commonly used is that the ability to recognize coving requires extensive practice. A review of the tracings in Chapter 9 is a beginning point for those who wish to recognize the presence of coving.

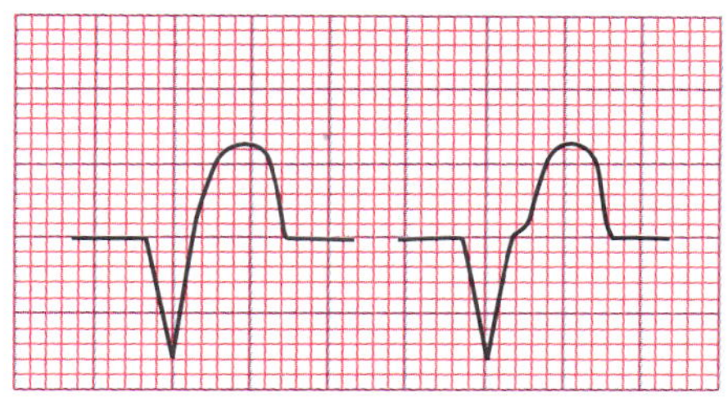

FIG. A-1 An example of coving.

Appendix B

V1 in Right Ventricular Infarction and an Additional Use for V4R

V1 IN RVI

Elevation of the ST segment in the right-sided chest leads is the recognition criteria for right ventricular infarction (RVI) described in the text. However, when looking retrospectively at tracings obtained from previous patients, the right-sided chest leads may not be available. In this situation, it is sometimes still possible to detect the presence of RVI by close examination of lead V1. Occasionally, V1 and V2 may show ST segment elevation from an RVI, because V1 is located in the same position as V2R, and V2 is also V1R.

In the instances when an inferior infarct exists and the ST segment is elevated in V1 and/or V2, an RVI is presumed to exist when the amount of ST segment elevation is greater in V1 than in V2. Conversely, when V1 and V2 show ST segment elevation due to a septal infarction, the amount of ST segment elevation is typically greater in V2 than in V1.

The use of V1 as an indicator for RVI is fairly specific but not very sensitive. Therefore, approximately only 20% of all RVIs will produce ST segment elevation in V1.

ADDITIONAL USE FOR V4R

In the majority of patients, it is the right coronary artery that supplies the right ventricle and the inferior wall of the left ventricle (see Fig. B-1). Therefore, a proximal occlusion of the right coronary artery can produce a more extensive infarct, one which affects both ventricles. If only one lead were used to detect an RVI, lead V4R is the single best lead. Elevation of this lead in the presence of an inferior infarction

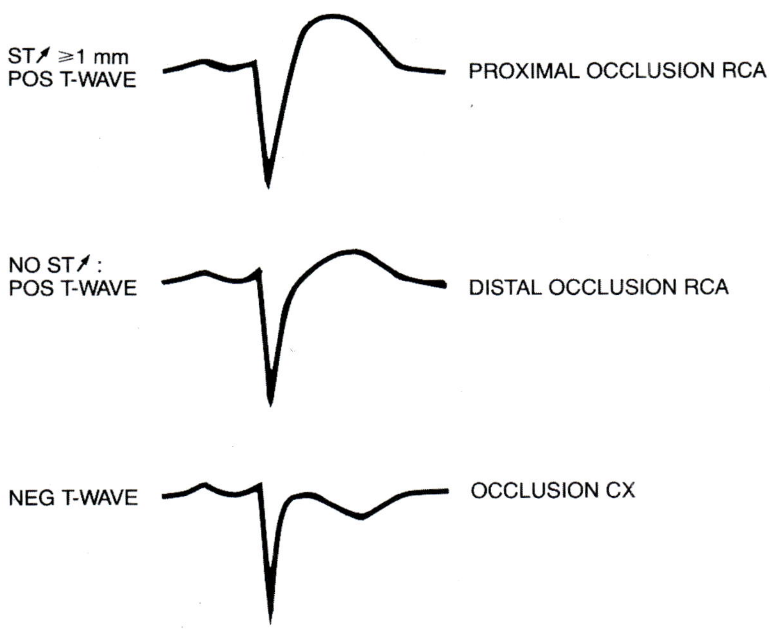

FIG. B-1 V4R leads. *(From Wellens/Conover. The ECG in Emergency Decision Making. Philadelphia: WB Saunders Co., 1992.)*

indicates a 90% probability that a simultaneous RVI exists.

This correlation between inferior wall infarctions and right ventricular infarctions is due to the fact that in 90% of the population, the right coronary artery supplies both areas. However, in 10% of the population the inferior wall is supplied by the left coronary artery (left coronary dominant). This pattern of coronary artery distribution may be identified by close inspection of lead V4R.

In the left coronary dominant patient experiencing an inferior wall infarction, the right ventricle is unlikely to be affected. Therefore, inspection of V4R is unlikely to reveal any ST segment elevation. However, in the presence of an inferior wall infarction, ST segment depression and an inverted T wave in V4R suggests a left coronary artery occlusion. An extension of this infarct is likely to involve the lateral wall, not the right ventricle.

Appendix C

Non-Q Wave Infarctions

A wide Q wave is the most conclusive ECG evidence of infarction. However, some patients with confirmed infarct never develop a Q wave. 20–25% of infarctions may not produce a Q wave, with a greater incidence among women.

There are a few possible explanations for the non-Q wave infarction. First, the infarct size is typically smaller compared to a Q wave infarction. This suggests that the reduced infarct size is difficult for the ECG to detect. Another factor which may interfere with the detection of a Q wave is that some areas of the myocardium are electrically silent, making analysis difficult. In many of these patients, a Q wave is detected when an ECG electrode is directly applied to the epicardium. Finally, because the goal of early treatment is to limit the infarct size, it offers another explanation of how a non-Q wave infarction may occur.

While they are not synonymous, Q wave infarction and non-Q wave infarction have generally replaced the previously used terms, transmural infarction and subendocardial infarction.

Appendix D

Unstable Angina

Unstable angina is suspected clinically when previous angina patients report an increase in the frequency and severity of chest pain, or when patients without a cardiac history report chest pain not associated with activity or exertion.

The label of unstable angina may be misinterpreted to mean that it is a severe case of typical angina. However, this assumption can lead to an underestimation of the patient's condition. Unstable angina can be thought of as "preinfarct angina," because the underlying conditions which produce the unstable angina are identical to those that produce myocardial infarction. In the setting of unstable angina, the coronary arteries have been narrowed by heart disease, and a blood clot may be present which worsens the occlusion. This occlusion is usually subtotal and some blood flow beyond the occlusion is possible.

If the tone of the coronary arteries increases, or the blood clot increases in size, infarct may result. The ECG criteria used for the recognition of unstable angina varies depending on the artery affected. Usually the criteria involve ST segment depression and T wave inversion. Despite the fact that these patients do not meet the objective ECG criteria for infarct recognition, they should be treated as high priority patients.

Appendix E

Prinzmetal's Angina

Unlike typical angina, which is the result of a narrowed coronary artery, Prinzmetal's angina is the result of coronary artery vasospasm. This variant angina may occur in otherwise healthy individuals, with little or no demonstrable coronary heart disease. The episode of coronary artery spasm usually lasts only a few minutes, but this may be long enough to produce a potentially lethal arrhythmia. If the spasm persists, infarct may result.

It can be difficult to suspect Prinzmetal's angina from the clinical presentation. These patients complain of chest pain, which is often relieved by nitroglycerin. However, while typical angina produces T segment depression, Prinzmetal's angina produces ST segment elevation. Because nitroglycerin is effective at relieving the coronary spasm, the ECG evidence of Prinzmetal's may be lost if no pretreatment ECG is obtained.

Below is a prehospital multilead ECG showing ST segment elevation in leads supplied by the left coronary artery (Fig. E-1). This tracing was

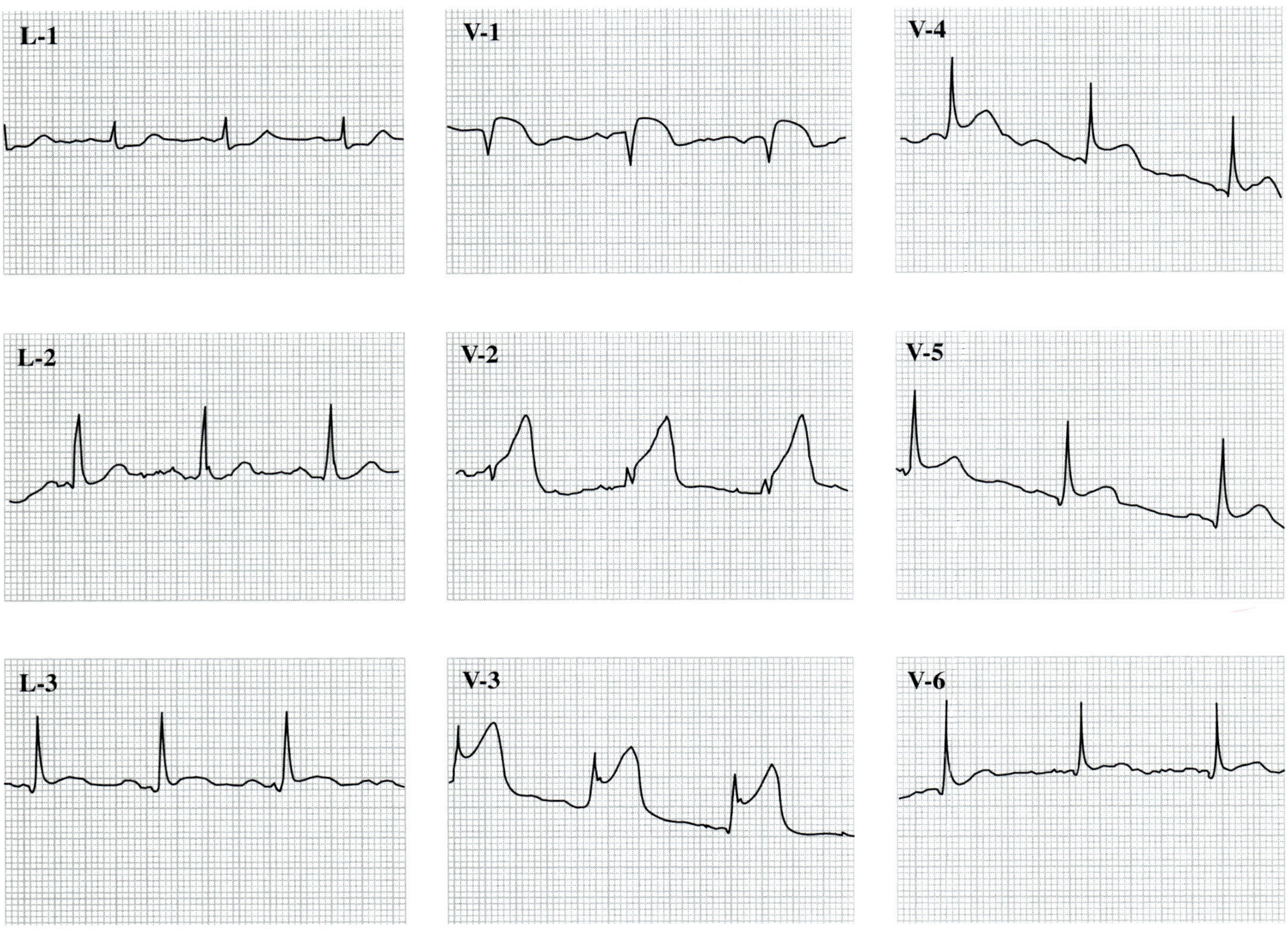

FIG. E-1 This lead was obtained before the administration of nitroglycerin.

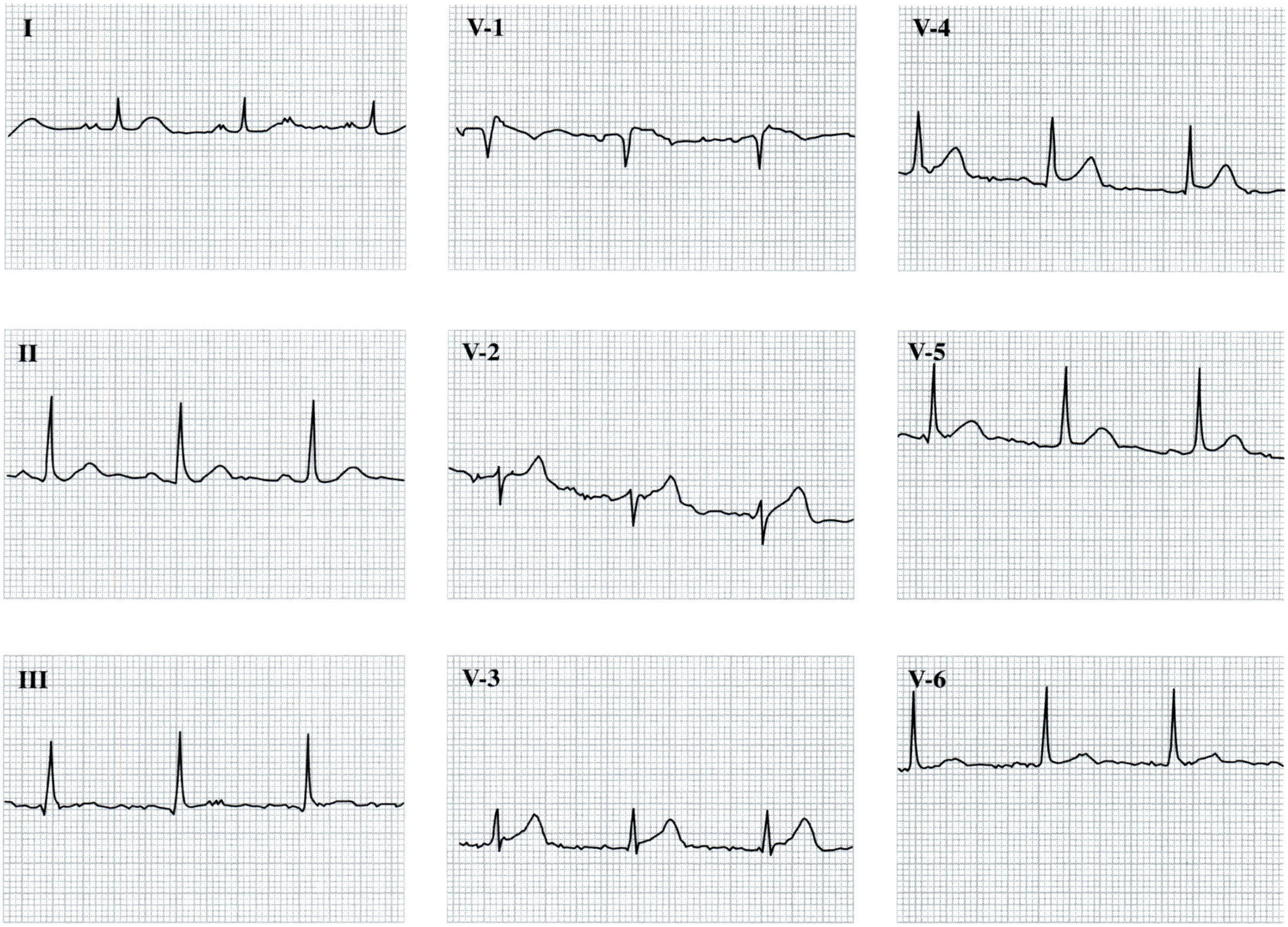

FIG. E-2 This lead was obtained after the patient was administered nitroglycerine.

obtained a few moments before the administration of nitroglycerin. The patient reported that the nitroglycerin had relieved the chest pain and a second tracing was then obtained. The obvious ST segment elevation noted in the first example is no longer present, suggesting the possibility of Prinzmetal's angina (Fig. E-2).

This type of evidence, obtained before and after treatment, can assist the physician in making the correct diagnosis.

Index

F

H

I

J

L

M

N

P

Q

R

S

T

U

V

W